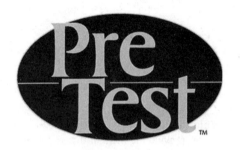

Medicine

PreTest™ Self-Assessment and Review

Notice

Medicine is an ever-changing science. As new research and clinical experience broaden our knowledge, changes in treatment and drug therapy are required. The authors and the publisher of this work have checked with sources believed to be reliable in their efforts to provide information that is complete and generally in accord with the standards accepted at the time of publication. However, in view of the possibility of human error or changes in medical sciences, neither the authors nor the publisher nor any other party who has been involved in the preparation or publication of this work warrants that the information contained herein is in every respect accurate or complete, and they disclaim all responsibility for any errors or omissions or for the results obtained from use of the information contained in this work. Readers are encouraged to confirm the information contained herein with other sources. For example and in particular, readers are advised to check the product information sheet included in the package of each drug they plan to administer to be certain that the information contained in this work is accurate and that changes have not been made in the recommended dose or in the contraindications for administration. This recommendation is of particular importance in connection with new or infrequently used drugs.

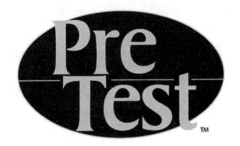

Medicine

PreTest™ Self-Assessment and Review
Twelfth Edition

Robert S. Urban, MD
Associate Professor
Department of Internal Medicine
Texas Tech University Health Sciences Center
School of Medicine
Amarillo, Texas

J. Rush Pierce, Jr., MD, MPH
Associate Professor
Department of Internal Medicine
Texas Tech University Health Sciences Center
School of Medicine
Amarillo, Texas

Marjorie R. Jenkins, MD
Associate Professor
Department of Internal Medicine
Executive Director, Laura W. Bush Institute for Women's Health
Texas Tech University Health Sciences Center
School of Medicine
Amarillo, Texas

Steven L. Berk, MD
Dean and Professor of Medicine
Texas Tech University Health Sciences Center
School of Medicine
Lubbock, Texas

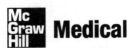 **Medical**

New York   Chicago   San Francisco   Lisbon   London   Madrid   Mexico City
Milan   New Delhi   San Juan   Seoul   Singapore   Sydney   Toronto

*The **McGraw·Hill** Companies*

Medicine: PreTest™ Self-Assessment and Review, Twelfth Edition

Copyright © 2009, 2006, 2003, 2001, 1998, 1995, 1992, 1989, 1987, 1985, 1982, 1978
by The McGraw-Hill Companies, Inc. All rights reserved. Printed in the United States of
America. Except as permitted under the United States Copyright Act of 1976, no part of this
publication may be reproduced or distributed in any form or by any means, or stored in a
data base or retrieval system, without the prior written permission of the publisher.

PreTest™ is a trademark of the McGraw-Hill Companies, Inc.

1 2 3 4 5 6 7 8 9 0   DOC/DOC   12 11 10 9

ISBN 978-0-07-160162-7
MHID 0-07-160162-7

This book was set in Berkeley by International Typesetting and Composition.
The editors were Kirsten Funk and Karen Davis.
The production supervisor was Sherri Souffrance.
Project management was provided by Gita Raman, International Typesetting and Composition.
RR Donnelley was printer and binder.

This book is printed on acid-free paper.

Library of Congress Cataloging-in-Publication Data

Medicine : PreTest self-assessment and review.—12th ed. / Robert S.
   Urban ... [et al.].
       p. ; cm.
   Includes bibliographical references and index.
   ISBN-13: 978-0-07-160162-7 (pbk.)
   ISBN-10: 0-07-160162-7
   1. Medicine—Examinations, questions, etc.   I. Urban, Robert S.
   [DNLM: 1. Medicine—Examination Questions. W 18.2 M4914 2009]
   R834.5.B38 2009
   616.0076—dc22   2008052477

Contributors

Todd Bell, MD
Assistant Professor, Internal Medicine
Texas Tech University School of Medicine, Amarillo
Hospital-Based Medicine, Cardiology

Harvey Richey, DO
Assistant Professor, Internal Medicine
Texas Tech University School of Medicine, Amarillo
Pulmonary Medicine

Joanna Wilson, DO
Assistant Professor, Internal Medicine
Chief, Division of Women's Health and Gender-Based Medicine
Texas Tech University School of Medicine, Amarillo
Women's Health

Student Reviewers

Miranda Boucher
Texas Tech University School of Medicine
Class of 2008

Anne Doughtie
Texas Tech University School of Medicine
Class of 2009

Edward Gould
SUNY Upstate Medical University
Class of 2009

Joshua Lynch
Lake Erie College of Osteopathic Medicine
Class of 2008

Reza Samad
SUNY Upstate Medical University
Class of 2009

Jay Yuan
Stony Brook University School of Medicine
Class of 2008

Contents

Introduction

Medicine: PreTest Self-Assessment and Review, Twelfth Edition, is intended to provide medical students, as well as house officers and physicians, with a convenient tool for assessing and improving their knowledge of medicine. The 500 questions in this book are similar in format and complexity to those included in Step 2 of the United States Medical Licensing Examination (USMLE). They may also be a useful study tool for Step 3.

For multiple-choice questions, the **one best** response to each question should be selected. For matching sets, a group of questions will be preceded by a list of lettered options. For each question in the matching set, select **one** lettered option that is **most** closely associated with the question. Each question in this book has a corresponding answer, a reference to a text that provides background to the answer, and a short discussion of various issues raised by the question and its answer. A listing of references for the entire book follows the last chapter.

To simulate the time constraints imposed by the qualifying examinations for which this book is intended as a practice guide, the student or physician should allot about one minute for each question. After answering all questions in a chapter, as much time as necessary should be spent in reviewing the explanations for each question at the end of the chapter. Attention should be given to all explanations, even if the examinee answered the question correctly. Those seeking more information on a subject should refer to the reference materials listed or to other standard texts in medicine.

Acknowledgments

We would like to offer special thanks to:

Joan Urban, David Urban,
Elizabeth Urban, Catherine Urban.

Diane Pierce, Read Pierce, Rebecca Pierce Martin,
Cason Pierce, and Susanna Pierce.

Stephen Jenkins, Katharine Jenkins,
Matthew Jenkins, Rebecca Jenkins.

Shirley Berk, Jeremy Berk, Justin Berk.

Cris Sheffield and Julie Schaef, for secretarial assistance.

To the medical students, residents, faculty, and staff
of Texas Tech University School of Medicine—
in pursuit of excellence.

Infectious Disease

Questions

1. A 30-year-old male patient complains of fever and sore throat for several days. The patient presents to you today with additional complaints of hoarseness, difficulty breathing, and drooling. On examination, the patient is febrile and has inspiratory stridor. Which of the following is the best course of action?

a. Begin outpatient treatment with ampicillin.
b. Culture throat for β-hemolytic streptococci.
c. Admit to intensive care unit and obtain otolaryngology consultation.
d. Schedule for chest x-ray.
e. Obtain Epstein-Barr serology.

2. A 70-year-old patient with long-standing type 2 diabetes mellitus presents with complaints of pain in the left ear with purulent drainage. On physical examination, the patient is afebrile. The pinna of the left ear is tender, and the external auditory canal is swollen and edematous. The white blood cell count is normal. Which of the following organisms is most likely to grow from the purulent drainage?

a. *Pseudomonas aeruginosa*
b. *Streptococcus pneumoniae*
c. *Candida albicans*
d. *Haemophilus influenzae*
e. *Moraxella catarrhalis*

3. A 25-year-old male student presents with the chief complaint of rash. He denies headache, fever, or myalgia. A slightly pruritic maculopapular rash is noted over the abdomen, trunk, palms of the hands, and soles of the feet. Inguinal, occipital, and cervical lymphadenopathy is also noted. Hypertrophic, flat, wartlike lesions are noted around the anal area. Laboratory studies show the following:

Hct: 40%
Hgb: 14 g/dL
WBC: 13,000/μL
Diff: 50% segmented neutrophils, 50% lymphocytes

Which of the following is the most useful laboratory test in this patient?

a. Weil-Felix titer
(b.) Venereal Disease Research Laboratory (VDRL) test
c. *Chlamydia* titer
d. Blood cultures
e. Biopsy of perianal lesions

4. A 35-year-old previously healthy male develops cough with purulent sputum over several days. On presentation to the emergency room, he is lethargic. Temperature is 39°C, pulse 110, and blood pressure 100/70. He has rales and dullness to percussion at the left base. There is no rash. Flexion of the patient's neck when supine results in spontaneous flexion of hip and knee. Neurologic examination is otherwise normal. There is no papilledema. A lumbar puncture is performed in the emergency room. The cerebrospinal fluid (CSF) shows 8000 leukocytes/μL, 90% of which are polys. Glucose is 30 mg/dL with a peripheral glucose of 80 mg/dL. CSF protein is elevated to 200 mg/dL. A CSF Gram stain shows gram-positive diplococci. Which of the following is the correct treatment option?

a. Begin acyclovir for herpes simplex encephalitis.
b. Obtain emergency MRI scan before beginning treatment.
(c) Begin ceftriaxone and vancomycin for pneumococcal meningitis.
d. Begin ceftriaxone, vancomycin, and ampicillin to cover both pneumococci and *Listeria*.
e. Begin high-dose penicillin for meningococcal meningitis.

5. A 20-year-old female college student presents with a 5-day history of cough, low-grade fever (temperature 37.8°C [100°F]), sore throat, and coryza. On examination, there is mild conjunctivitis and pharyngitis. Tympanic membranes are inflamed, and one bullous lesion is seen. Chest examination shows a few basilar rales. Sputum Gram stain shows white blood cells without organisms. Laboratory findings are as follows:

Hct: 31
WBC: 12,000/μL
Lymphocytes: 50%
Mean corpuscular volume (MCV): 94 nL
Reticulocytes: 9% of red cells
CXR: bilateral patchy lower lobe infiltrates

Which of the following is the best method for confirmation of the diagnosis?

a. High titers of antibody to adenovirus
b. High titers of IgM cold agglutinins or complement fixation test
c. Methenamine silver stain
d. Blood culture
e. Culture of sputum on chocolate media

6. A 22-year-old male, recently incarcerated and now homeless, has received one week of clarithromycin for low-grade fever and left upper-lobe pneumonia. He has not improved on antibiotics, with persistent cough productive of purulent sputum and flecks of blood. Repeat chest x-ray suggests a small cavity in the left upper lobe. Which of the following statements is correct?

a. The patient has anaerobic infection and needs outpatient clindamycin therapy.
b. The patient requires sputum smear and culture for acid fast bacilli.
c. The patient requires glove and gown contact precautions.
d. Isoniazid prophylaxis should be started if PPD is positive.
e. Drug resistant pneumococci may be causing this infection.

7. A 19-year-old male presents with a 1-week history of malaise and anorexia followed by fever and sore throat. On physical examination, the throat is inflamed without exudate. There are a few palatal petechiae. Cervical adenopathy is present. The liver span is 12 cm and the spleen is palpable.

Throat culture: negative for group A streptococci
Hgb: 12.5, Hct: 38%
Reticulocytes: 4%
WBC: 14, 000/μL
Segmented: 30%
Lymphocytes: 60%
Monocytes: 10%
Bilirubin total: 2.0 mg/dL (normal 0.2 to 1.2)
Lactic dehydrogenase (LDH) serum: 260 IU/L (normal 20 to 220)
Aspartate aminotransferase (AST): 40 U/L (normal 8 to 20 U/L)
Alanine aminotransferase (ALT): 35 U/L (normal 8 to 20 U/L)
Alkaline phosphatase: 40 IU/L (normal 35 to 125)

Which of the following is the most important initial test combination to order?

a. Liver biopsy and hepatitis antibody
b. Streptococcal screen and antistreptolysin O (ASO) titer
c. Peripheral blood smear and heterophile antibody
d. Toxoplasma IgG and stool sample
e. Lymph node biopsy and cytomegalovirus serology

8. A 30-year-old male presents with right upper quadrant pain. He has been well except for an episode of diarrhea that occurred 4 months ago, just after he returned from a missionary trip to Mexico. He has lost 7 pounds. He is not having diarrhea. His blood pressure is 140/70, pulse 80, and temperature 37.5°C (99.5°F). On physical examination there is right upper-quadrant tenderness without rebound. There is some radiation of the pain to the shoulder. The liver is percussed at 14 cm. There is no lower-quadrant tenderness. Bowel sounds are normal and active. Which of the following is the most appropriate next step in evaluation of the patient?

a. Serology and ultrasound
b. Stool for ova and parasite
c. Blood cultures
d. Diagnostic aspirate
e. Empiric broad-spectrum antibiotic therapy

9. An 80-year-old male complains of a 3-day history of a painful rash extending over the left half of his forehead and down to his left eyelid. There are weeping vesicular lesions on physical examination. Which of the following is the most likely diagnosis?

a. Impetigo
b. Adult chickenpox
c. Herpes zoster
d. Coxsackie A virus
e. Herpes simplex

10. A 28-year-old female presents to her internist with a 2-day history of low-grade fever and lower abdominal pain. She denies nausea, vomiting, or diarrhea. On physical examination, there is temperature of 38.3°C (100.9°F) and bilateral lower quadrant tenderness, without point or rebound tenderness. Bowel sounds are normal. On pelvic examination, an exudate is present and there is tenderness on motion of the cervix. Her white blood cell count is 15,000/μL and urinalysis shows no red or white blood cells. Serum β-hCG is undetectable. Which of the following is the best next step in management?

a. Treatment with ceftriaxone and doxycycline
b. Endometrial biopsy
c. Surgical exploration
d. Dilation and curettage
e. Aztreonam

11. A 35-year-old male complains of inability to close his right eye. Examination shows facial nerve weakness of the upper and lower halves of the face. There are no other cranial nerve abnormalities, and the rest of the neurological examination is normal. Examination of the heart, chest, abdomen, and skin show no additional abnormalities. There is no lymphadenopathy. About one month ago the patient was seen by a dermatologist for a bull's-eye skin rash. The patient lives in upstate New York and returned from a camping trip a few weeks before noting the rash. Which of the following is the most likely diagnosis?

a. Sarcoidosis
b. Idiopathic Bell palsy
c. Lyme disease
d. Syphilis
e. Lacunar infarct

12. A 25-year-old woman complains of dysuria, frequency, and suprapubic pain. She has not had previous symptoms of dysuria and is not on antibiotics. She is sexually active and on birth control pills. She has no fever, vaginal discharge or history of herpes infection. She denies back pain, nausea, or vomiting. On physical examination she appears well and has no costovertebral angle tenderness. A urinalysis shows 20 white blood cells per high power field. Which of the following statements is correct?

a. A 3-day regimen of trimethoprim-sulfamethoxazole is adequate therapy.
b. Quantitative urine culture with antimicrobial sensitivity testing is mandatory.
c. Obstruction resulting from renal stone should be ruled out by ultrasound.
d. Low-dose antibiotic therapy should be prescribed while the patient remains sexually active.
e. The etiologic agent is more likely to be sensitive to trimethoprim-sulfamethoxazole than to fluoroquinolones.

13. A 25-year-old woman is admitted with fever and hypotension. She has a 3-day history of feeling feverish. She has no history of chronic disease, but she uses tampons for heavy menses. She is acutely ill and, on physical examination, found to have a diffuse erythematous rash extending to palms and soles. She is confused. Initial blood tests are as follows:

White blood cell count: 22,000/μL
Na^+: 125 mEq/L
K^+: 3.0 mEq/L
Ca^{++}: 8.0 mEq/mL
Activated partial thromboplastin time (PTT): 65 (normal 21 to 36)
Prothrombin time (PT): 12s (normal < 15s)
Aspartate aminotransferase: 240 U/L (normal < 40)
Creatinine: 3.0 mg/dL
Antinuclear antibodies: negative
Anti-DNA antibodies: negative
Serologic tests for RMSF, leptospirosis, measles: negative

Which of the following best describes the pathophysiology of the disease process?

a. Acute bacteremia
b. Toxin-mediated inflammatory response syndrome
c. Exacerbation of connective tissue disease
d. Tick-borne rickettsial disease
e. Allergic reaction

14. You are a physician in charge of patients who reside in a nursing home. Several of the patients have developed influenza-like symptoms, and the community is in the midst of influenza A outbreak. None of the nursing home residents have received the influenza vaccine. Which course of action is most appropriate?

a. Give the influenza vaccine to all residents who do not have a contraindication to the vaccine (ie, allergy to eggs).
b. Give the influenza vaccine to all residents who do not have a contraindication to the vaccine; also give oseltamivir for 2 weeks to all residents.
c. Give amantadine alone to all residents.
d. Give azithromycin to all residents to prevent influenza-associated pneumonia.
e. Do not give any prophylactic regimen.

15. A 60-year-old male complains of low back pain, which has intensified over the past 3 months. He had experienced some fever at the onset of the pain. He was treated for acute pyelonephritis about 4 months ago. Physical examination shows tenderness over the L2-3 vertebra and paraspinal muscle spasm. Laboratory data show an erythrocyte sedimentation rate of 80 mm/h and elevated C-reactive protein. Which of the following statements is correct?

a. Hematogenous osteomyelitis rarely involves the vertebra in adults.
b. The most likely initial focus of infection was soft tissue.
c. Blood cultures will be positive in most patients with this process.
d. An MRI scan is both sensitive and specific in defining the process.
e. Surgery will be necessary if the patient has osteomyelitis.

16. A 30-year-old male with sickle cell anemia is admitted with cough, rusty sputum, and a single shaking chill. Physical examination reveals increased tactile fremitus and bronchial breath sounds in the left posterior chest. The patient is able to expectorate a purulent sample. Which of the following best describes the role of sputum Gram stain and culture?

a. Sputum Gram stain and culture lack the sensitivity and specificity to be of value in this setting.
b. If the sample is a good one, sputum culture is useful in determining the antibiotic sensitivity pattern of the organism, particularly *Streptococcus pneumoniae*.
c. Empirical use of antibiotics for pneumonia has made specific diagnosis unnecessary.
d. There is no characteristic Gram stain in a patient with pneumococcal pneumonia.
e. Gram-positive cocci in clusters suggest pneumococcal infection.

17. A recent outbreak of severe diarrhea is currently being investigated. Several adolescents developed bloody diarrhea, and one remains hospitalized with acute renal failure. A preliminary investigation has determined that all the affected ate at the same restaurant. The food they consumed was most likely to be which of the following?

a. Pork chops
b. Hamburger
c. Gefilte fish
d. Sushi
e. Soft-boiled eggs

18. A 40-year-old female nurse was admitted to the hospital because of fever to 39.4°C (103°F). Despite a thorough workup in the hospital for over 3 weeks, no etiology has been found, and she continues to have temperature spikes greater than 38.9°C (102°F). Which of the following statements about diagnosis is correct?

a. Chronic infection, malignancy, and collagen vascular disease are the most common explanations for this presentation.
b. Influenza may also present in this manner.
c. Lymphoma can be ruled out in the absence of palpable lymphadenopathy.
d. SLE is an increasing cause for this syndrome.
e. Factitious fever should be considered only in the patient with known psychopathology.

19. A 40-year-old school teacher develops nausea and vomiting at the beginning of the fall semester. Over the summer she had taught preschool children in a small town in Mexico. She is sexually active, but has not used intravenous drugs and has not received blood products. Physical examination reveals scleral icterus, right upper quadrant tenderness, and a palpable liver. Liver function tests show aspartate aminotransferase of 750 U/L (normal < 40) and alanine aminotransferase of 1020 U/L (normal < 45). The bilirubin is 13 mg/dL (normal < 1.4) and the alkaline phosphatase is normal. What further diagnostic test is most likely to be helpful?

a. Liver biopsy
b. Abdominal ultrasound
c. IgM antibody to hepatitis A
d. Antibody to hepatitis B surface antigen
e. Determination of hepatitis C RNA

20. A previously healthy 25-year-old music teacher develops fever and a rash over her face and chest. The rash is itchy and, on examination, involves multiple papules and vesicles in varying stages of development. One week later, she complains of cough and is found to have an infiltrate on x-ray. Which of the following is the most likely etiology of the infection?

a. *Streptococcus pneumoniae*
b. *Mycoplasma pneumoniae*
c. *Histoplasma capsulatum*
d. Varicella-zoster virus
e. *Chlamydia psittaci*

21. A 22-year-old male complains of fever and shortness of breath. There is no pleuritic chest pain or rigors and no sputum production. A chest x-ray shows diffuse perihilar infiltrates. The patient worsens while on erythromycin. A methenamine silver stain shows cystlike structures. Which of the following is correct?

a. Definitive diagnosis can be made by serology.
b. The organism will grow after 48 h.
c. History will likely provide important clues to the diagnosis.
d. Cavitary disease is likely to develop.
e. The infection will not recur.

22. A 40-year-old woman cut her finger while cooking in her kitchen. Two days later she became rapidly ill with fever and shaking chills. Her hand became painful and mildly erythematous. Later that evening her condition deteriorated as the erythema progressed and the hand became a dusky red. Bullae and decreased sensation to touch developed over the involved hand. What is the most important next step in the management of this patient?

a. Surgical consultation and exploration of the wound
b. Treatment with clindamycin for mixed aerobic-anaerobic infection
c. Treatment with penicillin for clostridia infection
d. Vancomycin to cover community-acquired methicillin-resistant *Staphylococcus*
e. Evaluation for acute osteomyelitis

23. A 25-year-old male from East Tennessee had been ill for 5 days with fever, chills, and headache when he noted a rash that developed on his palms and soles. In addition to macular lesions, petechiae are noted on the wrists and ankles. The patient has spent the summer camping. Which of the following is the most important fact to be determined in the history?

a. Exposure to contaminated springwater
b. Exposure to raw pork
c. Exposure to ticks
d. Exposure to prostitutes
e. Exposure to mosquitos

24. A 19-year-old male has a history of athlete's foot but is otherwise healthy when he develops sudden onset of fever and pain in the right foot and leg. On physical examination, the foot and leg are fiery red with a well-defined indurated margin that appears to be rapidly advancing. There is tender inguinal lymphadenopathy. The most likely organism to cause this infection is which of the following?

a. *Staphylococcus epidermidis*
b. *Tinea pedis*
c. *Streptococcus pyogenes*
d. Mixed anaerobic infection
e. Alpha-hemolytic streptococci

25. An 18-year-old male has been seen in the clinic for urethral discharge. He is treated with ceftriaxone, but the discharge has not resolved and the culture has returned as no growth. Which of the following is the most likely etiologic agent to cause this infection?

a. Ceftriaxone-resistant gonococci
b. *Chlamydia psittaci*
c. *Chlamydia trachomatis*
d. Herpes simplex
e. *Chlamydia pneumoniae*

26. A 70-year-old nursing home resident was admitted to the hospital for pneumonia and treated for 10 days with levofloxacin. On discharge she was improved but developed diarrhea one week later. She had low-grade fever and mild abdominal pain with 2 to 3 watery, nonbloody stools per day. A cell culture cytotoxicity test for *Clostridium difficile*–associated disease was positive. The patient was treated with oral metronidazole, but did not improve, even after 10 days. Diarrhea has increased and fever and abdominal pain continue. What is the best next step in the management of this patient?

a. Obtain *C difficile* enzyme immunoassay.
b. Continue metronidazole for at least two more weeks.
c. Switch treatment to oral vancomycin.
d. Hospitalize patient for fulminant *C difficile*–associated disease.
e. Use synthetic fecal bacterial enema.

27. A college wrestler develops cellulitis after abrading his skin during a match. He is afebrile and appears well but his arm is red and swollen with several draining pustules. Gram stain of the pus shows gram-positive cocci in clusters. Which of the following statements is correct?

a. The patient will require hospital admission and treatment with vancomycin.
b. The organism will almost always be sensitive to oxacillin.
c. The organism is likely to be sensitive to trimethoprim-sulfamethoxazole.
d. Community-acquired methicillin-resistant staphylococci have the same sensitivity pattern as hospital-acquired methicillin-resistant staphylococci.
e. The infection is likely caused by streptococci.

28. A 35-year-old male with documented HIV disease has completed his initial evaluation. He feels well but has a CD4 count of 198 μL and a viral load of 200,000 copies per mL. His physical examination has shown no evidence of opportunistic infection. PPD skin test, RPR, routine chemistry, CBC, lipid profile, and fasting blood sugar are all within normal limits. Which of the following is best advice?

a. The patient should begin treatment with either two nucleoside analogues and nonnucleoside reverse transcriptase inhibitor or two nucleoside analogues and a protease inhibitor.
b. The patient should make his own decision on beginning therapy since time of initiation does not affect mortality in an asymptomatic patient.
c. The patient should consider beginning new antiviral agents such as raltegravir or maraviroc.
d. Any new regimen should avoid abacavir because of its high incidence of hypersensitivity reactions.
e. Genotyping should not be obtained until the patient's first treatment failure.

29. A businessman traveling around the world asks about prevention of malaria. He will travel to India and the Middle East and plans to visit several small towns. What is the most appropriate advice for the traveler?

a. Common sense measures to avoid malaria such as use of insect repellants, bed nets, and suitable clothing have not really worked in preventing malaria.
b. The decision to use drugs effective against resistant *Plasmodium falciparum* malaria will depend upon the knowledge of local patterns of resistance and the patient's very specific travel plans.
c. Prophylaxis should be started the day of travel.
d. Chemoprophylaxis has been proven to be entirely reliable.
e. He should stay inside at the noon as this is the mosquito's peak feeding time.

Questions 30 to 33

Match the clinical description with the most likely organism. Each lettered option may be used once, more than once, or not at all.

a. *Streptococcus pneumoniae*
b. *Staphylococcus aureus*
c. Viridans streptococci
d. *Providencia stuartii*
e. *Actinomyces israelii*
f. *Haemophilus ducreyi*
g. *Neisseria meningitidis*
h. *Listeria monocytogenes*

30. A 30-year-old female with mitral valve prolapse and mitral regurgitant murmur develops fever, weight loss, and anorexia after undergoing a dental procedure.

31. An 80-year-old male, hospitalized for hip fracture, has a Foley catheter in place when he develops shaking chills, fever, and hypotension.

32. A young man develops a painless, fluctuant purplish lesion over the mandible. A cutaneous fistula is noted after several weeks.

33. A 47-year-old man who had a splenectomy after a childhood accident develops shaking chills and dies within 8 hours from refractory hypotension and respiratory failure.

Questions 34 to 36

Select the fungal agent most likely responsible for the disease process described. Each lettered option may be used once, more than once, or not at all.

a. *Histoplasma capsulatum*
b. *Blastomyces dermatitidis*
c. *Coccidioides immitis*
d. *Cryptococcus neoformans*
e. *Candida albicans*
f. *Aspergillus fumigatus*
g. Zygomycosis

34. A young, previously healthy male presents with verrucous skin lesions, bone pain, fever, cough, and weight loss. Chest x-ray shows nodular infiltrates.

35. A diabetic patient is admitted with elevated blood sugar and acidosis. The patient complains of headache and sinus tenderness and has black, necrotic material draining from the nares.   G

36. A young woman presents with asthma and eosinophilia. Fleeting pulmonary infiltrates occur with bronchial plugging.

F

Questions 37 to 40

Match each clinical description with the appropriate infectious agent. Each lettered option may be used once, more than once, or not at all.

a. Herpes simplex virus
b. Epstein-Barr virus
c. Parvovirus B19
d. *Staphylococcus aureus*
e. *Neisseria meningitidis*
f. *Listeria monocytogenes*
g. *Streptococcus viridans*
h. *Haemophilus influenzae*

37. Mother of a 5-year-old with sore throat and slapped-cheek rash also develops rash and arthralgia of small joints of the hand. *C*

38. A 30-year-old menstruating female has multisystem disease with hypotension, diffuse erythematous rash with desquamation of skin on hands and feet. *D*

39. An 18-year-old college student presents with fever, neck stiffness, and petechiae on his trunk. *E*

40. A 16-year-old has a sore throat and develops a diffuse rash after administration of ampicillin.

B

Questions 41 to 45

Match the clinical description with the most likely etiologic agent. Each lettered option may be used once, more than once, or not at all.

a. *Candida albicans*
b. *Aspergillus flavus*
c. *Coccidioides immitis*
d. Herpes simplex type 1
e. Herpes simplex type 2
f. Hantavirus
g. *Tropheryma whippelii*
h. Coxsackievirus B
i. *Histoplasma capsulatum*
j. Human parvovirus
k. *Cryptococcus neoformans*

41. An HIV-positive patient develops fever and dysphagia; endoscopic biopsy shows yeast and hyphae.   *A*

42. A 50-year-old develops sudden onset of bizarre behavior. CSF shows 80 lymphocytes; magnetic resonance imaging shows temporal lobe abnormalities.
D /E

43. A patient with a previous history of tuberculosis now complains of hemoptysis. There is an upper lobe mass with a cavity and a crescent-shaped air-fluid level.   *B*

44. A Filipino patient develops a pulmonary nodule after travel through the American Southwest.
C

45. A 35-year-old male who had a fever, cough, and sore throat develops chest pain after several days, with diffuse ST-segment elevations on ECG.
H

Infectious Disease

Answers

1. The answer is c. *(Fauci, pp 923-925.)* This patient, with the development of hoarseness, breathing difficulty, and stridor, is likely to have acute epiglottitis. Because of the possibility of impending airway obstruction, the patient should be admitted to an intensive care unit for close monitoring. The diagnosis can be confirmed by indirect laryngoscopy or soft tissue x-rays of the neck, which may show an enlarged epiglottis. Otolaryngology consult should be obtained. The most likely organism causing this infection is *H influenzae*. Many of these organisms are β-lactamase producing and would be resistant to ampicillin. Streptococcal pharyngitis can cause severe pain on swallowing but the infection does not descend to the hypopharynx and larynx. Lateral neck films would be more useful than a chest x-ray. Classic finding on lateral neck films would be the thumbprint sign. Infectious mononucleosis often causes exudative pharyngitis and cervical lymphadenopathy but not stridor.

2. The answer is a. *(Fauci, pp 949-956.)* Ear pain and drainage in an elderly diabetic patient must raise concern about malignant external otitis. The swelling and inflammation of the external auditory meatus strongly suggest this diagnosis. This infection usually occurs in older, poorly controlled diabetics and is almost always caused by *P aeruginosa*. It can invade contiguous structures including facial nerve or temporal bone and can even progress to meningitis. *S pneumoniae, H influenzae* and *M catarrhalis* frequently cause otitis media, but not external otitis. *Candida albicans* almost never affects the external ear.

3. The answer is b. *(Fauci, pp 1038-1046.)* The diffuse rash involving palms and soles would in itself suggest the possibility of secondary syphilis. The hypertrophic, wartlike lesions around the anal area, called *condylomata lata,* are specific for secondary syphilis. The VDRL slide test will be positive in all patients with secondary syphilis. The Weil-Felix titer has been used as a screening test for rickettsial infection. In this patient, who has condylomata and no systemic symptoms, Rocky Mountain spotted fever would be unlikely. No chlamydial infection would present in this way. Blood cultures might be drawn to rule out bacterial infection such as chronic meningococcemia; however, the clinical picture is not consistent with a systemic bacterial infection. Biopsy of the condyloma is not necessary in this setting, as regression of the lesion with treatment will distinguish it from genital wart (condyloma acuminatum) or squamous cell carcinoma.

4. The answer is c. *(Fauci, pp 908-914, 2621-2624.)* This previously healthy male has developed acute bacterial meningitis as evident by meningeal irritation with a positive Brudzinski sign, and a CSF profile typical for bacterial meningitis (elevated white blood cell count, high percentage of polymorphonuclear leukocytes, elevated protein, and low glucose). The patient likely has concomitant pneumonia. This combination suggests pneumococcal infection, and the CSF Gram stain confirms *S pneumoniae* as the etiologic agent. Because of the potential for beta-lactam resistance, the recommendation for therapy prior to availability of susceptibility data is ceftriaxone and vancomycin. Though herpes simplex is a common problem in young healthy patients, the clinical picture and CSF profile are not consistent with this infection. The CSF in herpes simplex encephalitis shows a lymphocytic predominance and normal glucose. *Listeria monocytogenes* meningitis is a concern in immunocompromised and elderly patients. Gram stain would show gram-positive rods. *Neisseria meningitidis* is the second commonest cause of bacterial meningitis but rarely causes pneumonia (the portal of entry is the nasopharynx). Gram stain of meningococci would show gram-negative diplococci. Because the patient has no papilledema and no focal neurologic findings, treatment should not be delayed to obtain an MRI scan.

5. The answer is b. *(Fauci, pp 1068-1070.)* This young woman presents with symptoms of both upper and lower respiratory infection. The combination of sore throat, bullous myringitis, and infiltrates on chest x-ray is consistent with infection caused by *M pneumoniae*. This minute organism is not seen on Gram stain. Neither *S pneumoniae* nor *H influenzae* would produce this combination of upper and lower respiratory tract symptoms. The patient is likely to have high titers of IgM cold agglutinins and a positive complement fixation test for mycoplasma. The low hematocrit and elevated reticulocyte count reflect a hemolytic anemia that can occur from *Mycoplasma* infection. These IgM-class antibodies are directed to the I antigen on the erythrocyte membrane. Adenovirus can cause upper respiratory symptoms, but pneumonia and bullous myringitis would be unusual with a viral infection. The methenamine silver stain is used for fungi and pneumocystis; these organisms do not cause bullous myringitis. *Mycoplasma* does not grow on blood or routine sputum cultures.

6. The answer is b. *(Fauci, pp 1006-1020).* The patient is high risk for tuberculosis due to his history of incarceration and homelessness. The location of the infiltrate in the upper lobe, as well as the formation of a cavity, further suggests reactivation tuberculosis. Sputum smear and culture for AFB are mandatory. The patient requires respiratory isolation precautions in a negative pressure room, not contact precautions. Anaerobic infection would be in the differential diagnosis of upper lobe infiltrate with cavity formation, but evaluation for tuberculosis is critical because of the risk of person-to-person spread. Single drug therapy with INH is a good prophylactic regimen but is inappropriate until active TB is excluded. Monotherapy for active TB leads to the rapid development of drug resistance. The pneumococcus rarely causes cavitary pneumonia.

7. The answer is c. *(Fauci, pp 1106-1109.)* This young man presents with classic signs and symptoms of infectious mononucleosis. In a young patient with fever, pharyngitis, lymphadenopathy, and lymphocytosis, the peripheral blood smear should be evaluated for atypical lymphocytes. A heterophile antibody test should be performed. The symptoms described in association with atypical lymphocytes and a positive heterophile test are virtually always caused by Epstein-Barr virus. Neither liver biopsy nor lymph node biopsy is necessary. Workup for toxoplasmosis or cytomegalovirus infection or hepatitis B and C would be considered in heterophile-negative patients. Hepatitis does not occur in the setting of rheumatic fever, and an anti-streptolysin O titer is not indicated.

8. The answer is a. *(Fauci, pp 1275-1279.)* The history and physical examination suggest amebic liver abscess. Symptoms usually occur 2 to 5 months after travel to an endemic area. Diarrhea usually occurs first but has usually resolved before the hepatic symptoms develop. The most common presentation for an amebic liver abscess is abdominal pain, usually RUQ. An indirect hemagglutination test is a sensitive assay and will be positive in 90% to 100% of patients. Ultrasound has a 75% to 85% sensitivity and shows abscess with well-defined margins. Stool will not show the trophozoite at this stage of the disease process. Blood cultures and broad-spectrum antibiotics would be ordered in cases of pyogenic liver abscess, but this patient's travel history, the chronicity of his illness, and his lack of clinical toxicity suggest *Entamoeba* *histolytica* as the probable cause. Aspiration is not necessary unless rupture of abscess is imminent. Metronidazole remains the drug of choice for amebic liver abscess.

9. The answer is c. *(Fauci, pp 1102-1105.)* A painful vesicular rash in a dermatomal distribution strongly suggests herpes zoster, although other viral pathogens may also cause vesicles. Herpes zoster may involve the eyelid when the first or second branch of the fifth cranial nerve is affected. Impetigo is a cellulitis caused by group A β-hemolytic streptococci. It often involves the face and can occur after an abrasion of the skin. Its distribution is not dermatomal, and while it may cause vesicles, they are usually small and are not weeping fluid. Chickenpox produces vesicles in various stages of development that are diffuse and produce more pruritus than pain. Coxsackievirus can produce a morbilliform vesiculopustular rash, often with a hemorrhagic component and with lesions of the throat, palms, and soles. Herpes simplex virus causes lesions of the lip (herpes labialis) and also does not spread in a dermatomal pattern.

10. The answer is a. *(Fauci, pp 829-831.)* This patient presents with the clinical picture of pelvic inflammatory disease (PID), including lower quadrant tenderness, cervical motion tenderness, and adnexal tenderness. Fever and mucopurulent discharge are additional evidence for the diagnosis. Treatment requires antibiotic therapy. Ceftriaxone and doxycycline are one recommended regimen that would cover both *Neisseria gonorrhoeae* and *C trachomatis*. Endometrial biopsy can provide definitive diagnosis, but it is unnecessary except when patients do not respond to therapy or have atypical presentations. Dilation and curettage, a more invasive procedure, would rarely be necessary. At times, surgical emergencies may mimic PID and even require hospitalization for further observation. The specific findings of cervical motion tenderness, discharge, and bilateral tenderness all distinguish PID from appendicitis in this patient. Aztreonam has good gram-negative coverage but does not adequately cover the sexually transmitted pathogens.

11. The answer is c. *(Fauci, pp 1055-1059.)* This patient's symptoms and time course are consistent with stage 2 Lyme disease. A few weeks after a camping trip and presumptive exposure to the *Ixodes* tick, the patient developed a rash consistent with erythema chronicum migrans (stage 1). Secondary neurologic, cardiac, or arthritic symptoms occur weeks to months after the rash. Facial nerve palsy is one of the more common signs of stage 2 Lyme disease; it may be unilateral (as in this case) or bilateral. Sarcoidosis can cause facial palsy, but there are no other signs or symptoms to suggest this disease. Idiopathic Bell palsy would not account for the previous rash or the exposure history. Syphilis always needs to be considered in the same differential with Lyme disease, but the rash described would be atypical, and the neurologic findings of secondary syphilis are usually associated with mild meningeal inflammation. The upper motor neuron involvement of lacunar infarct would spare the upper forehead.

12. The answer is a. (Fauci, pp 1820-1825.) The patient's presentation strongly suggests acute uncomplicated cystitis. Although some physicians still perform urine culture and sensitivity on all such patients, it is generally considered practical and appropriate to treat with empiric antibiotic therapy. A 3-day regimen of trimethoprim-sulfamethoxazole is recommended.

Workup for obstruction or kidney stone is not indicated in cystitis but may be necessary in the evaluation of pyelonephritis (especially recurrent disease). Low-dose antibiotic therapy has been used successfully in women with frequent (3 or more per year) urinary tract infections.

In regions where resistance to trimethoprim-sulfamethoxazole is greater than 20%, fluoroquinolones or nitrofurantoin may be used as empiric therapy instead. Fluoroquinolones have a better spectrum of activity than trimethoprim-sulfamethoxazole but are reserved for more serious or recurrent infections.

13. The answer is b. (Fauci, pp 877, 872-881.) The disease process described is most consistent with toxic shock syndrome, an inflammatory response syndrome characterized by hypotension, fever, and multiorgan involvement. It can occur in healthy women who use tampons. TSST-1 is a toxin produced by *S aureus* that is responsible for activating superantigens such as tumor necrosis factor and interleukin-1. Symptoms include confusion, as has occurred in this patient, in addition to diarrhea, myalgias, nausea and vomiting, and syncope. In addition to fever and hypotension there is a diffuse rash initially appearing on the trunk but spreading to palms of the hands and soles of the feet. Desquamation occurs a week after initial appearance of the rash. There are many potential laboratory abnormalities as manifestations of multiorgan involvement. These include azotemia, coagulopathy with abnormal aPTT, and electrolyte abnormalities, including hyponatremia, hypocalcemia, and hypokalemia. Liver function tests show hyperbilirubinemia and elevated alanine aminotransferase.

The disease is not a bacteremia, although it is precipitated by localized staphylococcal or sometimes streptococcal infection. Toxic shock syndrome sometimes mimics diseases that cause multiorgan involvement, such as systemic lupus or Rocky Mountain spotted fever. Serological studies for these diseases were negative in this patient. An allergic reaction would cause urticaria and would not account for the fever and the electrolyte abnormalities.

14. The answer is b. *(Fauci, pp 1127-1132.)* Influenza A is a potentially lethal disease in the elderly and chronically debilitated patient. In institutional settings such as nursing homes, outbreaks are likely to be particularly severe. Thus, prophylaxis is extremely important in this setting. All residents should receive the vaccine unless they have known egg allergy (patients can choose to decline the vaccine). Since protective antibodies to the vaccine will not develop for 2 weeks, oseltamivir can be used for protection against influenza A during the interim 2-week period. Because of increasing resistance, amantadine is no longer recommended for prophylaxis. The best way to prevent influenza-associated pneumonia is to prevent the outbreak in the first place.

15. The answer is d. *(Fauci, pp 803-807).* The presentation strongly suggests vertebral osteomyelitis. The vertebrae are a common site for hematogenous osteomyelitis. Prior urinary tract infection is often the primary mechanism for bacteremia and vertebral seeding. MRI is sensitive and specific for the diagnosis of vertebral osteomyelitis and is the diagnostic procedure of choice. Blood cultures at the time of presentation are positive in less than half of all cases. Treatment requires 6 to 8 weeks of antibiotics, but surgery is rarely required for cure.

16. The answer is b. *(Fauci, pp 881-890.)* The Infectious Disease Society of America's guidelines on the treatment of community-acquired pneumonia still recommend the use of sputum Gram stain and culture. This is particularly important in the era of multiantibiotic-resistant *S pneumoniae*. Sputum culture and sensitivity can direct specific antibiotic therapy for the patient as well as provide epidemiologic information for the community as a whole. A good sputum sample showing many polymorphonuclear leukocytes and few squamous epithelial cells can give important clues to etiology. A Gram stain that shows gram-positive lancet-shaped diplococci intracellularly is good evidence for pneumococcal infection. Gram-positive cocci in clusters would suggest staphylococcal infection, which would be uncommon in this setting. Empirical antibiotic therapy becomes more difficult in community-acquired pneumonia as more pathogens are recognized and as the pneumococcus develops resistance to penicillin, macrolides, and even quinolones.

17. The answer is b. *(Fauci, pp 940-942.)* The outbreak described is similar to those caused by *Escherichia coli* O157:H7. Ingestion of and infection with this organism may result in a spectrum of illnesses, including mild diarrhea, hemorrhagic colitis with bloody diarrhea, acute renal failure, and hemolytic uremic syndrome. Infection has been associated with ingestion of contaminated beef (in particular ground beef), ingestion of raw milk, and contamination via the fecal-oral route. Cooking ground beef until it is no longer pink is an effective means of preventing infection, as are hand washing and pasteurization of milk.

18. The answer is a. *(Fauci, pp 130-134.)* Patients may develop fever as a result of infectious or noninfectious diseases. The term *fever of unknown origin* (FUO) is applied when significant fever persists without a known cause after an adequate evaluation. Several studies have found the leading causes of FUO to include infections, malignancies, collagen vascular diseases, and granulomatous diseases. As the ability to more rapidly diagnose some of these diseases increases, their likelihood of causing undiagnosed persistent fever lessens. Infections such as intra-abdominal abscesses, tuberculosis, hepatobiliary disease, endocarditis (especially if the patient had previously taken antibiotics), and osteomyelitis may cause FUO. In immunocompromised patients, such as those infected with HIV, a number of opportunistic infections or lymphomas may cause fever and escape early diagnosis. Self-limited infections such as influenza should not cause fever that persists for many weeks. Neoplastic diseases such as lymphomas and some solid tumors (eg, hypernephroma and primary or metastatic disease of the liver) are associated with FUO. A number of collagen vascular diseases may cause FUO. Since conditions such as systemic lupus erythematosus are more easily diagnosed today, they are less frequent causes of this syndrome. Adult Still disease, however, is often difficult to diagnose. Other causes of FUO include granulomatous diseases (ie, giant cell arteritis, regional enteritis, sarcoidosis, and granulomatous hepatitis), drug fever, and peripheral pulmonary emboli. Factitious fever is most common among young adults employed in health-related positions. A prior psychiatric history or multiple hospitalizations at other institutions may be clues to this condition. Such patients may induce infections by self-injection of nonsterile material, with resultant multiple abscesses or polymicrobial infections. Alternatively, some patients may manipulate their thermometers. In these cases, a discrepancy between temperature and pulse or between oral temperature and witnessed rectal temperature will be observed.

19. The answer is c. *(Fauci, pp 1932-48.)* This patient has evidence for acute hepatitis as is suggested by the history, physical examination and laboratory data showing hepatocellular injury. The epidemiology favors acute hepatitis A; the patient's history of travel to Mexico and work as a teacher are risk factors for hepatitis A. The incubation period of about one month is also typical. Hepatitis B and C are less likely without evidence for drug abuse or blood transfusion. Antibody to hepatitis B surface antigen would not be evidence for acute hepatitis B. HCV RNA is the appropriate test for acute hepatitis C infection, but this disease typically causes mild transaminase elevation and rarely presents with icterus.. Liver biopsy is not indicated in acute hepatitis as the diagnosis is usually apparent from the examination, liver enzymes, and serological evidence of recent viral infection. Abdominal ultrasound would not be helpful as liver enzymes suggest hepatocellular damage, not biliary obstruction.

20. The answer is d. *(Fauci, pp 1102-1105.)* Varicella pneumonia develops in about 20% of adults with chickenpox. It occurs 3 to 7 days after the onset of the rash. The hallmarks of the chickenpox rash are papules, vesicles, and scabs in various stages of development. Fever, malaise, and itching are usually part of the clinical picture. The differential can include some coxsackievirus and echovirus infections, which might present with pneumonia and vesicular rash. Rickettsialpox, a rickettsial infection, has also been mistaken for chickenpox. Although the pneumococcus, *Mycoplasma,* and *Chlamydia* are common causes of community-acquired pneumonia in young adults, they would not account for the preceding vesicular rash. Histoplasmosis can cause acute pneumonitis after a large exposure but would not account for the rash.

21. The answer is c. *(Fauci, pp 1170, 1267-1269.)* Patients with *Pneumocystis jiroveci* (formerly *carinii*) frequently present with shortness of breath and no sputum production. The interstitial pattern of infiltrates on chest x-ray distinguishes the pneumonia from most bacterial infections. Diagnosis is made by review of methenamine silver stain. Serology is not sensitive or specific enough for routine use. The organism does not grow on any media. Cavitation can occur particularly in those who have received aerosolized pentamidine but is quite unusual. The history is likely to suggest a risk factor for HIV disease. The disease commonly recurs in patients with CD4 counts below 200 U/L.

22. The answer is a. *(Fauci p. 801.)* The striking features of this infection are its rapid onset and progression to a cellulitis characterized by dusky dark red erythema, bullae formation, and anesthesia over the area. These are clues to necrotizing fasciitis, a rapidly spreading deep soft tissue infection. The organism, usually *S pyogenes*, reaches the deep fascia from the site of penetrating trauma. Prompt surgical exploration down to fascia or muscle may be lifesaving. Necrotic tissue is Gram stained and cultured—streptococci, staphylococci, mixed anaerobic infection, or clostridia are all possible pathogens. Antibiotics to cover these organisms are important but not as important as prompt surgical debridement. Acute osteomyelitis is considered when cellulitis does not respond to antibiotic therapy, but would not present with this rapidity.

23. The answer is c. *(Fauci, pp 1061-1065.)* The rash of Rocky Mountain spotted fever (RMSF) occurs about 5 days into an illness characterized by fever, malaise, and headache. The rash may be macular or petechial, but almost always spreads from the ankles and wrists to the trunk. The disease is most common in spring and summer. North Carolina and East Tennessee have a relatively high incidence of disease. RMSF is a rickettsial disease with the tick as the vector. About 80% of patients will give a history of tick exposure. Doxycycline is considered the drug of choice, but chloramphenicol is preferred in pregnancy because of the effects of tetracycline on fetal bones and teeth. Overall mortality from the infection is now about 5%.

24. The answer is c. *(Fauci, pp 800, 884-886.)* Erysipelas, the cellulitis described, is typical of infection caused by *S pyogenes* (group A β-hemolytic streptococci). There is often a preceding event such as a cut in the skin, dermatitis, or superficial fungal infection that precedes this rapidly spreading cellulitis. *Staphylococcus epidermidis* does not cause rapidly progressive cellulitis. *Staphylococcus aureus* can cause cellulitis that is difficult to distinguish from erysipelas, but it is usually more focal and likely to produce furuncles, or abscesses. Tinea infections spread slowly and are confined to the epidermis; they would not cause fever, dermal edema, or tender lymphadenopathy. Anaerobic cellulitis is more often associated with underlying diabetes. Alpha-hemolytic streptococci rarely cause skin and soft tissue infections.

25. The answer is c. *(Fauci, pp 823-824.)* About half of all cases of non-gonococcal urethritis are caused by *C trachomatis*. *Ureaplasma urealyticum* and *Trichomonas vaginalis* are rarer causes of urethritis. Herpes simplex would present with vesicular lesions and pain. *C psittaci* is the etiologic agent in psittacosis. Almost all gonococci are susceptible to ceftriaxone at recommended doses.

26. The answer is c. *(Fauci, pp 818-821.)* The diagnosis is very consistent with *C difficile* disease. The patient is elderly, has been in both a nursing home and hospital setting and received more than a week of a fluoroquinolone antibiotic. Mild fever, abdominal pain, and watery diarrhea are all consistent with the diagnosis, and the cell culture cytotoxicity test is the most specific of diagnostic tests. Failure on metronidazole is increasingly reported with at least a 25% failure rate. Switch to oral vancomycin is recommended. The patient does not have fulminant disease which usually presents as an acute abdomen, sepsis, or toxic megacolon. Synthetic fecal bacterial enema is one potential treatment being studied for recurrent *C difficile* disease but is not standard treatment.

27. The answer is c. *(King MD, et al, pp 309-317.)* Community onset skin infection is often caused by methicillin-resistant staphylococci. Over 63% of *Staphylococcus* isolates from the community were methicillin-resistant in one study. However these isolates are different from the methicillin-resistant *Staphylococcus* seen in the hospital setting. In the King study, all of these community isolates were sensitive to trimethoprim-sulfamethoxazole and to clindamycin as well. They were resistant to beta lactams and erythromycin. In healthy individuals such as the wrestler described, hospitalization and treatment with vancomycin would not be necessary or appropriate. Linezolid and daptomycin are alternates to vancomycin in some circumstances for the management of hospital-acquired methicillin-resistant *Staphylococcus*. Streptococci usually cause a rapidly spreading cellulitis without pustule formation.

28. The answer is a. *(Fauci, pp 1189-1200.)* Guidelines for antiviral therapy are changing rapidly, but it is clear that the institution of antiviral therapy in patients with CD4 counts below 200 improves longevity even if the patient is asymptomatic. Recommendations now include instituting therapy even for CD4 counts between 200 and 350, although supporting data are somewhat less clear. There are several new antiviral drugs and new classes of drugs for HIV disease, but the approach to initial treatment with two nucleoside reverse transcriptase inhibitors (NRTIs) and a non-nucleoside reverse transcriptase inhibitor (NNRTI) or two NRTIs with a protease inhibitor is not likely to change any time soon. New categories of drugs such as raltegravir, an integrase inhibitor, and maraviroc, a CCR5 antagonist, are used to treat patients who have failed therapy. Genotyping is recommended even in the workup of treatment-naive patients, as resistant HIV strains are becoming more prevalent (about 15%, depending on geographic area). With the routine screening for HLA B5701 in patients being considered for abacavir treatment, this agent has become safer; hypersensitivity reactions are unlikely to occur in patients who are HLA B5701 negative.

29. The answer is b. (*Fauci, pp 1291-1293.*) Whether or not to use drugs such as atovaquone-proguanil, mefloquine, or primaquine for resistant *P falciparum* will depend upon knowledge of specific local patterns of drug sensitivity of plasmodia. Specific information can be obtained from the CDC malaria hotline or the CDC emergency operations center. The common sense measures described are extremely important and part of the overall worldwide plan to contain the spread of malaria. Prophylaxis should begin two days to two weeks before departure in order to have adequate levels of drug on arrival and to identify potential side effects before leaving. Mosquito peak feeding periods are dawn and dusk.

30 to 33. The answers are 30-c, 31-d, 32-e, 33-a. (*Fauci, pp 789-798,889.*) The 30-year-old female with mitral valve prolapse has developed subacute bacterial endocarditis. The likely etiologic agent is a viridans streptococci. Viridans streptococci cause most cases of subacute bacterial endocarditis. No other agent listed is likely to cause this infection. The 80-year-old male with a Foley catheter in place has developed a nosocomial infection likely secondary to urosepsis. *Providencia* species and other gram-negative rods frequently cause urinary tract infection in the hospitalized patient. The young man with a fluctuant lesion and fistula over the mandible presents a classic picture of cervicofacial actinomycosis. The man with fulminant post-splenectomy sepsis was unable to fight off an encapsulated organism once it reached the bloodstream. The pneumococcus is the most likely organism, although *H influenzae* and *Neisseria meningitidis* can cause the same syndrome.

34 to 36. The answers are 34-b, 35-g, 36-f. (*Fauci, pp 1249-1251, 1256-1260, 1261-1263.*) Blastomycosis presents with signs and symptoms of chronic respiratory infection. The organism has a tendency to produce skin lesions in exposed areas that become crusted, ulcerated, or verrucous. Bone pain is caused by osteolytic lesions. Mucormycosis is a zygomycosis that originates in the nose and paranasal sinuses. Sinus tenderness, bloody nasal discharge, and obtundation occur usually in the setting of diabetic ketoacidosis. *Aspergillus* can result in several different infectious processes, including aspergilloma, disseminated *Aspergillus* in the immunocompromised patient, or allergic bronchopulmonary aspergillosis. Bronchopulmonary aspergillosis is the most likely diagnosis in the young woman with asthma and eosinophilia. Bronchial plugs, often filled with hyphal forms, result in repeated infiltrates and exacerbation of wheezing.

37 to 40. The answers are 37-c, 38-d, 39-e, 40-b. *(Fauci, pp 124-129, 1106-1109, 1114-1117.)* Parvovirus B19 is the agent responsible for erythema infectiosum, also known as fifth disease. This disease most commonly affects children between the ages of 5 and 14 years, but it can also occur in adults. Adults can develop a polyarthropathy syndrome. The disease is characterized by a slapped-cheek rash in children, which may follow a prodrome of low-grade fever. A diffuse lacelike rash occurs in adults. Complications in adults also include aplastic crisis in patients with chronic hemolytic anemia, spontaneous abortion, and hydrops fetalis.

Desquamation of the skin usually occurs during or after recovery from toxic shock syndrome (associated with a toxin produced by *S aureus*). Peeling of the skin is also seen in Kawasaki disease, scarlet fever, and some severe drug reactions.

Petechial rashes are often seen with potentially life-threatening infections, including meningococcemia, gonococcemia, rickettsial disease, infective endocarditis, atypical measles, and disseminated intravascular coagulation (DIC) associated with sepsis.

Infectious mononucleosis is the usual manifestation of infection with Epstein-Barr virus. Since it is a viral disease, antibiotic therapy is not indicated. A diffuse maculopapular rash has been observed in over 90% of patients with infectious mononucleosis who are given ampicillin. The rash does not represent an allergic reaction to β-lactam antibiotics.

41 to 45. The answers are 41-a, 42-d, 43-b, 44-c, 45-h. *(Fauci, pp 1098-1099, 1173, 1174-1176, 1247-1249, 1256-1260.)* There are several causes for dysphagia in the HIV-positive patient, including *C albicans,* herpes simplex, and cytomegalovirus. The biopsy result in this patient confirms *Candida* infection with the typical picture of both yeast and hyphae seen on smear.

Herpes simplex encephalitis can occur in patients of any age—usually in immunocompetent patients. Most adults with HSV encephalitis have previous infection with mucocutaneous HSV-1. The bizarre behavior includes personality aberrations, hypersexuality, or sensory hallucinations. CSF shows lymphocytes with a near normal sugar and protein. Focal abnormalities are seen in the temporal lobe by CT scan, MRI, or EEG.

The patient who has had a previous history of tuberculosis and now complains of hemoptysis would be reevaluated for active tuberculosis. However, the chest x-ray described is characteristic of a fungus ball—almost always the result of an aspergilloma growing in a previous cavitary lesion.

The Filipino patient who has developed a pulmonary nodule after travel through the Southwest would be suspected of having developed coccidioidomycosis. Individuals from the Philippines have a higher incidence of the disease and are more likely to have complications of dissemination.

The 35-year-old with cough, sore throat, and fever went on to develop symptoms of myopericarditis with typical ECG findings. Coxsackievirus B infection is the most likely cause of URI symptoms that evolve into a picture of myopericarditis. Pericarditis may be asymptomatic or can present with chest pain, both pleuritic and ischemic-like. Enteroviruses rarely if ever attack the pericardium alone without involving the subepicardial myocardium.

Hospital-Based Medicine

Questions

46. A 72-year-old man presents with progressive abdominal pain over the last 2 days. He has had several loose stools, subjective fever, and decreased appetite. Past medical history is significant for hypertension, diet-controlled diabetes mellitus, and one admission to the hospital for heart failure 2 years ago. He takes a beta-blocker and loop diuretic faithfully as prescribed by his physician. Vital signs include heart rate 92 and blood pressure 126/64. Physical examination reveals mucosal stranding of the oropharynx, no JVD, no lower extremity edema, and tenderness to palpation of the left lower quadrant of the abdomen. CT scan with contrast of the abdomen has been ordered. What is the best next step in the management of this patient?

a. Administer low-dose aspirin for prophylaxis of venous thromboembolism.
b. Administer low-dose low-molecular-weight heparin for prophylaxis of venous thromboembolism.
c. Administer treatment dose of low-molecular-weight heparin for presumed ischemic colitis.
d. Administer 600-mg N-acetylcysteine for prevention of contrast-induced nephropathy.
e. Administer 150-mEq sodium bicarbonate in 1-L D5 water for prevention of contrast-induced nephropathy.

47. You respond to the cardiopulmonary arrest of a 72-year-old woman in the intensive care unit. She has no palpable pulse, but the cardiac monitor shows sinus tachycardia at 124/minute. Breath sounds are symmetric with bag-mask positive pressure ventilation. What is the best next step in evaluation or management of this patient?

a. Immediate electrical cardioversion
b. Immediate transthoracic cardiac pacing
c. Immediate administration of high-volume normal saline
d. Immediate large-bore pericardiocentesis
e. Immediate administration of extended spectrum antibiotics

48. A 64-year-old man presents with acute exacerbation of chronic obstructive pulmonary disease. The patient had a long smoking history before quitting 2 years ago. In spite of his poor baseline lung function, he has been able to maintain an independent lifestyle. The patient is in obvious respiratory distress and appears tired. He has difficulty greeting you secondary to shortness of breath. Respiratory rate is 32/minute. Auscultation of the lungs reveals minimal air movement. ABGs show pH = 7.28, $PaCO_2 = 77$, and $PaO_2 = 54$. One dose of IV methylprednisolone has already been administered. What is the best next step in the management of this patient's disease?

a. Urgent institution of BiPAP (bilevel positive airway pressure)
b. Urgent endotracheal intubation
c. Administration of 100% FiO_2 by face mask
d. Arrangement for admission to monitored ICU bed
e. IV levofloxacin

49. A 71-year-old woman is brought to the emergency room by her daughter because of sudden onset of right-sided weakness and slurred speech. The patient, a recent immigrant from Southeast Asia, has not seen a doctor in 2 decades. Her symptoms began 75 minutes ago while she was eating breakfast. A stat noncontrast CT scan of the head is normal. Labs are normal. Physical examination reveals an anxious appearing woman with dense hemiplegia of the R upper and lower extremities. Deep tendon reflexes are not discernible on the R side and 2+ on the left. Aspirin has been given. What is the best next step in management of this patient?

a. Immediate intravenous unfractionated heparin
b. Immediate thrombolytic therapy
c. Immediate administration of interferon-beta
d. Emergent MRI/MRA of head
e. Emergent cardiac catheterization

50. You are asked to see a 78-year-old woman prior to surgical repair of a femoral neck fracture. Her medical problems include hypertension, osteoporosis, and hypothyroidism. Morphine is the only medication ordered so far. She is comfortable at rest. Her BP is 136/82, HR 88, RR 16. Her cardiac examination is normal, and her lungs are clear. What is the best recommendation to prevent postoperative venous thrombosis?

a. Postoperative low-dose ASA
b. Postoperative SCDs (sequential compression devices)
c. Early mobilization and ambulation
d. Postoperative subcutaneous low-molecular-weight heparin
e. Postoperative intravenous unfractionated heparin

51. An 84-year-old woman develops confusion and agitation after surgery for hip fracture. Her family reports that prior to her hospitalization she functioned independently at home, although requiring help with balancing her checkbook and paying bills. Her current medications include intravenous fentanyl for pain control, lorazepam for control of her agitation, and DVT prophylaxis. She has also been started on ciprofloxacin for pyuria (culture pending). In addition to frequent reorientation of the patient, which of the following series of actions would best manage this patient's delirium?

a. Increase lorazepam to more effective dose, repeat urinalysis.
b. Discontinue lorazepam, remove Foley catheter, add haloperidol for severe agitation, and change to nonfluoroquinolone antibiotic.
c. Continue lorazepam at current dose, discontinue fentanyl, add soft restraints.
d. Continue lorazepam at current dose, add alprazolam 0.25 mg for severe agitation, repeat urinalysis, restrain patient to prevent self harm.
e. Discontinue lorazepam, remove Foley catheter, add alprazolam 0.25 mg for severe agitation, place the patient on telemetry.

52. You are caring for a 72-year-old male admitted to the hospital with an exacerbation of congestive heart failure. Two weeks prior to admission, he was able to ambulate two blocks before stopping because of dyspnea. He has now returned to baseline and is ready for discharge. His preadmission medications include aspirin, metoprolol, and furosemide. Systolic blood pressure has ranged from 110 mm Hg-128 mm Hg over the course of his hospitalization. Heart rate was in 120s at the time of presentation, but has been consistently around 70/minute over the past 24 hours. An echocardiogram performed during this hospitalization revealed global hypokinesis with an ejection fraction of 30%. Which of the following medications, when added to his preadmission regimen, would be most likely to decrease his risk of subsequent mortality?

a. Digoxin
b. Enalapril
c. Hydrochlorothiazide
d. Propranolol
e. Spironolactone

53. A 64-year-old woman presents to the emergency room with flank pain and fever. She noted dysuria over the past 3 days. Blood and urine cultures are obtained, and she is started on intravenous ciprofloxacin. Six hours after admission, she becomes tachycardic and her blood pressure drops. Her intravenous fluid is NS at 100 mL/h. Her current blood pressure is 79/43 mm Hg, heart rate is 128/minute, respiratory rate is 26/minute and temperature is 39.2°C (102.5°F). She seems drowsy yet uncomfortable. Extremities are warm with trace edema. What is the best next course of action?

a. Administer IV hydrocortisone at stress dose.
b. Begin norepinephrine infusion and titrate to mean arterial pressure greater than 65 mm Hg.
c. Add vancomycin to her antibiotic regimen for improved gram positive coverage.
d. Administer a bolus of normal saline.
e. Place a central venous line to monitor central venous oxygen saturation.

54. An 88-year-old resident of a local nursing home is transferred to your facility with shortness of breath. She has been coughing for the past 2 to 3 days. The patient has a history of mild dementia, but has had no witnessed episodes of coughing or choking when eating. Vital signs include a heart rate of 103/minute, respiratory rate of 22/minute, blood pressure 158/68 mm Hg, temperature of 37.9°C (100.2°F) with a weight of 52 kg. Upon examination, she is pleasant but disoriented. Chest auscultation reveals crackles in the left lower lung field. WBC count is 11,000, BUN is 32, and creatinine is 1.3. Chest radiograph shows an infiltrate in the left lower lobe, and induced sputum sample has been sent for Gram stain and culture. What is the best initial course of therapy for this patient?

a. Begin a third-generation cephalosporin and macrolide and admit her to the hospital.
b. Begin a renal-dosed third-generation cephalosporin and macrolide and admit her to the hospital.
c. Begin a respiratory fluoroquinolone and discharge her to the nursing home for follow-up.
d. Begin an antipseudomonal carbapenem, antipseudomonal respiratory fluoroquinolone, and glycopeptide and admit her to the hospital.
e. Begin a renal-dosed antipseudomonal carbapenem, antipseudomonal respiratory fluoroquinolone, and glycopeptide and admit her to the hospital.

55. A 78-year-old male presents to the emergency department with acute onset of bright red blood per rectum. Symptoms started 2 hours earlier, and he has had 3 bowel movements since then with copious amounts of blood. He denies prior episodes of rectal bleeding. He notes dizziness with standing but denies abdominal pain. He has had no vomiting or nausea. A nasogastric lavage is performed and shows no coffee ground emesis or blood. Lab evaluation reveals hemoglobin of 10.5 g/dL. What is the most likely source of the bleeding?

a. Internal hemorrhoids
b. Dreulofoy lesion
c. Diverticulosis
d. Mallory-Weiss tear
e. Sessile polyp

56. You are caring for a 52-year-old man with back and shoulder pain. He has a history of heavy smoking and occasionally uses marijuana. An admission chest radiograph suggests a lytic lesion in his right scapula and mediastinal lymphadenopathy. He currently is receiving 2 mg morphine IV every 4 hours but reports his pain remains an "8" on a pain scale of "1-10." What is the best next step in controlling his pain while his evaluation continues?

a. Bolus with 4 mg morphine and begin morphine patient controlled analgesia (PCA).
b. Begin morphine patient controlled analgesia (PCA).
c. Begin basal therapy with a transdermal fentanyl patch.
d. Begin adjunct therapy with oral gabapentin.
e. Change narcotic to meperidine at an equipotent dose.

57. A 48-year-old male is admitted to your service after an inhalational chemical exposure. He develops respiratory distress and requires endotracheal intubation and mechanical ventilation. Which of the following is most likely to decrease his risk of developing ventilator acquired pneumonia?

a. Daily interruption of sedation to assess respiratory status
b. Nasopharyngeal rather than oropharyngeal endotracheal intubation
c. Institution of protocol to keep bed flat during ventilation
d. Intermittent nasopharyngeal suctioning
e. Prophylactic narrow spectrum intravenous antibiotics

58. You have been asked to see a 58-year-old male admitted to the ICU after coronary artery bypass surgery yesterday. He has no history of diabetes, but his blood sugars have ranged from 59 to 225 over the past 24 hours. His nurse reports that he has been nauseated and ate very little of his clear liquid diet this morning. His current medications include "sliding scale" insulin, a beta-blocker, and a thiazide diuretic. What is the best next step in managing this patient's blood sugar?

a. Begin metformin 500-mg po bid.
b. Begin scheduled subcutaneous long-acting insulin and scheduled short-acting insulin with meals.
c. Begin intravenous insulin drip.
d. Continue sliding scale insulin and make patient NPO until blood sugars stabilize.
e. Continue sliding scale and stop the beta-blocker as this may mask signs of hypoglycemia.

59. A 78-year-old woman is admitted to the hospital after losing consciousness at home. She reports that she was walking from the kitchen to the bedroom and began to feel "light-headed." Within a few seconds, symptoms progressed to the point of unconsciousness and she fell to the floor. Her daughter, who witnessed the event, reports that she regained consciousness almost immediately after falling to the floor. She had one prior similar episode the week before. The patient has no significant past medical history except for hypertension, for which she takes hydrochlorothiazide and metoprolol. Blood pressure is 138/64 standing and 140/70 supine. Physical examination is otherwise unrevealing. ECG shows a sinus rhythm. An echocardiogram reveals no structural heart abnormality. What is the best next test to evaluate her sudden loss of consciousness?

a. Carotid ultrasound
b. Electroencephalogram (EEG)
c. Fasting glucose study
d. MRI of brain with contrast
e. Overnight observation with continuous cardiac monitoring

60. A 42-year-old male was admitted to the hospital with pneumonia. On the third day of his hospitalization he becomes agitated and confused. He reports feeling "spiders" crawling on his skin. You note that he has a blood pressure of 172/94 mm Hg, heart rate of 107/minute, and temperature of 38°C (100.4°F). With the exception of agitation and tremor, the remainder of his physical examination is unchanged from earlier in the day. What is the best initial step in management of this patient?

a. Emergent noncontrast CT scan of the brain
b. Emergent administration of intravenous haloperidol
c. Emergent administration of intravenous lorazepam
d. Emergent administration of intravenous labetalol
e. Placement of physical restraints for patient safety

Hospital-Based Medicine

Answers

46 The answer is e. (*Fauci, pp 1755, 2492.*) The patient likely has diverticulitis. He is also, however, at high risk of development of radiography-contrast-induced nephropathy from the CT scan. Volume depletion, diabetes mellitus, congestive heart failure, chronic kidney disease and multiple myeloma are all risk factors for contrast-induced kidney damage. The patient's renal risk can be reduced by correction of his volume status with IV fluids. In at-risk patients who are euvolemic, aggressive hydration with normal saline or iso-osmolar sodium bicarbonate infusion prior to and after contrast administration reduces renal damage. Risk may also be decreased by the use of low-osmolar, nonionic contrast agents. N-acetylcysteine is commonly used to decrease the risk of renal damage, but appropriate fluid resuscitation remains paramount. Prophylaxis of venous thromboembolism (VTE) would be important if the patient is hospitalized but would not take precedence over fluid resuscitation. Ischemic colitis is usually caused by low flow in a mesenteric vessel; even if this were the diagnosis (and diverticulitis is more likely), therapeutic doses of anticoagulants are not used in the treatment of ischemic colitis. Aspirin is not acceptable prophylaxis of VTE.

47. The answer is c. (*Fauci, pp 1707-1713.*) Pulseless electrical activity (PEA) is a common cause of cardiopulmonary arrest in the hospital setting. Etiologies of PEA include hypovolemia, hypoxia, hyperkalemia, severe acidosis, pulmonary embolism, cardiac tamponade, and tension pneumothorax. The loss of cardiac output results from decreased ventricular filling (hypovolemia, pulmonary embolism, cardiac tamponade, or tension pneumothorax) or electromechanical dissociation (hypoxia, hyperkalemia, or severe acidosis). Management of PEA arrest requires rapid establishment of vascular access, airway stabilization, and administration of IV fluids. Physical examination focuses on potential correctable etiologies. Electrical cardioversion will not benefit a patient in sinus rhythm. Similarly, cardiac pacing is unlikely to be successful. Sudden pericardial tamponade is uncommon, but if suspected (proper setting, jugular distension, low-voltage ECG) pericardiocentesis is performed. If sepsis is suspected, broad spectrum antibiotics would be appropriate, but antibiotic administration will not affect the immediate outcome of the cardiopulmonary arrest.

48. The answer is a. *(Fauci, pp 1665-1668, 1684-1688.)* Bilevel positive airway pressure (BiPAP) ventilation has found increased favor in acute lung or heart disease, especially in those with acute CO_2 retention. The use of BiPAP may prevent the need for endotracheal intubation with its concomitant risks. BiPAP is contraindicated in patients with severe respiratory acidosis, decreased level of consciousness, bradypnea, or hemodynamic instability, for whom endotracheal intubation is the best treatment. Although oxygen should never be withheld from a hypoxic patient, caution must be exercised in patients with chronic CO_2 retention. Overly aggressive oxygen therapy may actually increase $Paco_2$. In patients with chronic CO_2 retention, a targeted oxygen saturation of 88%-92% is appropriate. Admission to the ICU is appropriate, but the patient must be stabilized before transporting. Antibiotics are given for severe COPD exacerbations (especially if the patient is producing purulent sputum) but will not affect the immediate outcome of his respiratory failure.

49. The answer is b. *(Fauci, pp 2513-2531.)* This patient presents with an acute left middle cerebral artery stroke. Time is of the essence if thrombolytic therapy is to be beneficial. Intravenous thrombolytics may be administered up to 3 hours after the onset of symptoms. Fortunately, this patient was brought to the ER promptly. CT scan of the brain shows no evidence of bleed. Evidence of ischemia may not become apparent until 48-72 hours. A prior history of intracranial hemorrhage, recent surgery, bleeding diathesis, onset of symptoms greater than 3 hours prior to therapy and unknown time of onset of symptoms are contraindications to thrombolytic therapy. This patient should be given intravenous tissue-type plasminogen activator (t-PA).

Anticoagulation in acute stroke (answer a) is not currently recommended. In most trials of anticoagulation, any benefit of therapy is matched by an increase in hemorrhagic transformation. Interferon-beta (answer c) is used to treat multiple sclerosis, not ischemic stroke. Emergent scanning with MRI (answer d) wastes precious time and is not always available. Patients with acute stroke often have mild elevation in cardiac biomarkers. Cardiac catheterization (answer e) is unnecessary, and may very well prove harmful in the setting of a stroke.

50. The answer is d. *(Fauci, pp 731-735)*. After orthopedic injury, patients are at high risk of development of deep vein thrombosis. Other risk factors for DVT formation include advanced age, immobility, malignancy, hypercoagulable states, and prior history of DVT. Appropriate options for DVT prophylaxis after hip fracture include subcutaneous unfractionated or low-molecular-weight heparin. SCDs (answer b) may be used in addition to chemoprophylaxis, but SCDs by themselves are not effective in hip fracture patients. Early ambulation is recommended as tolerated for all patients at risk for DVT, but is not enough to fully attenuate risk after a hip fracture. Aspirin (answer a) is never recommended by itself for inpatient DVT prophylaxis. Intravenous heparin is used for DVT therapy, not prophylaxis.

51. The answer is b. *(Fauci, pp 158-162.)* Delirium is a common complication in the hospital setting. Delirium may be differentiated from dementia by its acute onset and waxing and waning mental state. Elderly patients, especially those with a history of dementia, and the severely ill are at greatest risk of developing delirium. Delirium may be precipitated by medications, postsurgical state, infection, or electrolyte imbalance. The management of delirium relies on nonpharmacologic approaches, including frequent reorientation, discontinuation of any unnecessary noxious stimuli (eg, urinary catheters, unnecessary oxygen delivery systems or telemetry monitors, and restraints), environmental modification to establish day/night sleep cycles, and discontinuation of all unnecessary medications. This patient likely will continue to need pain control, but the dose of fentanyl should be minimized to the smallest effective dose. Benzodiazepines frequently induce a delirium and their continued use or escalation may impair recovery. Fluoroquinolones can worsen mental status in the elderly. Physical or chemical restraints actually impair recovery from delirium and should be used only as last resort to prevent serious harm to self or others. A repeat urinalysis would provide no useful information since the original urine culture is still pending.

52. The answer is b. *(Fauci, pp 1443-1455.)* Inhibition of the renin-angiotensin-aldosterone system by either angiotensin converting enzyme inhibitors (ACEi) or angiotensin receptor blockers (ARB) has been proven to decrease mortality in patients with symptoms of congestive heart failure and a depressed ejection fraction. All patients with a history of congestive heart failure should be maintained on a beta-blocker and an ACEi or ARB. Most patients will require a diuretic for symptom control. Digitalis glycosides decrease rehospitalization rate but have not been shown to improve mortality. Thiazide diuretics are excellent medications for blood pressure control. Our patient, however, has well-controlled blood pressure. The patient is already on a selective beta-blocker and the addition of a nonselective beta-blocker is unlikely to be helpful. Spironolactone provides mortality benefit in patients with NYHA class III or IV heart failure. The patient in this scenario was able to walk 2 blocks prior to stopping and would be classified as NYHA class II.

53. The answer is d. *(Fauci, pp 1695-1702.)* This patient is septic, and immediate therapy should be directed at correcting her hemodynamic instability. Patients with sepsis require aggressive fluid resuscitation to compensate for capillary extravasation. This patient's vital signs suggest decreased effective circulating volume. Normal saline at 100 cc/h is insufficient volume replacement. The patient should be given a saline bolus of 2 L over 20 minutes, and then her blood pressure and clinical status should be reassessed. The elevated respiratory rate could be evidence of pulmonary edema or respiratory compensation of acidosis from decreased tissue perfusion. Even if the patient has evidence of pulmonary edema, fluid resuscitation remains the first intervention for hypotension from sepsis. She is more likely to die from hemodynamic collapse than from oxygenation issues related to pulmonary edema.

Stress doses of hydrocortisone and intravenous norepinephrine are both used in patients with shock refractory to volume resuscitation, but should be reserved until after the saline bolus. Vancomycin is a reasonable choice to cover enterococci, which can cause UTI-associated sepsis, but again would not address the immediate hemodynamic problem. If the patient does not improve, a central line (to measure filling pressures and mixed venous oxygen saturation) would allow the "early goal-directed" sepsis protocol to be used.

54. The answer is e. *(Fauci, pp 1619-1628.)* The term "healthcare-associated pneumonia" is used to describe patients with increased risk for drug-resistant etiologies of pneumonia. Residents of long-term care facilities as well as patients with recent antibiotic exposure, recent hospitalization, chronic dialysis, and home wound care are at greater risk of pneumonia from multidrug resistant (MDR) bacteria such as *Pseudomonas aeruginosa*, extended-spectrum beta-lactamase gram-negative bacilli, *Acinetobacter,* and methicillin-resistant *Staphylococcus aureus*. As such, it would be inappropriate to treat this patient in the same manner as a community dweller without risk factors for MDR. Instead of the typical community-acquired pneumonia (CAP) coverage (third-generation cephalosporin and macrolide or a respiratory fluoroquinolone as in answers a, b, and c), the patient should also be empirically treated for the MDR bacteria listed above. The carbapenem and fluoroquinolone would cover potentially resistant gram-negative rods; the glycopeptide (vancomycin is often used) would cover MRSA. Of note, the patient in this vignette has an estimated creatinine clearance of 25 mL/min. Renal dose adjustment of her antibiotics would be appropriate.

55. The answer is c. (*Fauci, pp 257-260.*) Bright red blood per rectum typically indicates a lower GI source of bleeding, although occasionally a high output upper GI bleed may result in bright red blood. Diverticular bleeds can be massive. Although 80% resolve spontaneously, bleeding recurs in one-fourth of patients. Colonoscopy would be the diagnostic method of choice if diverticular bleed is suspected, but bleeding has frequently stopped before visualization occurs. With recurrent diverticular bleed, hemicolectomy may be necessary. Although nasogastric lavage has lost favor as a diagnostic maneuver, in this case, a negative lavage decreases the likelihood of a significant bleed in the stomach or esophagus. Neither internal hemorrhoids nor sessile colonic polyps usually result in hemodynamically significant acute bleeding. A Dieulafoy vessel is a large caliber vessel close the mucosal surface, most commonly located on the greater curvature of the stomach. Mallory-Weiss tears occur as a result of traumatic injury at the gastroesophageal junction from forceful vomiting and may lead to large-volume blood loss. Both of these lesions would be associated with evidence of upper GI bleeding.

56. The answer is a. (*Fauci, pp 482-486.*) The patient's clinical findings and history are highly suspicious for metastatic cancer. The patient has experienced minimal relief with intermittent narcotic dosing. A larger bolus of narcotic will be necessary to reduce the pain to an acceptable level. None of the other therapies mentioned will promptly control his pain. Patient-controlled analgesia pumps deliver narcotics in small amounts and, without an additional bolus, would take hours to days to achieve pain relief. Transdermal delivery systems are useful for maintenance therapy, but are difficult to titrate to achieve acute control. Gabapentin is especially helpful in patients with neuropathic pain. Although a few patients note significant improvement with one narcotic over another, the relatively low dose of narcotic prescribed here would suggest failure of therapy secondary to dosing rather than a problem with the medication chosen. Meperidine use is limited by the production of an active metabolite (normeperidine) with increase risk of CNS toxicity including sedation, respiratory depression, and seizures.

57. The answer is a. *(Fauci, pp 1687-1688.)* Daily interruption of sedation ("sedation holiday") to assess readiness for extubation has been shown to decrease the risk of ventilator acquired pneumonia. Oropharyngeal (rather than nasopharyngeal) intubation, elevating the head of the bed (rather than keeping the patient flat), and subglottic secretion suctioning can also decrease ventilator acquired pneumonia. Nasopharyngeal and gastrointestinal tract bacterial flora modulation via topical or oral antibiotics may also decrease VAP risk, although it is not routinely recommended. Prophylactic intravenous antibiotics are not recommended.

58. The answer is c. *(Fauci, p 1678.)* Although there is no consensus for a universal target blood sugar in the intensive care unit, there is good evidence that surgical patients in the ICU benefit from tight blood sugar control. In particular, the poststernotomy patient with uncontrolled blood sugars is at increased risk of mediastinitis. Elevated blood sugars in this patient would be most rapidly controlled with an intravenous insulin drip. Metformin may increase the risk of lactic acidosis in the first 24-48 hours postsurgery or after the administration of intravenous radiographic contrast. Scheduled basal and preprandial insulin is the mainstay of blood sugar control in the hospital, but titration to target blood sugar takes longer than intravenous insulin. Sliding scale insulin alone is rarely the best choice of therapy in the hospitalized patient. Beta-blockers may mask the symptoms of hypoglycemia, but are an important component of post-coronary-artery bypass-surgery therapy. Discontinuing the patient's beta-blocker will not improve the patient's blood sugar control.

59. The answer is e. *(Fauci, pp 139-143.)* Syncope is usually caused by decreased blood flow to the brain. Although occasionally seizures and hypoglycemia can cause transient loss of consciousness, this patient's rapid onset of symptoms and rapid recovery once recumbent suggest decreased cerebral perfusion. She has no evidence of aortic stenosis or other structural heart disease on echocardiogram. It would be reasonable to monitor the patient's heart rhythm initially in the hospital. Carotid artery disease almost never causes transient syncope, although vertebral-basilar disease may. Therefore, carotid Doppler imaging is not recommended as part of the routine evaluation of syncope. Structural imaging of the brain and EEG are not part of the routine evaluation of syncope unless history or physical examination suggest seizure or a focal CNS lesion.

60. The answer is c. (*Fauci, p 2728.*) This patient exhibits several symptoms suggestive of acute alcoholic withdrawal syndrome. An acute intracranial event will usually be associated with head trauma (subdural hematoma) or focal neurological abnormalities. In addition, radiographic imaging may be difficult to perform while the patient is acutely agitated. Haloperidol is commonly used to treat acute psychosis, but benzodiazepines are better in the setting of alcohol withdrawal. The patient's blood pressure will likely improve with administration of benzodiazepine and beta-blockade may be unnecessary. Physical restraints should only be used as a therapy "of last resort" and do not take the place of treating the underlying disorder.

Rheumatology

Questions

61. A 40-year-old woman complains of 7 weeks of pain and swelling in both wrists and knees. She has several months of fatigue. After a period of rest, resistance to movement is more striking. On examination, the metacarpophalangeal joints and wrists are warm and tender. There are no other joint abnormalities. There is no alopecia, photosensitivity, kidney disease, or rash. Which of the following is correct?

a. The clinical picture suggests early rheumatoid arthritis, and a rheumatoid factor should be obtained.
b. The prodrome of lethargy suggests chronic fatigue syndrome.
c. Lack of systemic symptoms suggests osteoarthritis.
d. X-rays of the hand are likely to show joint space narrowing and erosion.
e. An aggressive search for occult malignancy is indicated.

62. A 70-year-old man complains of fever and pain in his left knee. Several days previously, he suffered an abrasion of his knee while working in his garage. The knee is red, warm, and swollen. An arthocentesis is performed, which shows 200,000 leukocytes/μL and a glucose of 20 mg/dL. No crystals are noted. Which of the following is the most important next step?

a. Gram stain and culture of joint fluid
b. Urethral culture
c. Uric acid level
d. Antinuclear antibody
e. Antineutrophil cytoplasmic antibody

63. A 60-year-old woman complains of dry mouth and a gritty sensation in her eyes. She states it is sometimes difficult to speak for more than a few minutes. There is no history of diabetes mellitus or neurologic disease. The patient is on no medications. On examination, the buccal mucosa appears dry and the salivary glands are enlarged bilaterally. Which of the following is the best next step in evaluation?

a. Lip biopsy
b. Schirmer test and measurement of autoantibodies
c. IgG antibody to mumps virus
d. A therapeutic trial of prednisone for 1 month
e. Administration of a benzodiazepine

64. A 40-year-old man complains of exquisite pain and tenderness in the left ankle. There is no history of trauma. The patient is taking hydrochlorothiazide for hypertension. On examination, the ankle is very swollen and tender. There are no other physical examination abnormalities. Which of the following is the best next step in management?

a. Begin colchicine and broad-spectrum antibiotics.
b. Perform arthrocentesis.
c. Begin allopurinol if uric acid level is elevated.
d. Obtain ankle x-ray to rule out fracture.
e. Apply a splint or removable cast.

65. A 48-year-old woman complains of joint pain and morning stiffness for 4 months. Examination reveals swelling of the wrists and MCPs as well as tenderness and joint effusion in both knees. The rheumatoid factor is positive, antibodies to cyclic citrullinated protein are present, and subcutaneous nodules are noted on the extensor surfaces of the forearm. Which of the following statements is correct?

a. Prednisone 60 mg per day should be started.
b. The patient has RA and should be evaluated for disease-modifying antirheumatic therapy.
c. A nonsteroidal antiinflammatory drug should be added to aspirin.
d. The patient's prognosis is highly favorable.
e. The patient should receive a 3-month trial of full-dose nonsteroidal anti-inflammatory agent before determining whether and/or what additional therapy is indicated.

66. A 45-year-old woman with long-standing, well-controlled rheumatoid arthritis develops severe pain and swelling in the left elbow over 2 days. She is not sexually active. Arthrocentesis reveals cloudy fluid. Synovial fluid analysis reveals >100,000 cells/mL; 98% of these are PMNs. What is the most likely organism to cause this scenario?

a. *Streptococcus pneumoniae*
b. *Neisseria gonorrhoeae*
c. *Escherichia coli*
d. *Staphylococcus aureus*
e. *Pseudomnonas aeruginosa*

67. A 66-year-old man complains of a 1-year history of low-back and buttock pain that worsens with walking and is relieved by sitting or bending forward. He has hypertension and takes hydrochlorothiazide but has otherwise been healthy. There is no history of back trauma, fever, or weight loss. On examination, the patient has a slightly stooped posture, pain on lumbar extension, and has a slightly wide base gait. Pedal pulses are normal and there are no femoral bruits. Examination of peripheral joints and skin is normal. What is the most likely cause for this patient's back and buttock pain?

a. Lumbar spinal stenosis
b. Herniated nucleus pulposus
c. Atherosclerotic peripheral vascular disease
d. Facet joint arthritis
e. Prostate cancer

68. A 60-year-old man complains of pain in both knees coming on gradually over the past 2 years. The pain is relieved by rest and worsened by movement. The patient is 5 ft 9 in. tall and weighs 210 lb. There is bony enlargement of the knees with mild warmth and small effusions. Crepitation is noted on motion of the knee joint bilaterally. There are no other findings except for bony enlargement at the distal interphalangeal joint. Which of the following is the best way to prevent disease progression?

a. Weight reduction
b. Calcium supplementation
c. Total knee replacement
d. Long-term nonsteroidal anti-inflammatory drug (NSAID) administration
e. Oral prednisone

69. A 22-year-old man develops the insidious onset of low-back pain improved with exercise and worsened by rest. There is no history of diarrhea, conjunctivitis, urethritis, rash, or nail changes. On examination, the patient has loss of mobility with respect to lumbar flexion and extension. He has a kyphotic posture. A plain film of the spine shows sclerosis of the sacroiliac joints. Calcification is noted in the anterior spinal ligament. Which of the following best characterizes this patient's disease process?

a. He is most likely to have acute lumbosacral back strain and requires bed rest.
b. The patient has a spondyloarthropathy, most likely ankylosing spondylitis.
c. The patient is likely to die from pulmonary fibrosis and extrathoracic restrictive lung disease.
d. A rheumatoid factor is likely to be positive.
e. A colonoscopy is likely to show Crohn disease.

70. A 20-year-old woman has developed low-grade fever, a malar rash, and arthralgias of the hands over several months. High titers of anti-DNA antibodies are noted, and complement levels are low. The patient's white blood cell count is 3000/µL, and platelet count is 90,000/µL. The patient is on no medications and has no signs of active infection. Which of the following statements is correct?

a. If glomerulonephritis, severe thrombocytopenia, or hemolytic anemia develops, high-dose glucocorticoid therapy would be indicated.
b. Central nervous system symptoms will occur within 10 years.
c. The patient can be expected to develop Raynaud phenomenon when exposed to cold.
d. Joint deformities will likely occur.
e. The disease process described is an absolute contraindication to pregnancy.

71. A 45-year-old woman has pain in her fingers on exposure to cold, arthralgias, and difficulty swallowing solid food. What is the best diagnostic test?

a. Rheumatoid factor
b. Antinucleolar antibody
c. ECG
d. BUN and creatinine
e. Reproduction of symptoms and findings by immersion of hands in cold water

72. A 20-year-old man complains of arthritis and eye irritation. He has a history of burning on urination. On examination, there is a joint effusion of the right knee and a rash of the glans penis. Which of the following is correct?

a. *Neisseria gonorrhoeae* is likely to be cultured from the glans penis.
b. The patient is likely to be rheumatoid factor—positive.
c. An infectious process of the GI tract may precipitate this disease.
d. An ANA is very likely to be positive.
e. CPK will be elevated.

73. Last week a 20-year-old college student developed acute wrist pain and swelling. This resolved in four days. Yesterday, he developed pain and swelling in his left knee. Two months ago he went on a backpacking trip in Rhode Island. A week or so later he developed an enlarging circular red spot that persisted for 2 weeks and then resolved. What is the most likely diagnosis?

a. Acute rheumatoid arthritis
b. Parvovirus infection
c. Psoriatic arthritis
d. Lyme disease
e. Inflammatory bowel disease

74. A 75-year-old man complains of headache. On one occasion he transiently lost vision in his right eye. He also complains of aching in the shoulders and neck. There are no focal neurologic findings. Carotid pulses are normal without bruits. Laboratory data show a mild anemia. Erythrocyte sedimentation rate (ESR) is 85. Which of the following is the best approach to management?

a. Begin glucocorticoid therapy and arrange for temporal artery biopsy.
b. Schedule temporal artery biopsy and begin corticosteroids based on biopsy results and clinical course.
c. Schedule carotid angiography.
d. Follow ESR and consider further studies if it remains elevated.
e. Start aspirin and defer any invasive studies unless further symptoms develop.

75. A 55-year-old man with psoriasis has been troubled by long-standing destructive arthritis involving the hands, wrists, shoulders, knees, and ankles. Hand films demonstrate pencil-in-cup deformities. He has been treated with naproxen 500 mg bid, sulfasalazine 1 g bid, prednisone 5 mg qd, and methotrexate 17.5 mg once a week without substantive improvement. Which of the following treatments is most likely to provide long-term benefit?

a. Cyclophosphamide
b. Addition of folic acid supplementation
c. Oral cyclosporine
d. Tumor necrosis factor alpha inhibitor
e. Higher-dose steroids in the range of 20 mg of prednisone per day

76. A 65-year-old man develops the onset of severe knee pain over 24 hours. The knee is red, swollen, and tender. He has a history of diabetes mellitus and cardiomyopathy. An x-ray of the knee shows linear calcification. Definitive diagnosis is best made by which of the following?

a. Serum uric acid
b. Serum calcium
c. Arthrocentesis and identification of positively birefringent rhomboid crystals
d. Rheumatoid factor
e. ANA

77. A 35-year-old woman complains of aching all over. She says she sleeps poorly and all her muscles and joints hurt. Her symptoms have progressed over several years. She reports she is desperate because pain and weakness often cause her to drop things. Physical examination shows multiple points of tenderness over the neck, shoulders, elbows, and wrists. There is no joint swelling or deformity. A complete blood count and erythrocyte sedimentation rate are normal. Rheumatoid factor is negative. Which of the following is the best therapeutic option in this patient?

a. Graded aerobic exercise
b. Prednisone
c. Weekly methotrexate
d. Hydroxychloroquine
e. A nonsteroidal antiinflammatory drug

78. A 38-year-old man has pain and stiffness of his right knee. This began 2-weeks ago after he fell while skiing. On two occasions he had the sense that his knee was locked in a semiflexed position for a few seconds. He has noted a popping sensation when he bends his knee. On examination there is tenderness over the medial joint line of the knee. Marked flexion and extension of the knee are painful. The Lachman test (anterior displacement of the lower leg with the knee at 20° of flexion) and the anterior drawer test are negative. What is the most likely diagnosis?

a. Medial meniscus tear
b. Osteoarthritis
c. Anterior cruciate ligament tear
d. Chondromalacia patella
e. Lumbosacral radiculopathy

79. Over the last six weeks a 45-year-old nurse has developed progressive difficulty getting out of chairs and climbing stairs. She can no longer get in and out of the bathtub. She has no muscle pain and takes no regular medications. She does not use alcohol and does not smoke cigarettes. On examination she has a purplish rash that involves both eyelids (see figure). There is weakness of the proximal leg muscles. What is the best next diagnostic test?

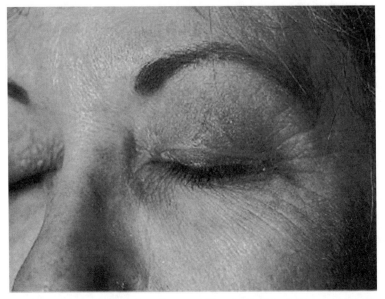

Reproduced, with permission, from Fitzpatrick T et al. *Color Atlas & Synopsis of Clinical Dermatology,* 4th ed. New York, NY: McGraw-Hill; 2001.

   a. Vitamin B_{12} level
   b. Chest x-ray
   c. HLAB27
   d. MRI scan of the lumbar spine
   e. CPK

80. A 63-year-old painter complains of severe right shoulder pain. The pain is located posteriorly over the scapula. These symptoms began after he fell from a ladder 2 weeks ago. The pain is especially bad at night and makes it difficult for him to sleep. In addition, he has had some pain in the right upper arm. Treatment with acetaminophen and ibuprofen has been unsuccessful in controlling his pain. On examination the patient appears uncomfortable. The right shoulder has full range of motion. Movement of the shoulder is not painful. There is no tenderness to palpation of the scapula. What is the most likely diagnosis?

a. Subdeltoid bursitis
b. Rotator cuff tendonitis
c. Adhesive capsulitis
d. Osteoarthritis
e. Cervical radiculopathy

81. A 50-year-old woman with rheumatoid arthritis has been treated with meloxicam (Mobic). You add hydroxychloroquine. Six weeks later her arthritis is mildly improved. The same joints are still involved but she now reports only 1-hour morning stiffness. She has, however, developed epigastric burning and melena for the past 3 days. Stool is strongly positive for occult blood. Which of the following is the most likely cause for the melena in this case?

a. Emotional stress over her illness resulting in acid peptic disease
b. Hydroxychloroquine-induced acid peptic disease
c. Gastric lymphoma associated with autoimmune disease
d. NSAID gastropathy
e. Meckel diverticulum

82. A 55-year-old woman with long-standing rheumatoid arthritis is on prednisone 5 mg daily and etanercept (Enbrel) 50 mg subcutaneously once a week. Her arthritis is well-controlled. However, she complains of a 2-day history of headaches, chills, and spiking fevers to 39.4°C (103°F). You suspect which of the following?

a. An allergic febrile reaction to etanercept
b. Fever related to her underlying autoimmune disease
c. A serious infection
d. A viral syndrome
e. An occult malignancy

83. A 32-year-old Japanese woman has a long history of recurrent aphthous oral ulcers. In the last 2 months she has had recurrent genital ulcers. She now presents with a red painful eye that was diagnosed as anterior uveitis. What is the most likely diagnosis?

a. Herpes simplex
b. HIV infection
c. Behçet disease
d. Diabetes mellitus
e. Systemic lupus erythematosus

84. A 53-year-old man presents with arthritis and bloody nasal discharge. Urinalysis reveals 4+ proteinuria, RBCs, and RBC casts. ANCA is positive in a cytoplasmic pattern. Antiproteinase 3 (PR3) antibodies are present, but antimyeloperoxidase (MPO) antibodies are absent. Which of the following is the most likely diagnosis?

a. Behçet syndrome
b. Sarcoidosis
c. Wegener granulomatosis
d. Henoch-Schönlein purpura
e. Classic polyarteritis nodosa

85. A 50-year-old white woman presents with aching and stiffness in the trunk, hip, and shoulders. There is widespread muscle pain after mild exertion. Symptoms are worse in the morning and improve during the day. They are also worsened by stress. The patient is always tired and exhausted. She has trouble sleeping at night. On examination, joints are normal. ESR is normal, and Lyme antibody and HIV test are negative. A diagnosis is best made by which of the following?

a. Trial of glucocorticoid
b. Muscle biopsy
c. Demonstration of 11 tender points
d. Psychiatric evaluation
e. Trial of an NSAID

86. A 35-year-old right-handed construction worker presents with complaints of nocturnal numbness and pain involving the right hand. Symptoms wake him and are then relieved by shaking his hand. There is some atrophy of the thenar eminence. Tinel sign is positive. Which of the following is the most likely diagnosis?

a. Carpal tunnel syndrome
b. De Quervain tenosynovitis
c. Amyotrophic lateral sclerosis
d. Rheumatoid arthritis of the wrist joint
e. Guillain-Barré syndrome

Questions 87 to 91

Select the most probable diagnosis for each patient. Each lettered option may be used once, more than once, or not at all.

a. Churg Strauss syndrome
b. Cryoglobulinemic vasculitis
c. Temporal arteritis
d. Wegener granulomatosis
e. Takayasu arteritis
f. Polyarteritis nodosa
g. Henoch-Schönlein purpura

87. A 78-year-old man presents with a 2-month history of fever and intermittent abdominal pain. He develops peritoneal signs and at laparotomy is found to have an area of infarcted bowel. Biopsy shows inflammation of small- to medium-sized muscular arteries.

88. An elderly male presents with pain in his shoulders and hips. Temporal arteries are tender to palpation. ESR is 105 mm/L.

89. A 45-year-old man has wheezing for several weeks and now presents with severe tingling of the hands and feet. There is wasting of the intrinsic muscles of the hands and loss of sensation in the feet. WBC is 13,000 with 28% eosinophils.

90. A 42-year-old woman with hepatitis C develops fatigue, joint aches, and palpable purplish spots on her legs. Serum creatinine is 2.1 mg/dL and a 24-hour urine protein collection is 750 mg.

91. A 20-year-old female competitive swimmer notes that her arms now ache after swimming one or two laps, and she is unable to continue. She has had night sweats and a 10-lb weight loss. Pulses in the upper extremity are difficult to palpate.

Questions 92 to 95

Match each description with the appropriate disease. Each lettered option may be used once, more than once, or not at all.

a. Plantar fasciitis
b. Metatarsal stress fracture
c. Charcot foot
d. Tarsal tunnel syndrome
e. Podagra
f. Hallux valgus
g. Morton neuroma

92. A 32-year-old runner has been training for her first marathon. She complains of 2 weeks of heel pain which is severe for the first few steps each morning and then goes away. She has no pain at night.

93. A 54-year-old woman complains of pain and burning over the bottom of the forefoot; her symptoms are relieved by going barefoot.

94. A 49-year-old sedentary man goes on an 8-mile hike with his son's scout troop, and awakens that night with severe pain, swelling, and redness of the first metatarsophalangeal joint.

95. Toward the end of her soccer season, a 17-year-old high school student suddenly develops pain in the top of the right foot. The pain is quite severe and she cannot run. Examination reveals point tenderness over the right third metatarsal. Radiographs of the foot are negative for fracture.

Rheumatology

Answers

61. The answer is a. *(Fauci, pp 2083-2089.)* The clinical picture of symmetrical swelling and tenderness of the metacarpophalangeal (MCP) and wrist joints lasting longer than 6 weeks strongly suggest rheumatoid arthritis. Rheumatoid factor, an immunoglobulin directed against the Fc portion of IgG, is positive in about two-thirds of cases and may be present early in the disease. The history of lethargy or fatigue is a common prodrome of RA. The inflammatory joint changes on examination are not consistent with chronic fatigue syndrome; furthermore, patients with CFS typically report fatigue existing for many years. The MCP-wrist distribution of joint symptoms makes osteoarthritis very unlikely. The x-ray changes described are characteristic of RA, but would occur later in the course of the disease. Although arthritis can occasionally be a manifestation of hematologic malignancies and, rarely, other malignancies, the only indicated screening would be a complete history and physical examination along with a CBC.

62. The answer is a. *(Stobo, pp 251-256; Fauci, pp 2169-2175.)* The clinical and laboratory picture suggests an acute septic arthritis. The most important first step is to determine the etiologic agent of the infection. Synovial leukocyte counts in gout typically range between 2000/μL and 50,000/μL; in addition, serum uric acid levels are often normal in acute gout. In the absence of negatively birefringent crystals in the synovial fluid, a uric acid level will not be helpful. There are no symptoms suggesting connective tissue disease. Gonococci can cause a septic arthritis, but a urethral culture in the absence of urethral discharge would not be helpful. Antineutrophil cytoplasmic antibodies are present in certain vasculitides. There is no indication of systemic vasculitis in this patient.

63. The answer is b. *(Fauci, pp 2107-2109.)* The complaints described are characteristic of Sjögren syndrome, an autoimmune disease with presenting symptoms of dry eyes and dry mouth. The disease is caused by lymphocytic infiltration and destruction of lacrimal and salivary glands. The Schirmer test, which assesses tear production by measuring the amount of wetness on a piece of filter paper placed in the lower eyelid for 5 minutes, is the appropriate screening test. Most patients with Sjögren syndrome produce autoantibodies, particularly anti-Ro (SSA). Lip biopsy is needed only to evaluate uncertain cases, such as when dry mouth occurs without dry eye symptoms. Mumps can cause bilateral parotitis, but would not explain the patient's complaint of a gritty sensation, which is the most typical symptom of dry eye syndrome. Corticosteroids are reserved for severe vasculitis or other serious complications. Although anxiety (for which a benzodiazepine could be administered) can cause a dry mouth, it would not cause either parotid swelling or dry eyes.

64. The answer is b. *(Fauci, pp 2165-2167.)* The sudden onset and severity of this monoarticular arthritis suggests acute gouty arthritis, especially in a patient on diuretic therapy. However, an arthrocentesis is indicated in the first episode to document gout by demonstrating needle-shaped, negatively birefringent crystals and to rule out other diagnoses such as infection. The level of serum uric acid during an episode of acute gouty arthritis may actually fall. Therefore, a normal serum uric acid does not exclude a diagnosis of gout. For most patients with acute gout, NSAIDs are the treatment of choice. Colchicine is also effective but causes nausea and diarrhea. Antibiotics should not be started for suspected septic arthritis before an arthrocentesis is performed. Treatment for hyperuricemia should not be initiated in the setting of an acute attack of gouty arthritis. Long-term goals of management are to control hyperuricemia, prevent further attacks, and prevent joint damage. Long-term prophylaxis with allopurinol is considered for repeated attacks of acute arthritis, urolithiasis, or formation of tophaceous deposits. X-ray of the ankle would likely be inconclusive in this patient with no trauma history. In the absence of trauma, there is no indication for immobilization.

65. The answer is b. *(Fauci, pp 2089-2092.)* The patient has more than four of the required signs or symptoms of RA, including morning stiffness, swelling of the wrist or MCP, simultaneous swelling of joints on both sides of body, subcutaneous nodules, and positive rheumatoid factor. Subcutaneous nodules and anti-CCP antibodies are poor prognostic signs for the activity of the disease, and disease-modifying antirheumatic drugs (DMARDs) such as methotrexate, antimalarials, sulfasalazine, leflunomide, anti-TNF agents, or a combination of these drugs should be instituted. Methotrexate has emerged as a cornerstone of most disease-modifying regimens, to which other agents are often added. Low-dose corticosteroids have recently been shown to reduce the progression of bony erosions and, although controversial, are considered by some to be appropriate disease-modifying agents for long-term therapy. High dose steroids, however, should be avoided. Use of anti-inflammatory doses of both aspirin and nonsteroidals together is not desirable because it will increase the risk of side effects. Given the aggressive nature of this woman's rheumatoid arthritis and negative prognostic signs, use of DMARDs is indicated. Significant joint damage has been shown by MRI to occur quite early in the course of disease.

66. The answer is d. (*Fauci, pp 2169-2170, 2174.*) *Staphylococcus aureus* is the most common organism to cause septic arthritis in adults. β-Hemolytic streptococci are the second most common. *N gonorrhoeae* can also produce septic arthritis, but would be less likely in this patient who is not sexually active. *S pneumoniae* and gram-negative rods such as *E coli or Pseudomonas aeruginosa* are rare causes of septic arthritis and usually occur secondary to a primary focus of infection. Septic arthritis commonly occurs in joints that are anatomically damaged, as in this case with prior rheumatoid arthritis. Any time a patient with arthritis develops a monoarticular flare out of proportion to the other joints, septic arthritis must be suspected.

67. The answer is a. (*Fauci, pp 110-113.*) Lumbar spinal stenosis is a frequent cause of back pain in the elderly. Patients typically have pain that radiates into the buttocks (and sometimes thighs) and that is aggravated by walking and by lumbar extension. Decreased vibratory sensation and a wide based gait may also be seen. Narrowing of the spinal canal is usually caused by age-related degenerative changes. A recent randomized controlled trial demonstrated that surgery was more effective than medical therapy in the relief of symptoms for patients with lumbar spinal stenosis. Symptoms often recur several years after surgery.

Disc herniation and facet joint arthropathy usually cause unilateral radicular symptoms. Leg pain associated with walking can also be caused by vascular disease, but the symptoms often are unilateral and usually occur in the distal leg. Normal pedal pulses and the classic history make vascular claudication an unlikely diagnosis in this patient. The bone pain of metastatic cancer is rarely positional and is usually unremitting, causing pain both day and night.

68. The answer is a. (*Fauci, pp 2158-2165.*) The clinical picture of pain in weight-bearing joints made worse by activity is suggestive of degenerative joint disease, also called osteoarthritis. Osteoarthritis may have a mild to moderate inflammatory component. Crepitation in the involved joints is characteristic, as is bony enlargement of the DIP joints. In this overweight patient, weight reduction is the best method to decrease the risk of further degenerative changes. Aspirin, other NSAIDs, or acetaminophen can be used as symptomatic treatment but do not affect the course of the disease. The long-term use of NSAIDs is limited by potential side effects including renal insufficiency and gastrointestinal bleeding. Calcium supplementation is relevant for osteoporosis, but does not treat osteoarthritis. Oral prednisone would not be indicated. Intraarticular corticosteroid injections may be given two to three times per year for symptom reduction. Knee replacement is the treatment of last resort, usually when symptoms are not controlled by medical regimens and/or activities are severely limited.

69. The answer is b. *(Fauci, pp 2109-2113.)* Insidious back pain occurring in a young male and improving with exercise suggests one of the spondyloarthropathies—ankylosing spondylitis, reactive arthritis (including Reiter syndrome), psoriatic arthritis, or enteropathic arthritis. In the absence of symptoms or findings to suggest one of the other conditions and in the presence of symmetrical sacroiliitis on x-ray, ankylosing spondylitis is the most likely diagnosis. Acute lumbosacral strain would not be relieved by exercise or worsened by rest. The prognosis in ankylosing spondylitis is generally very good, with only 6% dying of the disease itself. While pulmonary fibrosis and restrictive lung disease can occur, they are rarely a cause of death (cervical fracture, heart block, and amyloidosis are leading causes of death as a result of ankylosing spondylitis). Rheumatoid factor is negative in all the spondyloarthropathies. Crohn disease can cause an enteropathic arthritis, which may precede the gastrointestinal manifestations, but this diagnosis is far less likely in this case than ankylosing spondylitis.

70. The answer is a. *(Fauci, pp 2075-2083.)* The combination of fever, malar rash, and arthritis suggests systemic lupus erythematosus (SLE), and the patient's thrombocytopenia, leukopenia, and positive antibody to native DNA provide more than four criteria for a definitive diagnosis. Other criteria for the diagnosis of lupus include discoid rash, photosensitivity, oral ulcers, serositis, renal disorders (proteinuria or cellular casts), and neurologic disorder (seizures). High-dose corticosteroids would be indicated for severe or life-threatening complications of lupus such as described in item a. The arthritis in SLE is nondeforming. Patients with SLE have an unpredictable course. Few patients develop all signs or symptoms. Neuropsychiatric disease occurs at some time in about half of all SLE patients and Raynaud phenomenon in about 25%. Pregnancy is relatively safe in women with SLE who have controlled disease and are on less than 10 mg of prednisone.

71. The answer is b. (*Fauci, pp 2096-2106.*) The symptoms of Raynaud phenomenon, arthralgia, and dysphagia point toward the diagnosis of scleroderma. Scleroderma, or systemic sclerosis, is characterized by a systemic vasculopathy of small and medium-sized vessels, excessive collagen deposition in tissues, and an abnormal immune system. It is an uncommon multisystem disease affecting women more often than men. There are two variants of scleroderma—a relatively benign type called the CREST syndrome and a more severe, diffuse disease. Antinucleolar antibody occurs in only 20 to 30% of patients with the disease, but a positive test is highly specific. Cardiac involvement may occur, and an ECG could show heart block but is not at all specific. Renal failure can develop insidiously, but BUN and creatinine levels would not be diagnostically specific. Rheumatoid factor is nonspecific and present in 20% of patients with scleroderma. Reproduction of Raynaud phenomena is nonspecific and is not recommended as an office test.

72. The answer is c. (*Fauci, pp 1072, 2113-2115.*) Reactive arthritis (Reiter syndrome) is a reactive polyarthritis that develops several weeks after an infection such as nongonococcal urethritis or gastrointestinal infection caused by *Yersinia enterocolitica, Campylobacter jejuni,* or *Salmonella* or *Shigella* species. Reiter syndrome is characterized as a triad of oligoarticular arthritis, conjunctivitis, and urethritis. The disease is most common among young men and is associated with the histocompatibility antigen, HLA-B27. Circinate balanitis is a painless red rash on the glans penis that occurs in 25% to 40% of patients. Other clinical features may include keratodermia blennorrhagicum (a rash on the palms and soles indistinguishable from papular psoriasis) and spondylitis. ANA and rheumatoid factor are usually negative. CPK would be elevated in polymyositis or dermatomyositis but not in reactive arthritis. Gonorrhea can precipitate Reiter syndrome, but patients with the disease are culture negative.

73. The answer is d. (*Fauci, pp 1055-1059, 2172.*) This patient has Lyme disease. Lyme disease is caused by infection with a spirochete (*Borrelia burgdorferi*) that is transmitted to humans by the bite of an infected *Ixodes* tick. A majority of patients develop a circular rash (erythema migrans) at the site of the original tick bite three to 30 days later. One of the unusual characteristics of this rash is that it gradually enlarges over one to two weeks.

Dissemination of the spirochete results in involvement of multiple organ systems and may result in monoarticular arthritis (that is typically migratory), aseptic meningitis, facial nerve palsies, and conduction system disease of the heart. Lyme disease has a distinctive geographic location attributed to the habitat of the tick vector. Cases are typically seen in the Northeast and in Minnesota and Wisconsin. Most patients can be cured with oral antibiotics such as doxycycline or amoxicillin. Rheumatoid arthritis would not account for the rash or the epidemiologic history. Both RA and parvovirus infection tend to cause symmetric joint involvement. Rarely, joint involvement in psoriatic arthritis or IBD is the first sign of disease, but usually skin or GI involvement is well established when the joint symptoms develop.

74. The answer is a. (*Fauci, pp 2126-2127.*) Headache and transient unilateral visual loss (amaurosis fugax) in this elderly patient with polymyalgia rheumatica (PMR) symptoms suggest a diagnosis of temporal arteritis. The erythrocyte sedimentation rate is high in almost all cases. Temporal arteritis occurs most commonly in patients over the age of 55 and is highly associated with polymyalgia rheumatica. However, only about 25% of patients with PMR have giant cell arteritis. Older patients who complain of diffuse myalgias and joint stiffness, particularly of the shoulders and hips, should be evaluated for PMR with an ESR. Unilateral visual changes or even permanent visual loss may occur abruptly in patients with temporal arteritis. Biopsy results should not delay initiation of corticosteroid therapy. Biopsies may show vasculitis even after 14 days of glucocorticoid therapy. Delay risks permanent loss of sight. Once an episode of loss of vision occurs, workup must proceed as quickly as possible. Treatment for temporal arteritis requires relatively high doses of steroids, beginning with prednisone at 40 to 60 mg per day for about 1 month with subsequent tapering. Aspirin should be added because it decreases the risks of vascular occlusions but is not sufficient alone. The treatment for polymyalgia rheumatica without concomitant temporal arteritis requires much lower doses of steroids, in the range of 10 to 20 mg per day of prednisone. Carotid disease can cause amaurosis fugax but would not account for the headache, polymyalgia rheumatica, or the elevated sedimentation rate.

75. The answer is d. (*Fauci, pp 2115-2116.*) Psoriatic arthritis can be very aggressive and destructive. The radiographic pencil-in-cup deformity is a characteristic form of joint destruction in this condition. This man has failed conventional DMARD therapy. TNF blockers have shown dramatic benefit in regard to both the arthritis and the skin disease. Cyclophosphamide is used primarily for life-or organ-threatening vasculitis and is not indicated for arthritis alone. Although cyclosporine has been used for psoriatic arthritis with limited success, it is not as good a choice as a TNF blocking agent. Folic acid supplementation helps decrease the risk of some side effects of methotrexate. It does not improve its therapeutic effectiveness. Although low-dose steroids can be appropriate for inflammatory arthritis, doses higher than 10 mg per day should not be given for sustained periods because of the long-term side effects.

76. The answer is c. (*Fauci, pp 2167-2168.*) Acute monoarticular arthritis in association with linear calcification of the cartilage of the knee (chondrocalcinosis) suggests the diagnosis of pseudogout, a form of calcium pyrophosphate dihydrate deposition disease (CPPDD). In its acute manifestation the disease resembles gout. Positively birefringent crystals (looking blue or green when parallel to the axis of the red compensator on a polarizing microscope) can be demonstrated in joint fluid, although careful search is sometimes necessary. Serum uric acid and calcium levels are normal, as are rheumatoid factor and antinuclear antibodies. Pseudogout is about half as common as gout, but becomes more common after age 65. Calcium pyrophosphate dihydrate deposition disease is diagnosed in symptomatic patients by characteristic x-ray findings and crystals in synovial fluid. Pseudogout is treated with NSAIDs, colchicine, or steroids. Arthrocentesis and drainage with intraarticular steroid administration is also an effective treatment. Linear calcifications or chondrocalcinosis are often found in the joints of elderly patients who do not have symptomatic joint problems; such patients do not require treatment.

77. The answer is a. (*Fauci, pp 2175-2177.*) The patient's multiple tender points, associated sleep disturbance and lack of joint or muscle findings make fibromyalgia a likely diagnosis. Patients with fibromyalgia often report dropping things due to pain and weakness, but objective muscle weakness is not present on examination. The diagnosis hinges on the presence of multiple tender points in the absence of any other disease likely to cause musculoskeletal symptoms. CBC and ESR are characteristically normal. Cognitive behavioral therapy and graded aerobic exercise programs have been demonstrated to relieve symptoms. Tricyclic antidepressants may help restore sleep. Aspirin, other anti-inflammatory drugs (including corticosteroids), and DMARDs (such as methotrexate or hydroxychloroquine) are not helpful. Neither are simple stretching/flexibility exercises. Of note, rheumatoid factor and antinuclear antibodies occur in a small number of normal individuals. They are more frequent in women and increase in frequency with age. It is not uncommon for an individual with fibromyalgia and an incidentally positive RF or ANA to be misdiagnosed as having collagen vascular disease. Therefore, it is necessary to be careful to separate subjective tenderness on examination from objective musculoskeletal findings and to assiduously search for other criteria before diagnosing RA, SLE, or other collagen vascular disease.

78. The answer is a. (*Fauci, p 2154.*) This patient has a medial meniscus tear. This may occur after trauma, but sometimes occurs spontaneously. Patients complain of pain, stiffness and a popping sensation. A sensation of locking is very characteristic. On examination patients frequently have tenderness at the joint line and pain on flexion and extension. Routine x-rays are usually negative and the diagnosis is made by MRI scanning. Osteoarthritis usually occurs in patients older than age 50 unless the patient is very obese. OA pain typically comes on gradually, and physical examination may reveal patellofemoral crepitance. An anterior cruciate tear usually results from a twisting injury. It is a common injury in female soccer and basketball players. Frequently a large effusion occurs acutely. Chondromalacia patellae is a common problem in runners. The pain typically worsens when the patient walks down stairs. The physical examination demonstrates lateral displacement of the patella with knee extension. Pathology in the back and hip may be referred to the knee, but is not associated with physical examination abnormalities localized to the knee.

79. The answer is e. (*Fauci, p 2696-2703.*) This woman has classic dermatomyositis, which typically affects females aged 40 to 50. Patients present with progressive proximal myopathy and complain of difficulty arising from chairs, climbing stairs, and getting out of the bathtub. About half of patients with dermatomyositis have the classic heliotrope rash. Lung involvement is common but cardiac involvement is rare. Almost all patients have an elevated CPK. Patients may have the anemia of chronic disease, which is normocytic. The EMG is very characteristically abnormal with muscle fibrillations, spontaneous discharges and sharp waves. In a small percentage of patients, the EMG may be normal. Muscle biopsy is usually diagnostic. High-dose oral corticosteroids are the treatment of choice. Some patients require the addition of methotrexate or azathioprine. Only 25% of patients are cured and most will develop a chronic condition with significant morbidity. Vitamin B_{12} deficiency causes distal sensory findings (rather than this patient's proximal motor findings) and would not account for the heliotrope rash. Imaging studies would not focus on the primary process, which is in the musculature.

HLAB27 is diagnostically useful in the spondyloarthropathies such as ankylosing spondylitis; this patient has no back pain or morning stiffness to suggest this diagnosis.

80. The answer is e. *(Fauci, pp 115-117, 2154.)* Shoulder pain may be caused by inflammation of tendons or muscles in the shoulder girdle, intra-articular problems at the glenohumeral joint, or referred pain from a cervical radiculopathy. Posterior shoulder pain and a normal shoulder examination are clues to the correct diagnosis in this patient. The pain of cervical radiculopathy is often severe and worse at night. Extension of pain into the arm may occur, but this also occurs with other etiologies of shoulder pain. Shoulder pain is common, particularly in the elderly. Subdeltoid bursitis causes exquisite local tenderness. Rotator cuff tendonitis is frequently associated with pain on active but not passive movement of the joint. Weakness of the arm suggests rotator cuff tear. In adhesive capsulitis, range of motion is restricted. Crepitance on manipulation of the shoulder suggests osteoarthritis of the glenohumoral joint.

81. The answer is d. *(Fauci, pp 257-260.)* The patient's GI bleeding most likely results from NSAID gastropathy, an extremely common complication. It may occur without associated abdominal symptoms. It is more common in the elderly. Although she recently began hydroxychloroquine, that medicine does not cause GI bleeding. Emotional distress causing ulcer disease, lymphoma, and Meckel diverticulum are all possible, but there is nothing in this case history to suggest them, and they are much rarer than NSAID gastropathy.

82. The answer is c. *(Fauci, pp 2089-2091.)* Etanercept, infliximab, and adalimimab are TNF alpha inhibitors that have been shown to be highly efficacious DMARDs. Suppression of the action of TNF is associated with a significantly increased risk of serious infections, a complication requiring vigilance and timely action by physicians. Although all the other conditions listed can cause fever, the managing physician must first suspect and rule out a significant infection as a complication of immunosuppressant therapy. Tuberculosis, histoplasmosis, and coccidioidomycosis are common infectious complications. Tuberculin testing is recommended for patients who are to receive treatment with these agents.

83. The answer is c. *(Fauci, pp 2129, 2132.)* This patient has classic Behçet disease. This occurs more commonly in Asians. Behçet disease is a multisystem disorder that usually presents with recurrent oral and genital ulcers. One-fourth of patients develop superficial or deep vein thrombophlebitis. Iritis, uveitis, and nondeforming arthritis are common. Blindness, aseptic meningitis, and CNS vasculitis may occur. Rare complications include pulmonary artery aneurysms and GI inflammation which may lead to perforation. Mucocutaneous lesions are usually treated with topical corticosteroids. Immunosuppressive therapy is recommended for patients with threatened blindness or central nervous system disease. The oral lesions of herpes simplex infection occur over the lips; anterior uveitis would be very uncommon. The mucocutaneous lesions of HIV infection are usually caused by *Candida* and are easily distinguishable from aphthous ulcers. Neither diabetes nor lupus would cause this constellation of findings.

84. The answer is c. (*Fauci, pp 2121-2124.*) Wegener granulomatosis (WG) is a granulomatous vasculitis of small and medium sized arteries and veins. It affects the lungs, sinuses, nasopharynx, and kidneys, where it causes a focal and segmental glomerulonephritis. Other organs can also be damaged, including the skin, eyes, and nervous system. Most patients with the disease develop antibodies to certain proteins in the cytoplasm of neutrophils, called antineutrophil cytoplasmic antibodies (ANCA). The most common ANCA staining pattern seen in WG is cytoplasmic, C-ANCA. The C-ANCA pattern is usually caused by antibodies to proteinase-3. A perinuclear pattern, P-ANCA, is sometimes seen. P-ANCA is usually caused by antibodies to myeloperoxidase. Behçet syndrome is not associated with ANCA positivity. Henoch-Schönlein purpura and classic polyarteritis do not involve the upper airways. Sarcoidosis may involve the upper respiratory tract (20%), but it does not cause bloody nasal discharge and does not cause glomerulonephritis.

85. The answer is c. (*Fauci, pp 2175-2177.*) The signs and symptoms suggest fibromyalgia. Fibromyalgia is a very common disorder, particularly in middle-aged women, characterized by diffuse musculoskeletal pain, fatigue, and nonrestorative sleep. The American College of Rheumatology has established diagnostic criteria for the disease, which include a history of widespread pain in association with 11 of 18 specific tender point sites. In this patient with very characteristic signs and symptoms, the identification of 11 specific trigger points would be the best method of diagnosis. Polymyalgia rheumatica may sometimes be in the differential diagnosis. In this patient PMR would be particularly unlikely given the normal ESR. Fibromyalgia is distinct from inflammatory muscle disease like polymyositis or dermatomyositis. Patients with inflammatory muscle disease usually present with proximal muscle weakness and have elevated muscle enzymes, whereas patients with fibromyalgia usually complain predominantly of musculoskeletal pain and have normal muscle enzymes. Muscle pain is less prominent in inflammatory muscle disease. Fibromyalgia has been associated with other somatic syndromes, including irritable bladder, irritable bowel syndrome, headaches, and temporomandibular joint pain. Patients with fibromyalgia have an increased lifetime incidence of psychiatric disorders, particularly depression and panic disorder. However, there is convincing evidence that fibromyalgia is a disease of abnormal central nervous pain processing associated with amplification of nociceptive stimuli. This suggests that the demonstrated lower thresholds for noxious stimuli are caused by a CNS abnormality of as yet undetermined etiology. Psychiatric evaluation would, therefore, be useful only for other psychiatric symptoms, not for diagnosis of fibromyalgia itself. Steroids and NSAIDs have not been shown to be helpful in fibromyalgia and would not be expected to be so since there is no evidence of inflammation.

86. The answer is a. *(Fauci, pp 2153-2154.)* Carpal tunnel syndrome results from median nerve entrapment and is frequently associated with excessive use of the wrist. The process has also been associated with thickening of connective tissue, as in acromegaly, or with deposition of amyloid. It also occurs in hypothyroidism, rheumatoid arthritis, and diabetes mellitus. As in this patient, numbness is frequently worse at night and relieved by shaking the hand. Atrophy of the abductor pollicis brevis as evidenced by thenar wasting is a sign of advanced disease and an indication for surgery. Tinel sign (paresthesia induced in the median nerve distribution by tapping on the volar aspect of the wrist) is very characteristic but not specific. De Quervain tenosynovitis causes focal wrist pain on the radial aspect of the hand and results from inflammation of the tendon sheath of the abductor pollicis longus. It should not produce a positive Tinel sign or evidence of median nerve dysfunction. Amyotrophic lateral sclerosis may present with distal muscle weakness but does not cause pain. Diffuse atrophy and muscle fasciculation would be prominent. Rheumatoid arthritis would not produce these symptoms unless inflammation of the wrist was causing median nerve entrapment in the carpal tunnel. Guillain-Barré syndrome is a rapidly progressive polyneuropathy that typically presents with an ascending paralysis.

87 to 91. The answers are 87-f, 88-c, 89-a, 90-b, 91-e. *(Fauci, pp 2119-2132.)* The large vessel vasculitides include temporal (giant cell) arteritis and Takayasu arteritis. Temporal arteritis typically occurs in older patients and is accompanied by aching in the shoulders and hips, jaw claudication, and a markedly elevated ESR. Takayasu arteritis, a granulomatous inflammation of the aorta and its main branches, typically occurs in young women. Symptoms are attributed to local vascular occlusion and may produce arm or leg claudication. Systemic symptoms of arthralgia, fatigue, malaise, anorexia, and weight loss may precede the vascular symptoms. Surgery may be necessary to correct occlusive lesions.

The patient in question 87 has classic polyarteritis nodosa. It is a multi-system necrotizing medium-size vessel vasculitis that, prior to the use of steroids and cyclophosphamide, was uniformly fatal. Patients commonly present with signs of vascular insufficiency in the involved organs. Abdominal involvement is common. In 30% of patients, antecedent hepatitis B virus infection can be demonstrated; immune complexes containing the virus have been found in such patients and are likely pathogenic.

Small vessel vasculitides include Wegener granulomatosis, microscopic polyangitis, the Churg-Strauss syndrome, Henoch-Schönlein purpura, and cryoglobulinemic vasculitis. Wegener granulomatosis usually involves the sinuses, lungs, and kidneys. CXR may reveal cavities, infiltrates, or nodules. Many patients also develop glomerulonephritis which may result in acute renal failure. On biopsy, the vasculitis is necrotizing and granulomatous. Microscopic polyangiitis is a multisystem necrotizing vasculitis that typically results in glomerulonephritis, pulmonary hemorrhage, and fever. Lung biopsy shows inflammation of capillaries. Patients may also have mononeuritis multiplex and palpable purpura. Classic polyarteritis nodosa rarely involves the lungs.

The Churg-Strauss syndrome is characterized by wheezing, fever, eosinophilia and systemic vasculitis that may involve the peripheral nerves, central nervous system, heart, kidneys, or GI tract. Henoch-Schönlein purpura primarily occurs in children and presents with palpable purpura, arthritis, and glomerulonephritis. A third of the affected children will have a glomerulonephritis which occasionally results in renal failure. Cryoglobulinemia can be associated with a small vessel vasculitis. Patients typically present with palpable purpura, arthritis, and glomerulonephritis. Cryoglobulinemia is often associated with hepatitis C.

92 to 95. The answers are 92-a, 93-g, 94-e, 95-b. (*Fauci, pp 2154, 2165-2166, 2186, 2655.*) Primary care physicians frequently encounter patients with foot and ankle pain. Common causes of pain in the proximal foot include ankle sprains, plantar fasciitis, and tarsal tunnel syndrome. Ankle sprains result from trauma with stretching of the lateral ankle ligaments. Swelling and bruising distal to the lateral malleolus are common. Evidence-based guidelines (Ottawa rules) suggests that the only patients who need x-rays of the ankle are (1) those who cannot bear weight immediately after the injury or in the emergency department and (2) those with point tenderness over the medial or lateral malleolus. Plantar fasciitis typically causes heel pain that is worse for the first few steps in the morning or after sitting. This is a common condition of runners after an increase in exercise intensity. The tarsal tunnel is a pathway along the medial malleolus between bone and the flexor retinaculum. The posterior tibial nerve runs through this path. Inflammation in this area can result in nerve irritation which causes pain in the ankle and heel and numbness of the sole of the foot at night. This condition is referred to as tarsal tunnel syndrome.

Common causes of pain in the distal part of the foot include podagra (acute gout of the first metatarsal phalangeal joint, which comes on abruptly and is associated with swelling and redness), metatarsal stress fracture (which comes on abruptly, is made worse by weight-bearing, is associated with point tenderness, and may be associated with normal x-rays), hallux valgus (which is bunion formation as a result of lateral deviation of the great toe at the metatarsal joint) and Morton neuroma (which typically causes pain and numbness on the ball of the foot, and is made better by taking off shoes). Charcot joint is collapse of the arch of the associated with severe peripheral neuropathy.

Pulmonary Disease

Questions

96. A 50-year-old patient with long-standing chronic obstructive lung disease develops the insidious onset of aching in the distal extremities, particularly the wrists bilaterally. There is a 10-lb weight loss. The skin over the wrists is warm and erythematous. There is bilateral clubbing. Plain film is read as periosteal thickening, possible osteomyelitis. Which of the following is the most appropriate management of this patient?

a. Start ciprofloxacin.
b. Obtain chest x-ray.
c. Aspirate both wrists.
d. Begin methotrexate therapy.
e. Obtain erythrocyte sedimentation rate.

97. A patient with low-grade fever and weight loss has poor excursion on the right side of the chest with decreased fremitus, flatness to percussion, and decreased breath sounds all on the right. The trachea is deviated to the left. Which of the following is the most likely diagnosis?

a. Pneumothorax
b. Pleural effusion
c. Consolidated pneumonia
d. Atelectasis
e. Chronic obstructive lung disease

98. A 40-year-old alcoholic develops cough and fever. Chest x-ray, shown below, shows an air-fluid level in the superior segment of the right lower lobe. Which of the following is the most likely etiologic agent?

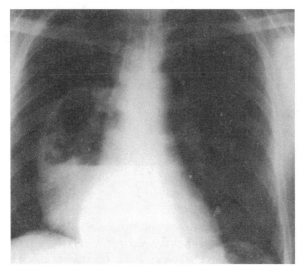

Reproduced, with permission, from Fauci A et al. *Harrison's Principles of Internal Medicine*, 17th ed. New York, NY: McGraw-Hill, 2008.

a. *Streptococcus pneumoniae*
b. *Haemophilus influenzae*
c. *Legionella pneumophila*
d. Anaerobes
e. *Mycoplasma pneumoniae*

99. A 30-year-old male is admitted to the hospital after a motorcycle accident that resulted in a fracture of the right femur. The fracture is managed with traction. Three days later the patient becomes confused and tachypneic. A petechial rash is noted over the chest. Lungs are clear to auscultation. Arterial blood gases show PO_2 of 50, PCO_2 of 28, and pH of 7.49. Which of the following is the most likely diagnosis?

a. Unilateral pulmonary edema
b. Hematoma of the chest
c. Fat embolism
d. Pulmonary embolism
e. Early *Staphylococcus aureus* pneumonia

100. A 70-year-old patient with chronic obstructive lung disease requires 2 L/min of nasal O_2 to treat his hypoxia, which is sometimes associated with angina. The patient develops pleuritic chest pain, fever, and purulent sputum. While using his oxygen at an increased flow of 5 L/min he becomes stuporous and develops a respiratory acidosis with CO_2 retention and worsening hypoxia. What would be the most appropriate next step in the management of this patient?

a. Stop oxygen.
b. Begin medroxyprogesterone.
c. Intubate and begin mechanical ventilation.
d. Observe patient 24 hours before changing therapy.
e. Begin sodium bicarbonate.

101. A 34-year-old black female presents to your office with symptoms of cough, dyspnea, and fatigue. Physical examination shows cervical adenopathy and hepatomegaly. Spleen tip is palpable. Her chest radiograph is shown below. Which of the following is the best approach in establishing a diagnosis?

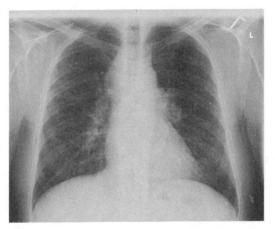

Reproduced, with permission, from Fauci A et al. *Harrison's Principles of Internal Medicine,* 17th ed. New York, NY: McGraw-Hill, 2008.

a. Open lung biopsy
b. Liver biopsy
c. Bronchoscopy and transbronchial lung biopsy
d. Scalene node biopsy
e. Serum angiotensin converting enzyme (ACE) level

102. A 64-year-old woman is found to have a right-sided pleural effusion on chest x-ray. Analysis of the pleural fluid reveals pleural fluid to serum protein ratio of 0.38, a lactate dehydrogenase (LDH) level of 110 IU (normal 100-190), and pleural fluid to serum LDH ratio of 0.46. Which of the following disorders is most likely in this patient?

a. Bronchogenic carcinoma
b. Congestive heart failure
c. Pulmonary embolism
d. Sarcoidosis
e. Systemic lupus erythematosus

103. A 25-year-old male presents to the clinic for evaluation of infertility. He has a life-long history of a productive cough and recurrent pulmonary infections. On his review of symptoms he has indicated chronic problems with abdominal pain, diarrhea, and difficulty gaining weight. He also has diabetes mellitus. His chest x-ray suggests bronchiectasis. Which is the most likely diagnosis?

a. COPD
b. Upper respiratory infections
c. Cystic fibrosis
d. Intrapulmonary hemorrhage
e. Asthma

104. A 28-year-old male with a long history of severe asthma presents to the emergency room with shortness of breath. He has previously required admission to the hospital and was once intubated for asthma. Which of the following findings on physical examination would predict a benign course?

a. Silent chest
b. Hypercapnia
c. Thoracoabdominal paradox (paradoxical respiration)
d. Pulsus paradoxus of 5 mm Hg
e. Altered mental status

105. A 40-year-old man without a significant past medical history comes to the emergency room with a 3-day history of fever and shaking chills, and a 15-minute episode of rigor. He also reports a nonproductive cough, anorexia, and the development of right-sided pleuritic chest pain. Shortness of breath has been present for the past 12 hours. Chest x-ray reveals a consolidated right middle lobe infiltrate, and CBC shows an elevated neutrophil count with many band forms present. Which of the following statements regarding pneumonia in this patient is correct?

a. If the sputum Gram stain shows multiple squamous epithelial cells and the culture is reported as mixed flora, the patient probably has a viral infection.
b. If the Gram stain reveals numerous gram-positive diplococci, numerous white blood cells, and few epithelial cells, *Streptococcus pneumoniae* is the most likely pathogen.
c. Although *S pneumoniae* is the agent most likely to be the cause of this patient's pneumonia, this diagnosis would be unlikely if blood cultures prove negative.
d. The absence of rigors would rule out a diagnosis of pneumococcal pneumonia.
e. Penicillin is still the drug of choice in pneumococcal pneumonia.

106. A 57-year-old man develops acute shortness of breath shortly after a 12-hour automobile ride. The patient is admitted to the hospital for shortness of breath. Findings on physical examination are normal except for tachypnea and tachycardia. He does not have edema or popliteal tenderness. An electrocardiogram reveals sinus tachycardia but is otherwise normal. Which of the following statements is correct?

a. A normal D-dimer level excludes pulmonary embolus.
b. The patient should be admitted to the hospital, and, if there is no contraindication to anticoagulation, full-dose heparin or enoxaparin should be started pending further testing.
c. Normal findings on examination of the lower extremities make pulmonary embolism unlikely.
d. Early treatment has little effect on overall mortality.
e. A normal lower extremity venous Doppler study will rule out a pulmonary embolus.

107. A 40-year-old woman has had increasing fatigue and shortness of breath for years. Chest x-ray shows right ventricular hypertrophy and enlargement of the central pulmonary arteries. Pulmonary embolus is ruled out by spiral CT scan. Other causes of pulmonary hypertension have also been ruled out. Right heart catheterization reveals a pulmonary artery pressure of 75/30 mm Hg. Which of the following is the best next step in the management of the patient?

a. Acute drug testing with short-acting pulmonary vasodilators
b. High-dose nifedipine
c. Intravenous prostacyclin
d. Lung transplantation
e. Empiric trial of sildenafil

108. A 65-year-old male with mild congestive heart failure is to receive total hip replacement. He has no other underlying diseases and no history of hypertension, recent surgery, or bleeding disorder. Which of the following is the best approach to prevention of pulmonary embolus in this patient?

a. Aspirin 75 mg/d
b. Aspirin 325 mg/d
c. Warfarin with INR of 2 to 3 or low-molecular-weight heparin
d. Early ambulation
e. Heparin 5000 units subcutaneously every 12 hours

109. An obese 50-year-old woman complains of insomnia, daytime sleepiness, and fatigue. During a sleep study she is found to have recurrent episodes of arterial desaturation—about 30 events per hour—with evidence of obstructive apnea. Which of the following is the treatment of choice for this patient?

a. Nasal continuous positive airway pressure
b. Uvulopalatopharyngoplasty
c. Hypocaloric diet
d. Tracheostomy
e. Oxygen via nasal cannula

110. A 30-year-old athlete presents to your office complaining of intermittent wheezing. This wheezing begins shortly after running. The patient admits to smoking 1-2 packs of cigarettes per day for 5 years. What finding would be consistent with asthma?

a. Hyperinflation present on chest x-ray
b. Improvement in FEV_1 after bronchodilator
c. Low oxygen saturation on finger oximetry
d. Decreased FVC on PFT testing
e. Dyspnea on assuming a supine position

111. A 60-year-old male has had a chronic cough with clear sputum production for over 5 years. He has smoked one pack of cigarettes per day for 20 years and continues to do so. X-ray of the chest shows hyperinflation without infiltrates. Arterial blood gases show a pH of 7.38, PCO_2 of 40 mm Hg, and PO_2 of 65 mm Hg. Spirometry shows an FEV_1/FVC of 45% without bronchodilator response. Which of the following is the most important treatment modality for this patient?

a. Oral corticosteroids
b. Home oxygen
c. Broad-spectrum antibiotics
d. Smoking cessation program
e. Oral theophylline

112. An anxious young woman who is taking birth control pills presents to the emergency room with shortness of breath. Which of the following physical findings would make the diagnosis of pulmonary embolus unlikely?

a. Wheezing
b. Pleuritic chest pain
c. Right-sided S_3 heart sound
d. Hemoptysis
e. Bibasilar rales

113. A 50-year-old male with emphysema develops the sudden onset of shortness of breath and left-sided pleuritic chest pain. Pneumothorax is suspected. Which of the following physical examination findings would be consistent with the diagnosis?

a. Localized wheezes at the left base
b. Hyper-resonance, decreased breath sounds in the left chest with trachea deviation to right
c. Increased tactile fremitus on the left side
d. Decreased breath sounds on the left side with deviation of the trachea to the left
e. Rales at the left base

114. A 30-year-old quadriplegic male presents to the emergency room with fever, dyspnea, and a cough. He has a chronic indwelling Foley catheter. Recurrent urinary tract infections have been a problem for a number of years. He has been on therapy to suppress the urinary tract infections. On examination, mild wheezing is audible over both lungs. A diffuse erythematous rash is noted. The chest x-ray shows a diffuse alveolar infiltrate. The CBC reveals a WBC of 13,500, with 50% segmented cells, 30% lymphocytes, and 20% eosinophils. Which of the following is the most likely diagnosis?

a. Sepsis with ARDS secondary to urinary tract infection
b. Healthcare-related pneumonia
c. A drug reaction to one of his medications
d. An acute exacerbation of COPD
e. Lymphocytic interstitial pneumonitis

115. A 35-year-old female complains of slowly progressive dyspnea. Her past history is negative, and there is no cough, sputum production, pleuritic chest pain, or thrombophlebitis. She has taken appetite suppressants at different times. Physical examination reveals jugular venous distention, a palpable right ventricular lift, and a loud P_2 heart sound. Chest x-ray shows clear lung fields. Oxygen saturation is 94%. ECG shows right axis deviation. A perfusion lung scan is normal, with no segmental deficits. Which of the following is the most likely diagnosis?

a. Primary pulmonary hypertension
b. Recurrent pulmonary emboli
c. Right-to-left cardiac shunt
d. Interstitial lung disease
e. Left ventricular diastolic dysfunction

116. A 60-year-old obese male complains of excessive daytime sleepiness. He has been in good health except for mild hypertension. He drinks alcohol in moderation. The patient's wife states that he snores at night and awakens frequently. Examination of the oropharynx is normal. Which of the following studies is most appropriate?

a. EEG to assess sleep patterns
b. Ventilation pattern to detect apnea
c. Arterial O_2 saturation
d. Study of muscles of respiration during sleep
e. Polysomnography

117. A 60-year-old male develops acute shortness of breath, tachypnea, and tachycardia while hospitalized for congestive heart failure. On physical examination there is no jugular venous distention and the lungs are clear to auscultation and percussion. There is a loud P_2 sound. Examination of the lower extremities shows no edema or tenderness. Which of the following is the most important diagnostic step?

a. Pulmonary angiogram
b. Thin cut chest CT pulmonary angiogram with contrast
c. D-dimer assay
d. Venous ultrasound
e. High resolution chest CT without contrast

118. A 60-year-old male complains of shortness of breath 2 days after a cholecystectomy. He denies fever, chills, sputum production, and pleuritic chest pain. On physical examination, temperature is 37.2°C (99°F); pulse is 75; respiratory rate is 20; and blood pressure is 120/70. There are diminished breath sounds and dullness over the left base. Trachea is shifted to the left side. A chest x-ray shows a retrocardiac opacity that silhouettes the left diaphragm. Which of the following is the most likely anatomical problem in this patient?

a. An acute process causing inflammation
b. A left lower lobe mass
c. Diminished lung volume in the left lower lobe, postoperative atelectasis
d. Acute bronchospasm caused by surgery
e. Acute pneumothorax

119. A 55-year-old woman with long-standing chronic lung disease and episodes of acute bronchitis complains of increasing sputum production, which is now on a daily basis. Sputum is thick, and daily sputum production has dramatically increased over several months. There are flecks of blood in the sputum. The patient has lost 8 lb. Fever and chills are absent, and sputum cultures have not revealed specific pathogens. Chest x-ray and CT are shown on page 78. Which of the following is the most likely cause of the patient's symptoms?

a. Pulmonary tuberculosis
b. Exacerbation of chronic lung disease
c. Bronchiectasis
d. Anaerobic lung abscess
e. Carcinoma of the lung

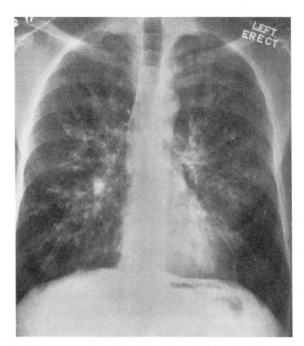

Reproduced, with permission, from Chen M et al. *Basic Radiology*. New York, NY: McGraw-Hill; 2003.

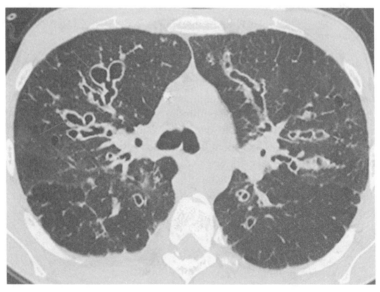

Reproduced, with permission, from Fauci A et al. *Harrison's Principles of Internal Medicine,* 17th ed. New York, NY: McGraw-Hill, 2008.

120. A 20-year-old fireman comes to the emergency room complaining of headache and dizziness after helping to put out a garage fire. He does not complain of shortness of breath, and the arterial blood gas shows a normal partial pressure of oxygen. Which of the following is the best first step in the management of this patient?

a. Begin oxygen therapy.
b. Obtain chest x-ray.
c. Obtain carboxyhemoglobin level.
d. Obtain CT scan.
e. Evaluate for anemia.

121. An 18-year-old male presents to your office. His family has noted a blue discoloration of his nose, ears, and fingers. This finding has only been noticed for a few weeks. Which of the following is true?

a. This patient has peripheral cyanosis.
b. Total hemoglobin is important in determining whether or not a patient will have cyanosis.
c. Central cyanosis with hypoxia suggests methemoglobinemia or sulfhemoglobinemia.
d. The presence of clubbing in a cyanotic patient confirms an acute cause of the cyanosis.
e. Large amounts of methemoglobin are required to produce cyanosis.

122. A 68-year-old woman with a prior diagnosis of asthma presents to your clinic for a routine clinic visit. She complains of occasional palpitations and tremor. Her dyspnea is well controlled. Her past medical history is remarkable for hospitalization for mild congestive heart failure 2 months ago; she notes occasional postprandial acid reflux. Her medications include lisinopril, digoxin, furosemide, an intermittent short-acting inhaled beta agonist, and theophylline. She uses an over-the-counter pill (whose name she cannot remember) for the reflux symptoms. On examination her heart rate is 112 beats per minute. S_1 and S_2 are normal; she has a mild tremor of the outstretched hands. What is the best next step in her management?

a. Chest x-ray to rule out congestive heart failure.
b. Theophylline level.
c. Spirometry before and after bronchodilator.
d. Intermittent lorazepam 0.5 mg po tid.
e. Discontinue beta agonist and substitute inhaled ipratropium.

Questions 123 to 128

Match the patient described with the type of pleural effusion. Each lettered option may be used once, more than once, or not at all.

a. Unilateral effusion, turbid, cell count 90,000 (95% polymorphonuclear cells), protein 4.5 g/dL (serum protein 5.2), LDH 255 U/L (serum LDH 290), pH 6.84, glucose 20 mg/dL. Culture and Gram stain pending.

b. Right-sided effusion, straw colored, cell count 150 (20% polys, 35% lymphocytes, 45% mesothelial cells), protein 1.4 g/L (serum protein 5.4), LDH 66 U/L (serum LDH 175), pH 7.42, glucose 100 mg/dL.

c. Bilateral effusions, slightly turbid, cell count 980 (10% polys, 30% lymphocytes, 60% mesothelial cells), protein 3.9 g/L (serum 3.8), LDH 225 U/L (serum 240), pH 7.52, glucose 5 mg/dL.

d. Bilateral effusions, straw colored, cell count 4200 (100% lymphocytes), protein 3 g/dL (serum 5.0), LDH 560 U/L (serum 450), pH 7.27, glucose 77 mg/dL.

e. Right-sided effusion, bloody, white cell count 1200 (15% polys, 5% lymphocytes, 80% "reactive" mesothelial cells), RBC 130,000, protein 4.2 g/L (serum 4.6), LDH 560 U/L (serum 226), pH 6.90, glucose 120 mg/dL.

f. Left-sided effusion, turbid, cell count 54,000 (92% polys, 8% lymphocytes), protein 5.2 g/L (serum 5.2), LDH 400 U/L (serum 200), pH 3.02, glucose 40 mg/dL.

g. Left-sided effusion, straw colored, cell count 2000 (80% polys, 10% lymphocytes, 10% mesothelial cells) protein 2.0 (serum 4.8), LDH 158 (serum 220), pH 7.52, Gram stain negative, amylase 32,000.

123. A 65-year-old male complains of shortness of breath at night and nocturnal dyspnea. On physical examination there is neck vein distention and bilateral rales at the bases. A chest x-ray shows bilateral pleural effusions, right larger than left, with cardiomegaly.

124. A 52-year-old alcoholic man develops left chest pain after repeated bouts of vomiting. On presentation he is diaphoretic with fever of 101.5, heart rate 126, BP 84/52. There are crackles and moderate dullness at the left base. The right lung is clear. He has subcutaneous emphysema over the left supraclavicular area.

125. A 72-year-old woman is admitted from the nursing home with fever and cough. Physical examination shows right basilar crackles and moderate dullness. CXR shows RLL pneumonia with moderate pleural effusion. She is treated with vancomycin and levofloxacin but remains febrile. Her shortness of breath worsens, and a follow-up chest x-ray shows enlarging pleural effusion.

126. A 52-year-old woman is admitted with abdominal pain and hyper-triglyceridemia. Amylase is elevated, and she is treated for pancreatitis with IV fluids and narcotics. Over the next several days she becomes more short of breath; left basilar dullness develops.

127. A 68-year-old retired construction worker has complained of right-sided chest pain and shortness of breath with dry cough. There is marked weight loss and anorexia. A chest x-ray shows right pleural effusion with pleural thickening.

Questions 128 to 131

Match the chest x-ray letter (see pages 82 and 83) with the most likely clinical description. Each lettered option may be used once, more than once, or not at all.

128. A 60-years-old man develops fever, chills, and productive cough while in the hospital after surgery. There is increased tactile fremitus in the right midlung field. Sputum Gram stain shows few squamous cells, many polys, and gram-positive cocci in clusters.

129. A 45-year-old male with known coronary artery disease develops short-ness of breath and awakens gasping for breath at night. There is dullness to percussion at the right base.

130. An 85-year-old male, newly arrived from Vietnam, has been complain-ing of cough and night sweats for more than a year. There are upper lobe crackles bilaterally.

131. A 50-year-old female has had long-standing hypertension that is poorly controlled. Physical examination shows the PMI to be displaced to the sixth intercostal space

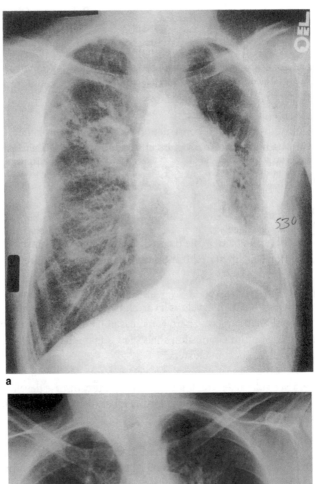

a

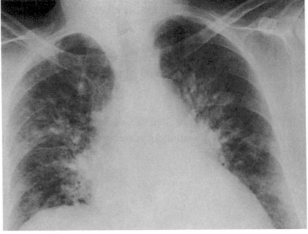

b

Reproduced, with permission, from Cheitlin MD, et al. *Clinical Cardiology,* 6th ed.
Stamford, CT: Appleton & Lange, McGraw-Hill; 1993.

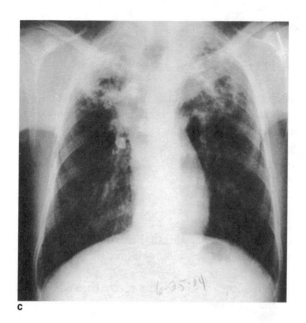

c

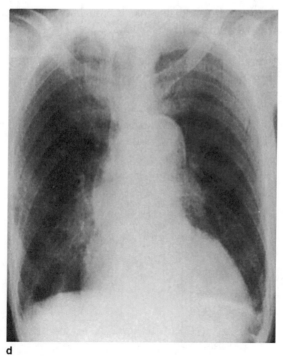

d

Reproduced, with permission, from Chen M et al. *Basic Radiology.* New York, NY: McGraw-Hill; 2003.

Questions 132 to 136

For each clinical situation, select the arterial blood gas and pH values with which it is most likely to be associated. Each lettered option may be used once, more than once, or not at all.

a. pH 7.50, P_{O_2} 75, P_{CO_2} 28
b. pH 7.14, P_{O_2} 78, P_{CO_2} 95
c. pH 7.06, P_{O_2} 36, P_{CO_2} 95
d. pH 7.06, P_{O_2} 108, P_{CO_2} 13
e. pH 7.37, P_{O_2} 48, P_{CO_2} 54

132. A 30-year-old obese female bus driver develops sudden pleuritic left-sided chest pain, hemoptysis, and dyspnea.

133. A 60-year-old heavy smoker has severe chronic bronchitis, peripheral edema, and cyanosis.

134. A 22-year-old drug-addicted man is brought to the emergency room by friends who were unable to awaken him.

135. A 62-year-old man with chronic bronchitis develops chest pain and is given oxygen via mask in the ambulance en route to the hospital. He becomes lethargic in the emergency room.

136. A 20-year-old man with diabetes mellitus comes to the emergency room with diffuse abdominal pain, tachypnea, and fever.

Questions 137 to 139

For each set of patients below, select the most likely diagnosis. Each lettered option may be used once, more than once, or not at all.

a. Small cell carcinoma of the lung
b. Bronchoalveolar carcinoma of the lung
c. Silicosis
d. Pneumonia
e. Cystic fibrosis
f. Hodgkin disease
g. Asbestosis
h. Hypersensitivity pneumonitis

137. A 20-year-old male has a cough and history of bronchitis with thick greenish sputum. There is no history of cigarette smoking. The patient has also been treated for abdominal cramping and malabsorption.

138. A 40-year-old construction worker has noted increasing shortness of breath and cough over many years. On physical examination bilateral inspiratory crackles are heard. Chest x-ray shows egg shell calcifications in hilar adenopathy and bilateral small nodular interstitial markings in the upper lobes.

139. A 42-year-old male is evaluated for fever, night sweats, and pruritus. There is a 2-cm firm rubbery supraclavicular node on physical examination as well as bilateral axillary nodes. Chest x-ray shows mediastinal lymphadenopathy.

Questions 140 to 142

For each of the clinical situations below, select the most likely diagnosis. Each lettered option may be used once, more than once, or not at all.

a. Tuberculosis
b. Primary lung tumor
c. Pulmonary embolus
d. Metastatic lung cancer
e. Asbestosis
f. Histoplasmosis
g. Idiopathic pulmonary fibrosis

140. A 32-year-old male has cough with yellow, blood-tinged sputum. He also has a history of night sweats and a 10-lb weight loss. The patient was born in India. On physical examination there is dullness to percussion above both clavicles. Chest x-ray shows bilateral upper lobe infiltrates with cavity formation.

141. A 55-year-old woman who is a heavy cigarette smoker complains of cough with small amounts of bright red blood. She has also noted loss of appetite and a 12-lb weight loss. A 3-cm pulmonary nodule with shaggy margins is seen on chest x-ray.

142. A 65-year-old who is retiring from work as a plumber has complained of a dry cough. He has also had some shortness of breath on walking. On physical examination there are bilateral crackling rales at both lung bases. Bilateral clubbing is also noted. On chest x-ray, bilateral linear infiltrates are seen at the lung bases. Pleural scarring is noted on CT scan.

Pulmonary Disease

Answers

96. The answer is b. (*Fauci, pp 2181-2183.*) The clinical picture suggests hypertrophic osteoarthropathy. This process, the pathogenesis of which is unknown, is characterized by clubbing of digits, periosteal new bone formation, and arthritis. Hypertrophic osteoarthropathy is associated with intrathoracic malignancy, suppurative lung disease, and congenital heart problems. Treatment is directed at the underlying disease process. While x-rays may suggest osteomyelitis, the process is usually bilateral and easily distinguishable from osteomyelitis. The first step in evaluation of this patient is to obtain a chest x-ray looking for lung infection and carcinoma. Although there is warmth over the wrists, the clubbing and periosteal changes would not be seen in rheumatoid arthritis; so wrist aspiration and methotrexate therapy would not address the underlying problem. An elevated sedimentation rate could be seen in neoplasm, infection, and inflammatory arthritis and would therefore be of little diagnostic value. Empiric antibiotic therapy is not warranted in this patient.

97. The answer is b. (*Fauci, pp 1584-1585.*) The diagnosis in this patient is suggested by the physical examination findings. The findings of poor excursion, flatness of percussion, and decreased fremitus on the right side are all consistent with a right-sided pleural effusion. A large right-sided effusion may shift the trachea to the left. A pneumothorax should result in hyper-resonance of the affected side. Atelectasis on the right side would shift the trachea to the right. A consolidated pneumonia would characteristically result in increased fremitus, flatness to percussion, and bronchial breath sounds, and would not cause tracheal deviation. COPD would not cause flatness to percussion or tracheal deviation. The distant breath sounds and hyper-resonance of COPD would be bilateral and symmetric.

98. The answer is d. (*Fauci, pp 1619-1628.*) The chest x-ray shows a pulmonary abscess in the right lower lobe with an air-fluid level. This is characteristic of an anaerobic infection. These are usually associated with a period of loss of consciousness and poor oral hygiene. The location of the infiltrate suggests aspiration, also making anaerobic infection most likely. The superior segment of the right lower lobe is the segment most likely to develop aspiration pneumonia. Of the organisms listed, only anaerobic infections are likely to cause a necrotizing process. *S pneumoniae* capsular type III pneumococci have been reported to cause cavitary disease, but this is unusual.

99. The answer is c. *(Fauci, p 334.)* Because clinical signs of neurologic deterioration and a petechial rash have occurred in the setting of fracture and hypoxia, fat embolism is the most likely diagnosis. This process occurs when neutral fat is introduced into the venous circulation after bone trauma or fracture. The latent period is 12 to 36 hours. A pulmonary embolus usually has a longer latent period. In addition pulmonary embolus would not cause the petechiae rash. The confusion out of proportion to the degree of hypoxemia is also seen with fat emboli. Unilateral pulmonary edema can be seen with aspiration and after rapid expansion of a pneumothorax, but not with fat embolism. Hematoma of the chest wall can occur after trauma, but does not cause hypoxemia and confusion. An early pneumonia would not be associated with a petechial rash.

100. The answer is c. *(Fauci, pp 1635-1643.)* This patient presents with severe COPD and hypoxemia. Chronic CO_2 retention has blunted his hypercarbic drive to breathe; he is dependent on mild hypoxia to stimulate respiration. An inappropriately high oxygen delivery has decreased even that drive, with resulting acute respiratory acidosis and CO_2 narcosis. However, stopping the oxygen will result in severe hypoxemia. Medroxyprogesterone has only a mild stimulatory effect on the respiratory centers, and is not appropriate therapy in this case. The patient has declared a deteriorating course. Continuing to monitor his status before beginning intervention would probably be fatal. Of the choices listed, the initiation of mechanical ventilation is the only acceptable choice. If the patient's mental status were better, noninvasive ventilation (BiPAP) might be considered. This patient has respiratory (not metabolic) acidosis. Bicarbonate plays no role in this acidosis. The correct therapy is to improve the patient's ventilation.

101. The answer is c. *(Fauci, pp 2135-2142.)* Sarcoidosis is a systemic illness of unknown etiology. There is a higher prevalence in female patients and in the African American population. Most patients have respiratory symptoms, including cough and dyspnea. Hilar and peripheral lymphadenopathy is common, and 20% to 30% of patients have hepatomegaly. The chest x-ray shows symmetrical hilar lymphadenopathy. The diagnostic method of choice is fiberoptic bronchoscopy with transbronchial biopsy, which will show a mononuclear cell granulomatous inflammatory process. While liver and scalene node biopsies are often positive, noncaseating granulomas are so frequent in these sites that they are not considered acceptable for primary diagnosis. ACE levels are elevated in two-thirds of patients, but false-positive values are common in other granulomatous disease processes. Open lung biopsy is more invasive and would only be considered if fiberoptic bronchoscopy failed to yield a diagnosis.

102. The answer is b. *(Fauci, pp 1658-1661.)* Classifying a pleural effusion as either a transudate or an exudate is useful in identifying the underlying disorder. Pleural fluid is exudative if it has any one of the following three properties: a ratio of concentration of total protein in pleural fluid to serum greater than 0.5, an absolute LDH greater than 2/3 the upper normal in serum or a ratio of LDH concentration in pleural fluid to serum greater than 0.6. Causes of exudative effusions include malignancy, pulmonary embolism, pneumonia, tuberculosis, abdominal disease, collagen vascular diseases, sarcoidosis, uremia, Dressler syndrome, and chylothorax. Exudative effusions may also be drug induced. If none of the aforementioned properties are met, the effusion is a transudate. Differential diagnosis for a transudative effusion includes congestive heart failure, nephrotic syndrome, cirrhosis, Meigs syndrome (benign ovarian neoplasm with effusion), and hydronephrosis. Exudative effusions are the result of an inflammatory process causing proteins to leak across the capillary membrane.

103. The answer is c. *(Fauci, pp 1632-1635.)* Patients with cystic fibrosis are now surviving into adulthood. The median survival is approximately age 41. Most cases are diagnosed in childhood; however, because of variable penetration of the genetic defect, approximately 7% are not found until the patient is an adult. Most male patients (>95%) are azoospermic. Chronic pulmonary infections occur, and bronchiectasis frequently develops. Diabetes mellitus and gastrointestinal problems indicate pancreatic insufficiency. COPD or emphysema at this age would be unusual unless the patient was deficient in alpha$_1$ antitrypsin. The patient's course is too prolonged for a simple upper respiratory tract infection. He has provided no history of hemoptysis or anemia to suggest a pulmonary hemorrhage syndrome. Asthma would not cause the abdominal symptoms, diabetes, or changes of bronchiectasis.

104. The answer is d. (*Fauci pp 1596-1607.*) It is important to accurately determine the severity of an exacerbation of asthma, since the major cause of death from asthma is the underestimation of the severity of a particular episode by either the patient or the physician. Silent chest is a particularly ominous finding, because the airway constriction is so great that airflow is insufficient to generate wheezing. Hypercapnia and thoracoabdominal paradox are almost always indicative of exhaustion and respiratory muscle failure or fatigue and generally need to be aggressively treated with mechanical ventilation. Altered mental status suggests severe hypoxia or hypercapnia, and ventilatory support is usually required. An increased pulsus paradoxus may also be a sign of severe asthma, as it increases with greater respiratory effort and generation of negative intrathoracic pressures during inspiration. However, pulsus paradoxus up to 8 to 10 mm Hg is considered normal; thus, a value of 5 mm Hg would not suggest a severe episode of asthma.

105. The answer is b. (*Fauci, pp 1619-1628.*) Pneumonia is a common disorder and is a major cause of death, particularly in hospitalized elderly patients. Before choosing empiric therapy for presumed pneumonia, it is necessary to know the age of the patient, whether the infection is community acquired or healthcare facility acquired, and whether there are any underlying debilitating illnesses. Community-acquired pneumonias in patients over the age of 35 are most likely caused by *S pneumoniae, Legionella pneumophila,* other atypical agents such as *Mycoplasma pneumoniae* and *Chlamydia pneumoniae, Moraxella catarrhalis,* and *Haemophilus influenzae.* In the case outlined, the history is strongly consistent with pneumococcal pneumonia, manifested by a short prodrome, shaking chills with rigor, pleuritic chest pain, and a consolidated lobar infiltrate on chest x-ray. The most reliable method of diagnosing pneumococcal pneumonia is seeing gram-positive diplococci on an adequate sputum (many white cells, few squamous epithelial cells). Sputum culture is also important in the era of penicillin-resistant pneumococci, but is not helpful in initial diagnosis. Blood cultures are positive in only about 20% of patients, and, when positive, are indicative of a more severe case. Although rigors may suggest pneumococcal bacteremia, the absence of rigors does not rule out the diagnosis. About 25% to 50% of pneumococci in the United States are partially or completely resistant to penicillin owing to chromosomal mutations resulting in penicillin-binding protein changes. Penicillin is no longer the empiric regimen of choice for pneumococcal pneumonia. A respiratory fluoroquinolone or ceftriaxone is widely used as initial therapy for pneumococcal pneumonia.

106. The answer is b. *(Fauci, pp 1651-1657.)* The clinical situation strongly suggests pulmonary embolism. In greater than 80% of cases, pulmonary emboli arise from thromboses in the deep venous circulation (DVTs) of the lower extremities, but a normal lower extremity Doppler does not exclude the diagnosis. DVTs often begin in the calf, where they rarely if ever cause clinically significant pulmonary embolic disease. However, thromboses that begin below the knee frequently "grow," or propagate, above the knee; clots that dislodge from above the knee cause clinically significant pulmonary emboli. Untreated pulmonary embolism is associated with a 30% mortality rate. Interestingly, only about 50% of patients with DVT of the lower extremities have clinical findings of swelling, warmth, erythema, pain, or palpable "cord." When a clot does dislodge from the deep venous system and travels into the pulmonary vasculature, the most common clinical findings are tachypnea and tachycardia; chest pain is less likely and is more indicative of concomitant pulmonary infarction. The ABG is usually abnormal, and a high percentage of patients exhibit low P_{CO_2} with respiratory alkalosis, and a widening of the alveolar-arterial oxygen gradient. The ECG is frequently abnormal in pulmonary embolic disease. The most common finding is sinus tachycardia, but atrial fibrillation, pseudoinfarction in the inferior leads, and acute right heart strain are also occasionally seen. Initial treatment for suspected pulmonary embolic disease includes prompt hospitalization and institution of intravenous heparin or therapeutic dose subcutaneous low-molecular-weight heparin. It is particularly important to make an early diagnosis of pulmonary embolus, as intervention can decrease the mortality rate from 30% down to 5%. A normal D-dimer level helps exclude pulmonary embolus in the low-risk setting. This patient, however, has a high pretest probability of PE; further testing (CT pulmonary angiogram, V/Q lung scan) must be done to exclude this important diagnosis.

107. The answer is a. *(Fauci, pp 1577-1579.)* In all patients in whom primary pulmonary hypertension is confirmed, acute drug testing with a pulmonary vasodilator is necessary to assess the extent of pulmonary vascular reactivity. Inhaled nitric oxide, intravenous adenosine, and intravenous prostacyclin have all been used. Patients who have a good response to the short-acting vasodilator are tried on a long-acting calcium channel antagonist under direct hemodynamic monitoring. Prostacyclin given via the pulmonary artery through a right heart catheter has been approved for patients who are functional class III or IV and have not responded to calcium channel antagonists. Sildenafil (a selective phosphodiesterase-5 inhibitor), treprostinil (a prostacyclin) and bosentan (an endothelin receptor antagonist) have also recently been approved for class III and IV disease. These drugs are not usually used empirically. Lung transplantation is reserved for late stages of the disease when patients are unresponsive to prostacyclin. The disease does not appear to recur after transplantation.

108. The answer is c. *(Fauci, pp 1655-1657.)* Warfarin is recommended for the prophylaxis of acute pulmonary embolus in patients who receive total hip replacement. Warfarin is started preoperatively, and the daily dose is adjusted to maintain an international normalized ratio (INR) of 2 to 2.5. Low-molecular-weight heparin given twice daily subcutaneously is also a recommended regimen. Aspirin alone is not effective in prevention of pulmonary embolus. Early ambulation and elastic stockings provide some additional benefit, but are not adequate in themselves in this high-risk situation. Warfarin is more effective than low-dose subcutaneous heparin in this setting.

109. The answer is a. *(Fauci, p 1667.)* This patient with multiple episodes of desaturation has obstructive sleep apnea. Continuous positive airway pressure is the recommended therapy. At present fewer than 5 apneic episodes per hour are considered normal. The severity of sleep apnea is graded using the apnea/hypopnea index. Mild sleep apnea is 5 to 15 events per hour; moderate sleep apnea is 15 to 30; severe apnea is greater than 30 events per hour. Awakenings from sleep apnea are associated with hypertension, insulin resistance, and multiple medical problems. Weight loss is often helpful and should be recommended as well. However, weight loss alone will take significant time and may not be sufficient. Uvulopalatopharyngoplasty, when applied to unselected patients, is effective in less than 50%. A trial of CPAP is usually tried before surgical therapy. Tracheostomy is a course of last resort that does provide immediate relief. Oxygen alone is less effective than CPAP.

110. The answer is b. *(Fauci, pp 1600-1601.)* Asthma is an inflammatory process with reversible air flow obstruction. This patient's presentation suggests exercise-induced asthma. Asthma is an incompletely understood disease that involves the lower airways and results in bronchoconstriction and excess production of mucus. This, in turn, leads to increased airway resistance and occasionally respiratory failure and death. In any obstructive lung diseases such as chronic obstructive pulmonary disease, hyperinflation may be present on chest x-ray and FEV_1 would be decreased. Only in asthma is the airway obstruction fully reversible. Hypoxia would be unusual in exercise-induced asthma and would suggest an alternative diagnosis. Reduced forced vital capacity (FVC) characterizes restrictive lung disease, not obstructive (airways) disease. Dyspnea on assuming a supine position would suggest congestive heart failure.

111. The answer is d. *(Fauci, pp 1635-1643.)* This patient's chronic cough, hyperinflated lungs, abnormal pulmonary function tests, and smoking history are all consistent with chronic bronchitis. A smoking cessation program can decrease the rate of lung deterioration and is successful in as many as 40% of patients, particularly when the physician gives a strong antismoking message and uses both counseling and nicotine replacement. Continuous low-flow oxygen becomes beneficial when arterial oxygen concentration falls below 55 mm Hg. Inhaled beta agonists or anticholinergics such as ipratropium or tiotropium are the cornerstones of symptomatic therapy but do not prevent progression of airways obstruction. Antibiotics are indicated only for acute exacerbations of chronic lung disease, which present with fever, change sputum color, and increasing shortness of breath. Oral corticosteroids are helpful in acute exacerbations but their side effect profile is significant in chronic use. Theophylline is a fourth-line treatment in COPD.

112. The answer is e. *(Fauci, p 1651-1654.)* All of these signs except bibasilar rales may occur in acute pulmonary embolism. Rales indicate alveolar fluid or interstitial inflammation, neither of which occurs in PE. The presence of prominent rales would suggest an alternative diagnosis such as congestive heart failure or pneumonia. Tachypnea is by far the most common physical finding in pulmonary embolism, occurring in more than 90%. Pleuritic chest pain occurs in about half of patients and is less common in the elderly and those with underlying heart disease. Hemoptysis and wheezing occur in less than half of patients. A right-sided S_3 is associated with large emboli that result in acute pulmonary hypertension.

113. The answer is b. *(Fauci, p 1660.)* The most characteristic findings of pneumothorax are hyper-resonance and decreased breath sounds. Occasionally hyperexpansion of the ipsilateral chest or subcutaneous emphysema may occur. A tension pneumothorax may displace the mediastinum and trachea to the unaffected side. Tactile fremitus would be decreased in the patient with a pneumothorax; increased fremitus suggests lung consolidation. Neither rales (suggesting alveolar fluid) nor a localized wheeze (suggesting airway narrowing) would be anticipated in pneumothorax.

114. The answer is c. (*Fauci, p 383, 1610*) The clues to this diagnosis are recurrent urinary tract infections and the use of suppressive therapy to control these infections. Nitrofurantoin is commonly used for this purpose. Nitrofurantoin can cause an acute hypersensitivity pneumonitis. This condition can progress to a chronic alveolitis with pulmonary fibrosis. The presenting symptoms are fever, chills, cough, and bronchospasm. In addition, the patient may experience arthralgias, myalgias, and an erythematous rash. The chest x-ray will show interstitial or alveolar infiltrates. CBC often shows leukocytosis with a high percentage of eosinophils. The treatment is to discontinue the nitrofurantoin, and begin corticosteroids. Sepsis secondary to a urinary tract infection, and a healthcare-related pneumonia might be considered. However, these would not present with a diffuse erythroderma or eosinophilia. Acute bacterial infections cause a neutrophilic leukocytosis; eosinophils are usually undetectable owing to the stress effect of catecholamines and cortisol. COPD rarely presents in a 30 year old. Lymphocytic interstitial pneumonia is a rare disease. Lung biopsy to establish the diagnosis of an interstitial lung disease would be considered only after the potentially offending drug had been discontinued.

115. The answer is a. (*Fauci, pp 1576-1581.*) Although a difficult diagnosis to make, primary pulmonary hypertension is the most likely diagnosis in this young woman who has used appetite suppressants. Primary pulmonary hypertension in the United States has been associated with fenfluramines. The predominant symptom is dyspnea, which is usually not apparent until the disease has advanced. When physical findings, chest x-ray, or echocardiography suggest pulmonary hypertension, recurrent pulmonary emboli must be ruled out. In this case, a normal perfusion lung scan makes pulmonary angiography unnecessary. Right-to-left cardiac shunts cause hypoxia (oxygen desaturation) that characteristically does not improve with oxygen supplementation. Restrictive lung disease should be ruled out with pulmonary function testing but is unlikely with a normal chest x-ray. An echocardiogram will show right ventricular enlargement and a reduction in the left ventricle size consistent with right ventricular pressure overload. Left ventricular diastolic dysfunction can cause pulmonary edema but not pulmonary hypertension.

116. The answer is e. (*Fauci, pp 1665-1668.*) With the history of daytime sleepiness and snoring at night, the patient requires evaluation for obstructive sleep apnea syndrome. Frequent awakenings are actually more suggestive of central sleep apnea. Polysomnography is required to assess which type of sleep apnea syndrome is present. EEG variables are recorded to identify various stages of sleep. Arterial oxygen saturation is monitored by finger or ear oximetry. Heart rate is monitored. The respiratory pattern is monitored to detect apnea and whether it is central or obstructive. Ambulatory sleep monitoring with oxygen saturation studies alone might identify multiple episodes of desaturation, but negative results would not rule out a sleep apnea syndrome. Overnight oximetry alone can be used in some patients when the index of suspicion for obstructive sleep apnea is high. Polysomnography includes all of these and is the best choice.

117. The answer is b. *(Fauci, pp 1653-1654.)* For suspected pulmonary embolism, CT with intravenous contrast is surpassing the ventilation-perfusion scan as the diagnostic method of choice. New multislice scanners can detect peripheral as well as central clots. Lung scanning may be useful in selected circumstances. The diagnosis is very unlikely in patients with normal or near-normal scans, and is highly likely in patients with high-probability scans. In patients with a high clinical index of suspicion for pulmonary embolus but low-probability scan, the diagnosis becomes more difficult. About two-thirds of patients with pulmonary embolus have evidence of deep venous disease on venous ultrasound. Therefore, pulmonary embolus cannot be excluded by a normal study. The quantitative D-dimer enzyme-linked immunosorbent assay is positive in 90% of patients with pulmonary embolus. It has been used to rule out pulmonary embolus in patients with a low- or intermediate-probability scan. A contrast CT study is needed to diagnose pulmonary embolism.

118. The answer is c. *(Fauci, pp 866-868, 1661-1665.)* Postoperative atelectasis or volume loss is a very common complication of surgery. General anesthesia and surgical manipulation lead to atelectasis by causing diaphragmatic immobilization. Atelectasis is usually basilar. On physical examination, shift of the trachea to the affected side suggests volume loss. On chest x-ray in this patient, loss of the left hemidiaphragm, increased density, and shift of the hilum downward would all suggest left lower lobe collapse. Atelectasis needs to be distinguished from acute consolidation of pneumonia, in which case fever, chills, and purulent sputum are more pronounced and consolidation is present without volume loss. Volume loss would not be a feature of a space-occupying mass, bronchospasm, or pneumothorax.

119. The answer is c. *(Fauci, pp 1629-1632.)* While symptoms such as sputum production and cough are nonspecific, particularly in a patient with known chronic lung disease, the high volume of daily sputum production suggests bronchiectasis. In this process, an abnormal and permanent dilatation of bronchi occurs as the muscular and elastic components of the bronchi are damaged. Clearance of secretions becomes a major problem, contributing to a cycle of bronchial inflammation and further deterioration. High-resolution CT scan, the diagnostic test of choice for this disease, shows prominent dilated bronchi and the signet ring sign of a dilated bronchus adjacent to a pulmonary artery. This CT scan picture is pathognomonic for bronchiectasis. Tuberculosis usually causes upper lobe cavitary disease. COPD causes hyperexpansion, upper lobe bullae, and nonspecific bronchial wall thickening. CT scan in anaerobic lung abscess would show an air-fluid level, usually within a shaggy inflammatory infiltrate. This CT scan shows no nodule or mass to suggest lung cancer.

120. The answer is c. *(Fauci, pp 229-231, 639-640, 1586-1592, 1723-1724.)* With symptoms of headache and dizziness in a fireman, the diagnosis of carbon monoxide poisoning must be addressed quickly. A venous or arterial measure of carboxyhemoglobin must first be obtained, if possible, before oxygen therapy is begun. The use of supplementary oxygen prior to obtaining the test may be a confounding factor in interpreting blood levels. Oxygen or even hyperbaric oxygen is given after blood for carboxyhemoglobin is drawn. Chest x-ray should also be obtained. It may be normal or show a pattern of nonpulmonary edema, or aspiration in severe cases. Central nervous system imaging would not be indicated; and there are no diagnostic patterns that are specific to carbon monoxide poisoning. Anemia might cause dizziness but the symptom would not occur as acutely as in this case.

121. The answer is b. *(Fauci, pp 229-231.)* Cyanosis, a bluish discoloration of the skin and/or mucous membranes, can indicate oxygen desaturation or other serious disease. The first step in evaluating cyanosis is to determine if the condition is new or has been present for a long period of time. Cyanosis present since infancy may be secondary to congenital heart disease. The presence of clubbing suggests chronic hypoxemia. The next step is to decide if cyanosis is peripheral or central. Peripheral cyanosis is secondary to slow blood flow through the digits. It may indicate vasoconstriction caused by cold exposure or may suggest more serious conditions such as shock or Raynaud phenomenon. In peripheral cyanosis, the mucous membranes and lips will be normal in color. Central cyanosis will usually be detectable if the absolute amount of reduced (desaturated) hemoglobin exceeds 4 g/dL. Therefore, the total hemoglobin concentration is important in determining whether the patient will display cyanosis. The COPD patient with a hemoglobin of 20 g/dL (owing to chronic hypoxia) will display central cyanosis with an O_2 saturation of 80%, whereas an anemic patient with hemoglobin of 10 g/dL requires an O_2 saturation of 60%. The next step in the evaluation of cyanosis, therefore, is to determine PaO_2 and SaO_2. Cyanosis in the absence of hypoxemia should prompt testing for methemoglobin (uncommon) and sulfhemoglobin (rare). Cyanosis can be produced by small amounts of methemoglobin and smaller amounts of sulfhemoglobin.

122. The answer is b. *(Fauci, pp 36-43,1602-1603.)* Theophylline has been used as a bronchodilator for a number of years. It has been less commonly used in recent years owing to its narrow therapeutic window. The drug is metabolized in the liver. A drug or process that interferes with the activity the cytochrome P450 system will slow the metabolism of theophylline and may lead to the accumulation of toxic levels in the blood. The metabolism of theophylline is slowed by age, infection, CHF (resulting from decreased hepatic blood flow), and a number of drugs. Commonly used drugs that impair the metabolism of theophylline include cimetidine, erythromycin, ciprofloxacin, allopurinol, and zafirlukast. This patient has probably been using over-the-counter cimetidine to treat her reflux symptoms. Stopping theophylline until the drug level has returned will probably relieve her palpitations and tremor. In the absence of dyspnea, wheezing, or clinical signs of CHF, chest film and spirometry would not be helpful. Using a benzodiazepine to treat her tremor would leave a potentially serious theophylline toxicity undetected. Finally beta agonists are more effective bronchodilators in asthma than is theophylline; the tremulousness associated with beta agonist use is usually short lived.

123 to 127. The answers are 123-b, 124-f, 125-a, 126-g, 127-e. *(Fauci, pp 1658-1661.)* The first step in determining the cause of a pleural effusion is to categorize it as either a transudate or exudate. Transudative effusions are caused by alteration in Starling forces (usually elevated hydrostatic pressure as in CHF or low plasma oncotic pressure as in hypoalbuminemia). The relatively low pleural fluid protein value means that capillary permeability is normal and that only small molecules (ie, salt and water) can leak out. Exudative effusions occur when an inflammatory (or neoplastic) process allows large molecules to enter the pleural space. According to the Light criteria, exudative effusions have one of the following characteristics: pleural fluid protein to serum protein ratio greater than 0.5, pleural fluid LDH to serum LDH ratio greater than 0.6, or pleural fluid LDH more than two-thirds the normal upper limit for serum.

The 65-year-old male with shortness of breath and paroxysmal nocturnal dyspnea has congestive heart failure. CHF usually produces a right-sided pleural effusion. Of all pleural fluid values, it is the only transudate. Cirrhosis and nephrotic syndrome are other common causes of transudative pleural effusions.

The alcoholic patient with repetitive nausea and vomiting has ruptured his esophagus (Boerhaave syndrome). Gastric contents enter the left pleural space and cause an inflammatory (ie, exudative) effusion. The very low pH is a tip-off that gastric acid is present and will distinguish Boerhaave syndrome from the more usual empyema.

The elderly woman with pneumonia has developed empyema, a bacterial infection of the pleural space. Empyema is characterized by a very high white cell count, turbid fluid, and pH less then 7.2. Antibiotics alone will not cure empyema. Pleural fluid drainage, either with a chest tube (if the effusion is free flowing) or surgical drainage (if the fluid is loculated), is necessary to fully eradicate the infection.

The patient with abdominal pain has developed a pleural effusion resulting from pancreatitis. Many peripancreatic effusions simply occur in response to nearby inflammation of the pancreas (so-called sympathetic effusion). Occasionally, as in this case, a pancreatico-pleural fistula will form, leading to an exudate with very high amylase level. Such effusions often require chest tube drainage. Almost all effusions resulting from pancreatitis are left-sided exudates.

The 68-year-old retired construction worker presents with characteristic features of mesothelioma. Mesotheliomas are primary tumors that arise from mesothelial cells that line the pleural cavity. They produce a hemorrhagic effusion; a bloody effusion in the absence of acute trauma always suggests malignancy. Thoracoscopy with pleural biopsy is usually necessary to make a definitive diagnosis.

128 to 131. The answers are 128-a, 129-b, 130-c, 131-d. (*Fauci, pp 1010-1015, 1446-1447, 1619-1628.*) The 60-year-old male has developed nosocomial pneumonia. A sputum Gram stain showing gram-positive cocci in clusters will grow *Staphylococcus aureus*. Chest x-ray **a** shows a necrotizing pneumonia characteristic of this infection. Cavities develop in association with lung infection when necrotic lung tissue is discharged into airways. Cavities greater than 2 cm are described as lung abscesses.

The 45-year-old with shortness of breath and paroxysmal nocturnal dyspnea has symptoms suggesting congestive heart failure. Chest x-ray **b** shows signs of congestive heart failure, including cardiomegaly, bilateral infiltrates, and cephalization. Cephalization occurs when long-standing venous hypertension causes the upper lobe vessels become more prominent owing to redistribution of pulmonary blood flow. When pulmonary edema becomes severe, fluid extends out from both hila in a bat-wing distribution.

The elderly Vietnamese patient with fever and night sweats has chest x-ray **c**. This x-ray shows characteristic changes of tuberculosis, including extensive apical and upper lobe scarring. When the lung is involved with tuberculosis, the range of abnormalities is broad. Cavitary infiltrates in the posterior apical segments are very common. Mass lesions, interstitial infiltrates, and noncavitary infiltrates also occur.

The woman with long-standing hypertension has chest x-ray **d**, with evidence for left ventricular hypertrophy. The cardiac silhouette is enlarged and takes on a boot-shaped configuration.

132 to 136. The answers are 132-a, 133-e, 134-c, 135-b, 136-d. *(Fauci, pp 1591-1592.)* The blood gas values associated with pulmonary embolism in the 30-year-old obese bus driver would be expected to show acute respiratory alkalosis. It is important to note that hypoxemia, although frequently found, need not be present.

The 60-year-old smoker has severe chronic lung disease. The presence of hypercapnia leads to a compensatory increase in serum bicarbonate. Thus, significant hypercapnia may be present with an arterial pH close to normal, but will never be completely corrected. Compensated respiratory acidosis suggests a long-standing problem.

The 22-year-old addict has a drug overdose. Acute respiratory acidosis may occur secondary to respiratory depression after drug overdose. Sudden hypoventilation is associated with hypoxia, hypercapnia, and uncompensated acidosis. Such severe acidosis implies that the serum bicarbonate is near normal, ie, the kidneys have not had enough time to compensate by retaining bicarbonate. Acute respiratory acidosis is a life-threatening condition. If this patient does not respond to naloxone, intubation and mechanical ventilation will be necessary.

In the presence of long-standing lung disease as in the patient in question 135, respiration may become regulated by hypoxia rather than by altered carbon dioxide tension and arterial pH, as in normal people. Thus, the unmonitored administration of oxygen may lead to respiratory suppression. In this patient high flow oxygen has resulted in acute on chronic respiratory acidosis. The Po_2 is higher than would be predicted by the alveolar gas equation. Therefore, this patient (unlike the patient in question 134 who has equally severe

CO_2 retention) is receiving supplemental oxygen. In addition, this patient's chronic hypercarbia has given the kidneys an opportunity to retain bicarbonate; therefore, his pH is not as low as that of the patient in question 134.

Young patients with type 1 diabetes mellitus may present with rapid onset of diabetic ketoacidosis (DKA), often secondary to a systemic infection. These patients usually are maximally ventilating, as indicated by a very low P_{CO_2}; however, they remain acidotic secondary to the severe metabolic ketoacidosis associated with this process. In general, patients are not hypoxic unless the underlying infection is pneumonia.

137 to 139. The answers are 137-e, 138-c, 139-f. (*Fauci, pp 551-562, 698-699, 1611-1619, 1632-1635.*) The 20-year-old male has evidence of chronic airway infection not associated with cigarette smoking. Cystic fibrosis is a multisystem disease with signs and symptoms usually beginning in childhood. However, 7% of patients are diagnosed as adults. This is an autosomal recessive disease with a gene mutation on chromosome 7. In addition to respiratory tract infection, there are intestinal complications and exocrine pancreatic insufficiency. This results in malabsorption with bulky stools.

The 40-year-old construction worker is an example of environmental lung disease. Silicosis is caused by the inhalation of crystalline silica. Occupations typically at risk include cement workers and sandblasters. These workers should be provided with respiratory protection such as a respirator. Usually, a latency period of 10 to 15 years from first exposure is required for the disease process to become evident. Asbestosis, another occupational lung disease, affects lower lobes (rather than the predominantly upper lobe involvement of silicosis). Asbestosis causes pleural disease, whereas silicosis causes lymphadenopathy.

The 42-year-old with fever, night sweats, and pruritus gives symptoms very characteristic of Hodgkin disease. Most patients present with palpable lymphadenopathy, and more than half will have mediastinal lymphadenopathy on presentation. About half will have symptoms of fever, night sweats, or weight loss. There may be unexplained itching as well as cutaneous lesions such as erythema nodosum or ichthyosis.

140 to 142. The answers are 140-a, 141-b, 142-e. (*Fauci, pp 225-228, 1010-1019, 1611-1619.*) The 32-year-old male has signs and symptoms of chronic tuberculosis. The disease presents with productive cough, hemoptysis, and weight loss. Night sweats are particularly characteristic of tuberculosis. Chronic cavitary disease usually involves the upper lobes.

The woman who is a heavy cigarette smoker is most likely to have a primary lung tumor. The symptom of hemoptysis in association with weight loss and loss of appetite is particularly concerning. A pulmonary nodule greater than 3 cm is most often malignant, and the shaggy border of the lesion also suggests malignancy. Metastases to the lung are more sharply defined and are usually multiple.

Asbestosis is a risk for those such as construction workers, shipbuilders, and plumbers who may have long-standing history of exposure to asbestos-containing materials. Symptoms are usually subtle and include an annoying dry cough and dyspnea on exertion. Asbestosis on chest x-ray produces a linear interstitial process at the lung bases. Pleural fibrosis and pleural plaques may also be noted, especially on CT scan.

Cardiology

Questions

143. A 60-year-old male patient is receiving aspirin, an angiotensin-converting enzyme inhibitor, nitrates, and a beta-blocker for chronic stable angina. He presents to the ER with an episode of more severe and long-lasting anginal chest pain each day over the past 3 days. His ECG and cardiac enzymes are normal. Which of the following is the best course of action?

a. Admit the patient and add intravenous digoxin.
b. Admit the patient and begin low-molecular-weight heparin.
c. Admit the patient for thrombolytic therapy.
d. Admit the patient for observation with no change in medication.
e. Increase the doses of current medications and follow closely as an outpatient.

144. You have been asked to evaluate a 42-year-old white male smoker who presented to the emergency department with sudden onset of crushing substernal chest pain, nausea, diaphoresis and shortness of breath. His initial ECG revealed ST segment elevation in the anterior-septal leads. Cardiac enzymes were normal. The patient underwent emergent cardiac catheterization, which revealed only a 25% stenosis of the left anterior descending (LAD) artery. No percutaneous intervention was performed. Which of the following interventions would most likely reduce his risk of similar episodes in the future?

a. Placement of a percutaneous drug-eluting coronary artery stent.
b. Placement of a percutaneous non-drug-eluting coronary artery stent.
c. Beginning therapy with an ACE inhibitor.
d. Beginning therapy with a beta-blocker.
e. Beginning therapy with a calcium-channel blocker.

145. A 15-year-old male presents to your office on the advice of his football coach. The patient started playing football this year and suffered a syncopal episode at practice yesterday. He reports that he was sprinting with the rest of the team and became lightheaded. He lost consciousness and fell to the ground, regaining consciousness within one or two minutes. He suffered no trauma during the event. He has no prior history of head injury or recent illness. He has had no prior episodes of syncope. The patient is adopted and family history unavailable. Physical examination is unremarkable. What is the best course of action regarding this patient's syncopal episode?

a. Perform an ECG and echocardiogram. The patient may not return to competitive sports until results are available.
b. Perform an ECG. The patient may not return to competitive sports until results are available.
c. Perform an ECG. The patient may return to competitive sports pending the results.
d. Reassurance. The patient may return to competitive sports provided he increases his water consumption during practice times.
e. Reassurance. The patient may return to competitive sports with no restrictions.

146. An 82-year-old white female is admitted to the hospital for observation after presenting to the emergency department with dizziness. After being placed on a cardiac monitor in the ER, the rhythm strip below was recorded. There is no past history of cardiac disease, diabetes, or hypertension. With prompting, the patient discloses several prior episodes of transient dizziness and one episode of brief syncope in the past. Physical examination is unremarkable. Which of the following is the best plan of care?

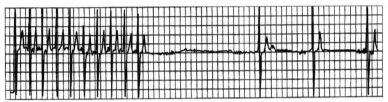

Reproduced, with permission, from Kasper DL et al. *Harrison's Principles of Internal Medicine,* 15th ed. New York, NY: McGraw-Hill, 2001.

a. Reassurance. This is a benign condition, and no direct therapy is needed.
b. Reassurance. The patient may not drive until she is symptom free, but otherwise no direct therapy is needed.
c. Nuclear cardiac stress testing; treatment depending on results.
d. Begin therapy with aspirin.
e. Arrange placement of a permanent pacemaker.

147. Two weeks after hospital discharge for documented myocardial infarction, a 65-year-old returns to your office concerned about low-grade fever and pleuritic chest pain. There is no associated shortness of breath. Lungs are clear to auscultation and the heart is free of murmur, gallop, or rub. ECG is unchanged from the last one in the hospital. Which therapy is most likely to be effective?

a. Antibiotics
b. Anticoagulation with warfarin (Coumadin)
c. An anti-inflammatory agent
d. An increase in antianginal medication
e. An anxiolytic agent

148. A 55-year-old patient presents to you after a 3-day hospital stay for gradually increasing shortness of breath and leg swelling while away on a business trip. He was told that he had congestive heart failure, but is asymptomatic now, with normal vital signs and physical examination. An echocardiogram shows an estimated ejection fraction of 38%. The patient likes to keep medications to a minimum. He is currently on aspirin and simvastatin. Which would be the most appropriate additional treatment?

a. Begin an ACE inhibitor and then add a beta-blocker on a scheduled basis.
b. Begin digoxin plus furosemide on a scheduled basis.
c. Begin spironolactone on a scheduled basis.
d. Begin furosemide plus nitroglycerin.
e. Given his preferences, no other medication is needed unless shortness of breath and swelling recur.

149. A 34-year-old woman is referred by an OB-GYN colleague for the onset of fatigue and dyspnea on exertion 1 month after her second vaginal delivery. Physical examination reveals a laterally displaced PMI, elevated jugular venous pressure and 2+ pitting lower extremity edema. Echocardiogram shows systolic dysfunction with an ejection fraction of 30%. Which statement most accurately describes her condition?

a. This disease may occur unexpectedly years after pregnancy and delivery.
b. About half of similar patients will recover completely.
c. The condition is idiosyncratic; the risk of recurrence with a future pregnancy is no greater than average.
d. This condition will require a different therapeutic approach than the typical dilated cardiomyopathy.
e. This condition will require endomyocardial biopsy for diagnosis.

150. Yesterday you admitted a 55-year-old white male to the hospital for an episode of chest pain, and you are seeking to rule out MI plus assess for any underlying coronary artery disease. The patient tends to be anxious about his health. On admission, his lungs were clear, but his heart revealed a grade 1/6 early systolic murmur at the upper left sternal border without radiation. Blood pressure readings have consistently been in the 140/90 to 150/100 range. Cardiac enzymes are normal. A resting ECG shows only left ventricular hypertrophy with secondary ST-T changes ("LVH with strain"). Why would a treadmill ECG stress test not be an appropriate test in this patient?

a. Anticipated difficulty with the patient's anxiety (ie, he might falsely claim chest pain during the test)
b. Increased risk associated with high blood pressure readings
c. Concern about the heart murmur, a relative contraindication to stress testing
d. The presence of LVH with ST-T changes on baseline ECG
e. Concern that this represents the onset of unstable angina with unacceptable risk of MI with stress testing

151. A 75-year-old patient presents to the ER after a syncopal episode. He is again alert and in retrospect describes occasional substernal chest pressure and shortness of breath on exertion. His blood pressure is 110/80 and lungs have a few bibasilar rales. Which auscultatory finding would best explain his findings?

a. A harsh systolic crescendo-decrescendo murmur heard best at the upper right sternal border
b. A diastolic decrescendo murmur heard at the mid-left sternal border
c. A holosystolic murmur heard best at the apex
d. A midsystolic click
e. A pericardial rub

152. A 72-year-old Caucasian male presents with shortness of breath that awakens him at night. At baseline he is able to walk less than a block before stopping to catch his breath. Physical examination findings include bilateral basilar rales and neck vein distention. The patient has a known history of congestive heart failure, and his last echocardiogram revealed an ejection fraction of 25%. The patient is compliant with a medication regimen including an ACE inhibitor, beta-blocker, and loop diuretic. Blood pressure is well controlled. What additional treatment should you begin next?

a. Spironolactone
b. Aspirin
c. Amlodipine
d. Warfarin
e. Hydralazine and isosorbide dinitrate

153. A 72-year-old male comes to the office with intermittent symptoms of dyspnea on exertion, palpitations, and cough occasionally productive of blood. On cardiac auscultation, a low-pitched diastolic rumbling murmur is faintly heard at the apex. What is the most likely cause of the murmur?

a. Rheumatic fever as a youth
b. Long-standing hypertension
c. A silent MI within the past year
d. A congenital anomaly
e. Anemia from chronic blood loss

154. You are helping with school sports physicals and see a 16-year-old boy who has had trouble keeping up with his peers. Which of the following auscultatory findings suggests a previously undiagnosed ventricular septal defect?

a. A systolic crescendo-decrescendo murmur heard best at the upper right sternal border with radiation to the carotids; the murmur is augmented with exercise.
b. A systolic murmur at the pulmonic area and a diastolic rumble along the left sternal border.
c. A holosystolic murmur at the mid-left sternal border.
d. A diastolic decrescendo murmur at the mid-left sternal border.
e. A continuous murmur through systole and diastole at the upper left sternal border.

155. A 68-year-old male was intubated in the emergency room because of pulmonary edema. Stat echocardiogram reveals an ejection fraction of 45% and severe mitral regurgitation. In spite of aggressive diuresis with furosemide, the patient continues to require mechanical ventilation secondary to pulmonary edema. What is the best next step in treating this patient?

a. Arrange for mitral valve replacement surgery.
b. Place an intra-aortic balloon pump.
c. Begin metoprolol.
d. Begin a second loop diuretic.
e. Begin intravenous enalapril.

156. A 30-year-old female presents with a chief complaint of palpitations. A 24-hour Holter monitor shows occasional unifocal premature ventricular contractions and premature atrial contractions. Which of the following is the best management for this patient?

a. Anxiolytic therapy
b. Beta-blocker therapy
c. Digoxin
d. Quinidine
e. Reassurance, no medication

157. An active 78-year-old female with history of hypertension presents with the new onset of left hemiparesis. Cardiac monitoring reveals atrial fibrillation. She had been in sinus rhythm on checkup 3 months earlier. Optimal management at discharge includes a review of antihypertensive therapy, a ventricular rate control agent, and which of the following?

a. Automated implanted cardioverter-defibrillator (AICD)/permanent pacemaker to avoid the need for anticoagulation
b. Immediate direct-current cardioversion
c. Antiplatelet therapy such as aspirin, without warfarin
d. Antiplatelet therapy plus warfarin with a target INR of 1.5
e. Warfarin with a target INR of 2.0 to 3.0.

158. A 72-year-old male with a history of poorly controlled hypertension develops a viral upper respiratory infection. On his second day of symptoms he experiences palpitations and presents to the emergency room. His blood pressure is 118/78. The following rhythm strip is obtained. What is the best next step in the management of this patient?

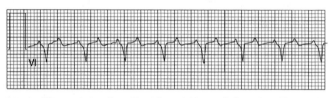

Reproduced, with permission, from Fauci A et al. *Harrison's Principles of Internal Medicine*, 17th ed. New York, NY: McGraw-Hill, 2008.

a. Administration of intravenous metoprolol
b. Administration of intravenous adenosine
c. Administration of intravenous amiodarone
d. Emergent electrical cardioversion
e. Initiation of chest compressions and preparation for semielective intubation

159. A 67-year-old male presents to your office after community ultrasound screening revealed an aortic aneurysm measuring 3.0 × 3.5 cm. Physical examination confirms a palpable, pulsatile, nontender abdominal mass just above the umbilicus. The patient's medical conditions include hypertension, hyperlipidemia, and tobacco use. What is the best recommendation for the patient to consider?

a. Watchful waiting is the best course until the first onset of abdominal pain.
b. Surgery is indicated except for the excess operative risk represented by the patient's risk factors.
c. Serial follow-up with ultrasound, CT, or MRI is indicated, with the major determinant for surgery being aneurysmal size greater than 5 to 6 cm.
d. Serial follow-up with ultrasound, CT, or MRI is indicated, with the major determinant for surgery being involvement of a renal artery.
e. Unlike stents in coronary artery disease, endovascular stent grafts have proven unsuccessful in the management of AAAs.

160. An otherwise asymptomatic 65-year-old man with diabetes presents to the ER with a sports-related right shoulder injury. His heart rate is noted to be irregular, and this ECG is obtained. Which of the following is the best immediate therapy?

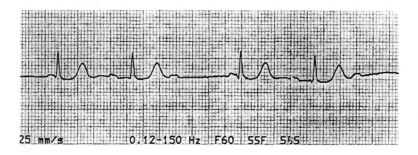

a. Atropine
b. Isoproterenol
c. Pacemaker placement
d. Electrical cardioversion
e. Observation

161. In the ICU, a patient suddenly becomes pulseless and unresponsive, with cardiac monitor indicating ventricular tachycardia. The crash cart is immediately available. What is the best first therapy?

a. Amiodarone 150-mg IV push
b. Lidocaine 1.5-mg/kg IV push
c. Epinephrine 1-mg IV push
d. Defibrillation at 200 J
e. Defibrillation at 360 J

162. A 70-year-old female has been healthy except for hypertension treated with a thiazide diuretic. She presents with sudden onset of a severe, tearing chest pain, which radiates to the back and is associated with dyspnea and diaphoresis. Blood pressure is 210/94. Lung auscultation reveals bilateral basilar rales. A faint murmur of aortic insufficiency is heard. The BNP level is elevated at 550 pg/mL (Normal < 100). ECG shows nonspecific ST-T changes. Chest x-ray suggests a widened mediastinum. Which of the following choices represents the best initial management?

a. IV furosemide plus IV loading dose of digoxin
b. Percutaneous coronary intervention with consideration of angioplasty and/or stenting
c. Blood cultures and rapid initiation of vancomycin plus gentamicin, followed by echocardiography
d. IV beta-blocker to control heart rate, IV nitroprusside to control blood pressure, transesophageal echocardiogram
e. IV heparin followed by CT pulmonary angiography

163. A 55-year-old African American female presents to the ER with lethargy and blood pressure of 250/150. Her family members indicate that she was complaining of severe headache and visual disturbance earlier in the day. They report a past history of asthma but no known kidney disease. On physical examination, retinal hemorrhages are present. Which of the following is the best approach?

a. Intravenous labetalol therapy
b. Continuous-infusion nitroprusside
c. Clonidine by mouth to lower blood pressure
d. Nifedipine sublingually to lower blood pressure
e. Intravenous loop diuretic

164. An 18-year-old male complains of fever and transient pain in both knees and elbows. The right knee was red and swollen for 1 day during the week prior to presentation. On physical examination, the patient has a low-grade fever. He has a III/VI, high pitched, apical systolic murmur with radiation to the axilla, as well as a soft, mid-diastolic murmur heard at the base. A tender nodule is palpated over an extensor tendon of the hand. There are pink erythematous lesions over the abdomen, some with central clearing. The following laboratory values are obtained:

Hct: 42
WBC: 12,000/µL with 80% polymorphonuclear leukocytes, 20% lymphocytes
ESR: 60 mm/h

The patient's ECG is shown below. Which of the following tests is most critical to diagnosis?

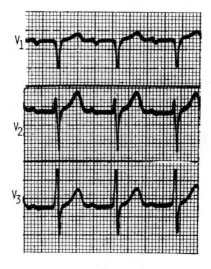

a. Blood cultures
b. Antistreptolysin O antibody
c. Echocardiogram
d. Antinuclear antibodies
e. Creatine kinase

165. A 36-year-old male presents with the sensation of a racing heart. His blood pressure is 110/70, respiratory rate 14/minute, and O_2 saturation 98%. His ECG shows a narrow QRS complex tachycardia with rate 180, which you correctly diagnose as paroxysmal atrial tachycardia. Carotid massage and Valsalva maneuver do not improve the heart rate. Which of the following is the initial therapy of choice?

a. Adenosine 6-mg rapid IV bolus
b. Verapamil 2.5 to 5 mg IV over 1 to 2 min
c. Diltiazem 0.25-mg/kg IV over 2 min
d. Digoxin 0.5 mg IV slowly
e. Electrical cardioversion at 50 J

166. A patient has been in the coronary care unit for the past 24 hours with an acute anterior myocardial infarction. He develops the abnormal rhythm shown below, although blood pressure remains stable at 110/68. Which of the following is the best next step in therapy?

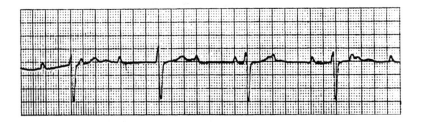

a. Perform cardioversion.
b. Arrange for pacemaker placement.
c. Give digoxin.
d. Give propranolol.
e. Give lidocaine.

167. A 70-year-old male with a history of coronary artery disease presents to the emergency department with 2 hours of substernal chest pressure, diaphoresis, and nausea. He reports difficulty "catching his breath." An electrocardiogram shows septal T-wave inversion. The patient is given 325-mg aspirin and sublingual nitroglycerin while awaiting the results of his blood work. His troponin I is 0.65 ng/mL (normal < 0.04 ng/mL). The physician in the emergency department starts the patient on low-molecular-weight heparin. His pain is 3/10. Blood pressure is currently 154/78 and heart rate is 72. You are asked to assume care of this patient. What is the best next step in management?

a. Arrange for emergent cardiac catheterization.
b. Begin intravenous thrombolytic therapy.
c. Admit the patient to a monitored cardiac bed and repeat cardiac enzymes and ECG in 6 hours.
d. Begin intravenous beta-blocker therapy.
e. Begin clopidogrel 300 mg po each day.

168. A 55-year-old obese woman develops pressure-like substernal chest pain lasting 1 hour. She works as a housekeeper; lifting and exertion have precipitated similar pain in the recent past. There is a positive family history of gallstones (mother and sister). Her ECG is shown below. Which of the following is the most likely diagnosis?

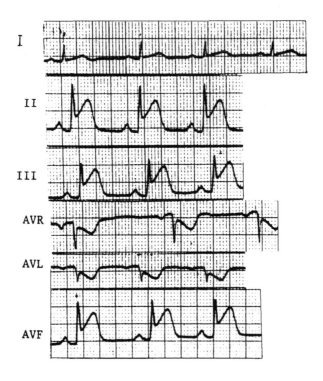

a. Costochondritis
b. Acute anterior myocardial infarction
c. Acute inferior myocardial infarction
d. Pericarditis
e. Gastroesophageal reflux

169. A 50-year-old construction worker continues to have elevated blood pressure of 160/95 even after a third agent is added to his antihypertensive regimen. Physical examination is normal, electrolytes are normal, and the patient is taking no over-the-counter medications. Which of the following is the best next step for this patient?

a. Check pill count.
b. Evaluate for Cushing syndrome.
c. Check chest x-ray for coarctation of the aorta.
d. Obtain a renal angiogram.
e. Obtain an adrenal CT scan.

170. A 35-year-old male complains of substernal chest pain aggravated by inspiration and relieved by sitting up. Lung fields are clear to auscultation, and heart sounds are somewhat distant. Chest x-ray shows an enlarged cardiac silhouette. Which of the following is the best next step in evaluation?

a. Right lateral decubitus chest x-ray
b. Cardiac catheterization
c. Echocardiogram
d. Serial ECGs
e. Thallium stress test

171. A 42-year-old female with acute pericarditis develops jugular venous distention and hypotension. The ECG shows electrical alternans. Which of the following is the most likely additional physical finding?

a. Basilar rales halfway up both posterior lung fields
b. S_3 gallop
c. Pulsus paradoxus
d. Strong apical beat
e. Epigastric tenderness

172. A 43-year-old woman with a 1-year history of episodic leg edema and dyspnea is noted to have clubbing of the fingers. Her ECG is shown below. Which of the following is the most likely diagnosis?

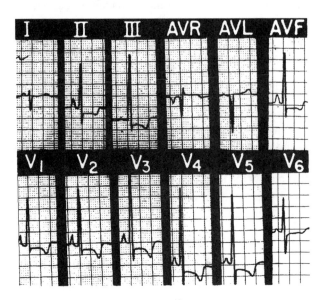

a. ST segment-elevation inferior wall myocardial infarction
b. Right bundle branch block
c. Acute pericarditis
d. Wolff-Parkinson-White syndrome
e. Cor pulmonale

173. A 62-year-old male with underlying COPD develops a viral upper respiratory infection and begins taking an over-the-counter decongestant. Shortly thereafter he experiences palpitations and presents to the emergency room, where the following rhythm strip is obtained. What is the most likely diagnosis?

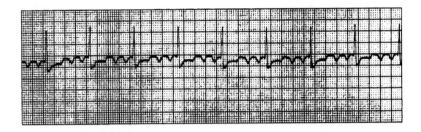

a. Normal sinus rhythm
b. Junctional rhythm
c. Atrial flutter with 4:1 atrioventricular block
d. Paroxysmal atrial tachycardia with 2:1 atrioventricular block
e. Complete heart block with 2:1 atrioventricular block

174. A 32-year-old male presents to your office with concern about progressive fatigue and lower extremity edema. He has experienced decreased exercise tolerance over the past few months, and occasionally awakens coughing at night. Past medical history is significant for sickle cell anemia and diabetes mellitus. He has had multiple admissions to the hospital secondary to vaso-occlusive crises since the age of three. Physical examination reveals a displaced PMI, but is otherwise unremarkable. ECG shows a first degree AV block and low voltage. Chest x-ray shows an enlarged cardiac silhouette with clear lung fields. Which of the following would be the best initial diagnostic approach?

a. Order serum iron, iron-binding capacity, and ferritin level.
b. Order brain-natriuretic peptide (BNP)
c. Order CT scan of the chest.
d. Arrange for placement of a 24-hour ambulatory cardiac monitor.
e. Arrange for cardiac catheterization.

175. You are volunteering with a dental colleague in a community indigent clinic. A nurse has prepared a list of patients who are scheduled for a dental procedure and may need antibiotic prophylaxis beforehand. Of the patients listed below, who would be most likely to benefit from antibiotic prophylaxis to prevent infective endocarditis?

a. 17-year-old male with coarctation of the aorta
b. 26-year-old female with a ventricular septal defect repaired in childhood
c. 42-year-old female with mitral valve prolapse
d. 65-year-old male with prosthetic aortic valve
e. 72-year-old female with aortic stenosis

176. An 80-year-old woman was admitted to your service for dizziness. Cardiac monitoring initially revealed atrial fibrillation with rapid ventricular response. Her ventricular rate was controlled with beta-blocker. An echocardiogram revealed an enlarged left atrium and an ejection fraction of 50%. No evidence of diastolic heart dysfunction was noted. She is now asymptomatic, with blood pressure 130/80, heart rhythm irregularly irregular, and heart rate around 80/minute. Which of the following is the best management strategy of this patient's arrhythmia?

a. Electrical cardioversion plus prolonged anticoagulation
b. Electrical cardioversion without anticoagulation
c. Chemical cardioversion plus prolonged anticoagulation
d. Chemical cardioversion without anticoagulation
e. Continued rate control plus prolonged anticoagulation

177. You are performing medical screening of new military recruits when an 18-year-old male reports several episodes of palpitation and syncope over the past several years. Physical examination is unremarkable. An ECG is obtained with excerpts shown below. What is the most likely diagnosis?

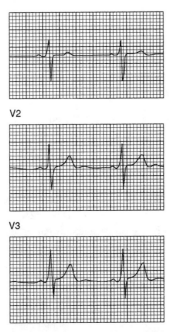

Reproduced, with permission, from Fauci A et al. *Harrison's Principles of Internal Medicine,* 17th ed. New York, NY: McGraw-Hill, 2008.

a. Prior myocardial infarction secondary to coronary artery disease
b. Congenital prolonged QT syndrome
c. Hypertrophic obstructive cardiomyopathy (HOCM)
d. Preexcitation syndrome (Wolff-Parkinson-White)
e. Rheumatic mitral stenosis

178. You are seeing a 45-year-old female patient of your partner for the first time in your clinic. A quick review of the patient's medical record shows that her systolic blood pressure was greater than 140 mm Hg at both of her last clinic appointments. Her medical history is otherwise significant only for diabetes mellitus. Her blood pressure today is 164/92. What is the best next step in her blood pressure management?

a. Ask the patient to keep a written record of her blood pressure and bring with her to a return appointment.
b. Advise the patient to begin a heart healthy, low sodium diet and refer to a nutritionist.
c. Prescribe an ACE inhibitor in addition to heart healthy diet.
d. Prescribe a dihydropyridine calcium-channel blocker in addition to a heart healthy diet.
e. Arrange for echocardiogram to assess for end-organ damage.

179. A 67-year-old male presents to your clinic to establish primary care; he is asymptomatic. He has a history of hypertension for which he takes hydrochlorothiazide. His father had a myocardial infarction at age 62. The patient smoked until 5 years ago, but has been abstinent from tobacco since then. His blood pressure in the office today is 132/78. Aside from being overweight, the remainder of the physical examination is unremarkable. Which of the following preventive health interventions would be most appropriately offered to him today?

a. Carotid ultrasound to evaluate for carotid artery stenosis
b. Abdominal ultrasound to evaluate for aortic aneurysm
c. Lipoprotein(a) assay to evaluate coronary heart disease risk
d. Exercise (treadmill) stress testing to evaluate for coronary artery disease
e. Homocysteine level to evaluate coronary heart disease risk

180. A 68-year-old male complains of pain in his calves while walking. He notes bilateral foot pain, which awakens him at night. His blood pressure is 117/68. Physical examination reveals diminished bilateral lower extremity pulses. An ankle:brachial index measures 0.6. The patient's current medications include aspirin and hydrochlorothiazide. Which of the following is the best initial management plan for this patient's complaint?

a. Smoking cessation therapy, warfarin
b. Smoking cessation therapy, graduated exercise regimen, cilostazol
c. Smoking cessation therapy, schedule an arteriogram
d. Smoking cessation therapy, warfarin, peripherally acting calcium-channel blocker
e. Smoking cessation therapy, consultation with a vascular surgeon

181. A 70-year-old male with a history of mild chronic kidney disease, diabetes mellitus, and CHF is admitted to your inpatient service with decreased urine output, weakness, and shortness of breath. He takes several medications but cannot remember their names. Labs are pending; his ECG is shown below. Based on the information available, what is the best initial step in management?

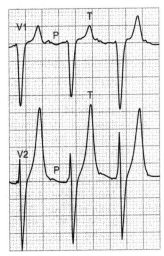

Reproduced, with permission, from Fauci A et al. *Harrison's Principles of Internal Medicine,* 17th ed. New York, NY: McGraw-Hill, 2008.

a. Administration of intravenous insulin
b. Administration of intravenous sodium bicarbonate
c. Administration of intravenous 3% hypertonic saline
d. Administration of oral sodium polystyrene sulfonate
e. Administration of intravenous calcium gluconate

182. You are called by a surgical colleague to evaluate a 54-year-old woman with ECG abnormalities one day after a subtotal thyroidectomy for a toxic multinodular goiter. Her only medication is fentanyl for postoperative pain control. The patient denies any history of syncope, and has no family history of sudden cardiac death. Physical examination is unremarkable except for a clean postoperative incision at the base of the neck. Her ECG is reproduced below. What is the best next step in evaluation and management of this patient?

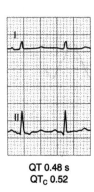

QT 0.48 s
QT$_C$ 0.52

Reproduced, with permission, from Fauci A et al. *Harrison's Principles of Internal Medicine,* 17th ed. New York, NY: McGraw-Hill, 2008.

a. Administration of intravenous magnesium sulfate
b. Measurement of serum ionized calcium
c. Stat noncontrast CT scan of the brain
d. Formal auditory testing
e. Reassure the patient that her ECG is normal for a woman her age

183. A 48-year-old male with a history of hypercholesterolemia presents to the ER after 1 hour of substernal chest pain, nausea, and sweating. His ECG is shown below. There is no history of hypertension, stroke, or any other serious illness. Which of the following is most appropriate at this time?

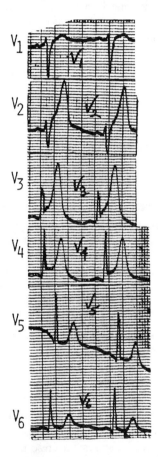

a. Aspirin, calcium-channel blocker, morphine, primary percutaneous coronary intervention
b. Aspirin, beta-blocker, morphine
c. Aspirin, beta-blocker, morphine, primary percutaneous coronary intervention
d. Aspirin, morphine, primary percutaneous coronary intervention
e. Aspirin, beta-blocker

Questions 184 to 186

You are working in the university student health clinic, seeing adolescents and young adults for urgent care problems, but you remain attuned to the possibility of more serious underlying disease. For each of the numbered cases below, select the associated valvular or related heart disease. Each lettered option may be used once, more than once, or not at all.

a. Tricuspid stenosis
b. Tricuspid regurgitation
c. Mitral stenosis
d. Mitral regurgitation
e. Aortic regurgitation (insufficiency)
f. Aortic stenosis
g. Hypertrophic cardiomyopathy
h. Pulmonic stenosis
i. Pulmonic regurgitation (insufficiency)

184. This tall, thin 19-year-old white female with little previous health care complains primarily of decreased vision. You note a strong pulse, blood pressure of 180/70, and a high-pitched, blowing, diastolic decrescendo murmur.

185. A 23-year-old graduate student complains of extreme fatigue and a vague sense of feeling ill the past few weeks. He has been under a lot of stress recently and is slightly agitated. On examination, BP is 110/70, pulse is 100, and temperature is 100.5°F (38.0°C). The neck veins are distended with prominent v waves. A holosystolic murmur is heard at the left sternal border; the murmur intensifies on inspiration.

186. An 18-year-old male is sent over from his physical education class owing to his symptoms of dizziness and palpitations after exercise. The instructor thinks he may be faking this to get out of future activities. Vital signs are within normal limits. A rapidly rising carotid pulse is noted. On auscultation an S_4 is heard along with a harsh systolic crescendo-decrescendo murmur, beginning well after S_1, best noted at the lower left sternal border.

Questions 187 to 189

While on call in the hospital, you become involved in the following emergent situations. For each case, choose the best next step in antiarrhythmic management. Each lettered option may be used once, more than once, or not at all.

a. Amiodarone
b. Atropine
c. Digoxin
d. Diltiazem
e. Isoproterenol
f. Lidocaine
g. Metoprolol
h. Quinidine
i. Observation

187. A 72-year-old male presents with a 2-hour history of chest pain, acute ST segment elevation in leads II, III, and a VF, and sinus bradycardia at a rate of 40. His blood pressure is 80/40 mm Hg.

188. A 58-year-old female smoker is admitted to the ICU with respiratory distress owing to pneumonia. Her course is complicated by an anterior myocardial infarction, with management including cautious use of beta-blockers. She now develops 10 to 12 PVCs per hour, occasional couplets, and a few short runs of ventricular tachycardia, although blood pressure and oxygen saturation remain stable.

189. A 60-year-old male during his first day post-myocardial infarction in the CCU develops an accelerated idioventricular rhythm, with rate of 80.

Cardiology

Answers

143. The answer is b. *(Fauci, pp1529-1531, Anderson et al, pp e12-19, e 45-61)* This patient presents with acute coronary syndrome, a change from the previous chronic stable state in that his chest pain has become more frequent and more severe. Antithrombotic therapy with intravenous heparin is indicated, along with additional antiplatelet therapy using clopidogrel. Subcutaneous administration of low-molecular-weight heparin (such as enoxaparin) is an alternative. There is no role for digoxin, as this may increase myocardial oxygen consumption and exacerbate the situation. Thrombolytic therapy is reserved for the treatment for ST-segment elevation myocardial infarction, and does not reduce cardiac events in the setting of unstable angina. The patient is at high risk for myocardial necrosis and should be admitted to the hospital for stabilization, but simple observation and failure to intensify his treatment would be inappropriate. A more aggressive approach is early interventional cardiac catheterization with angioplasty and/or stent placement, possibly in conjunction with glycoprotein IIb/IIIa inhibitors.

144. The answer is e. *(Fauci, pp1531-1532.)* This patient's presentation and minimal coronary artery disease are most consistent with Prinzmetal variant angina. Prinzmetal angina is caused by severe spasm of an epicardial coronary artery. The area of vasospasm is often near a nonhemodynamically significant atherosclerotic lesion. Patients tend to be smokers and are often younger than patients who present with atherosclerotic coronary artery disease. In this case, the patient's mild LAD stenosis does not explain the degree of ischemia evidenced by the ST segment elevation. Percutaneous intervention has not been shown to be useful in management of Prinzmetal angina, as the culprit is transient vasospasm rather than fixed obstruction. Calcium-channel blockers are the mainstay of therapy to prevent recurrence of spasm. ACE inhibitors and beta-blockers do not prevent acute vasospasm. Of course, the patient should also be counseled to abstain from smoking.

145. The answer is a. *(Fauci, pp 1484.)* This patient is at risk of sudden cardiac death. Although syncope associated with strenuous activity is not an uncommon event in adolescence, benign syncope typically occurs after the exercise has finished. Syncope during exercise should raise the specter of hypertrophic obstructive cardiomyopathy. This uncommon anatomic abnormality results in restricted flow through the left ventricular outflow tract. Physiologic changes that increase contractility (exercise), decrease preload (dehydration), or decrease afterload may increase the pressure gradient across the outflow tract. An ECG may reveal LV hypertrophy although the sensitivity of ECG for diagnosis of LVH is relatively poor. Echocardiogram will reveal symmetric or asymmetric hypertrophy of the ventricle, with the septum most commonly involved. If the patient's ECG and echocardiogram are normal, consideration could be given to pursuing an electrophysiological study. Until the results of the ECG and echocardiogram are available, the patient may not return to sports.

146. The answer is e. *(Fauci, pp1417-1419.)* The patient in question has symptomatic tachycardia-bradycardia syndrome. Sinus node automaticity is suppressed by the tachyarrhythmia and results in a prolonged sinus pause following termination of the tachycardia. The patient in this case is symptomatic, and pacemaker placement is warranted; reassurance would put the patient at risk of further syncopal episodes and bodily harm from fall or accident. Although a pacemaker will prevent bradycardia, it does not prevent tachycardia. The patient may need medication to prevent tachycardia if she continues to be symptomatic after pacemaker placement. It is unlikely that any positive findings on a stress test could be correlated with her ECG findings. The tachy-brady syndrome does increase the patient's risk of cardioembolic event, and anticoagulation should be considered. Aspirin, however, is not an appropriate agent to prevent cardioembolic disease.

147. The answer is c. *(Fauci, pp 1489-1493.)* The history and physical examination are consistent with post–cardiac injury syndrome (in the past also known as Dressler syndrome, or postmyocardial infarction syndrome). This benign, self-limited syndrome comprises an autoimmune pleuritis or pericarditis characterized by fever and pleuritic chest pain. Onset occurs days to 6 weeks after cardiac injury, especially with blood in the pericardial cavity, as after a cardiac operation, cardiac trauma, or ST elevation MI. The most effective therapy is a nonsteroidal anti-inflammatory drug or occasionally a glucocorticoid. Infection such as bacterial pneumonia, which would require antibiotics, would typically cause dyspnea, cough with sputum production, and rales on lung auscultation. Pulmonary embolism, which would require anticoagulation, would cause dyspnea and tachypnea, often in conjunction with physical findings of heat, swelling, and pain in the leg consistent with deep vein thrombosis. Angina or recurrent myocardial infarction is usually what the patient fears in this situation, but the nature of the pain—here pleuritic rather than pressure-like—and the unchanged ECG are reassuring and mitigate against an increase in antianginal therapy. Anxiety would not cause fever or pleuritic pain.

148. The answer is a. *(Fauci, pp1448-1453)* Angiotensin-converting enzyme inhibitors have been shown to prevent or retard the development of heart failure (HF) in patients with left ventricular dysfunction and to reduce long-term mortality when begun shortly after an MI. They play a central role in heart failure management. An angiotensin II receptor blocker may be substituted. Beta-blockers are typically the next addition, with evidence of fewer rehospitalizations for HF and future cardiac events. Loop or thiazide diuretics are administered to those with fluid accumulation. The aldosterone antagonist spironolactone is indicated in more advanced (NYHA III or IV) heart failure. Digoxin is reserved for those with symptomatic systolic dysfunction, especially with atrial flutter or fibrillation and rapid ventricular response. Nitrates relieve symptoms of angina but do not prolong survival or prevent hospitalization in patients with HF. General therapeutic measures include salt restriction and regular moderate exercise. Patient preferences are important to consider but should not keep you from giving your best medical recommendation, which the patient can then decide to accept or not.

149. The answer is b. *(Fauci, pp1482.)* Although peripartum (or postpartum) cardiomyopathy may occur during the last trimester of pregnancy or within 6 months of delivery, it most commonly develops in the month before or after delivery. The most common demographics are multiparity, African American race, and age greater than 30. About half of patients will recover completely, with most of the rest improving, although the mortality rate is 10% to 20%. These women should avoid future pregnancies due to the risk of recurrence. Treatment is as for other dilated cardiomyopathies, except that ACE inhibitors are contraindicated in pregnancy. Diagnosis can typically be made without invasive testing.

150. The answer is d. *(Fauci, pp1517-1519.)* Left ventricular hypertrophy and, in particular, preexisting ST-segment depression greater than 1 mm from any cause (such as bundle branch block, a paced rhythm, or WPW) preclude routine stress testing. New ST-segment depression is the most common stress test-induced evidence of myocardial ischemia and would be difficult to assess if the ST segment is already abnormal. Nuclear imaging would be indicated instead. Anxiety, mildly elevated blood pressure, or suspected angina do not preclude a stress test. Cardiac auscultation in this case suggests an innocent flow murmur. Pathologic murmurs, however, warrant caution. Aortic stenosis, in particular, would be a contraindication to stress testing. The murmur of aortic stenosis is classically harsh systolic crescendo-decrescendo murmur, usually heard best at the upper right sternal border with radiation to the carotids.

151. The answer is a. *(Fauci, pp1473-1474.)* The classic triad of symptoms in aortic stenosis are exertional dyspnea, angina pectoris, and syncope. Physical findings include a narrow pulse pressure and systolic murmur. The remaining answers describe aortic insufficiency murmur, mitral regurgitation murmur, mitral valve prolapse click, and a rub associated with pericarditis. These conditions are not associated with syncope as a presenting symptom.

152. The answer is a. *(Fauci, pp1448-1453.)* ACE inhibitors and beta-blockers are the basic regimen for patients with CHF and a depressed ejection fraction. The addition of spironolactone has been shown to be beneficial in management of CHF in patients with New York Heart Association Class III or IV heart failure and an ejection fraction less than 35%. NYHA Class III patients have marked limitation, with symptoms on less than usual activities. NYHA Class IV patients are dyspneic at rest. Although aspirin, warfarin, or amlodipine may be given for other indications, they are unlikely to improve his CHF symptoms. The combination of hydralazine and isosorbide dinitrate has been shown to be advantageous in African Americans who remain symptomatic on ACEIs and beta-blockers.

153. The answer is a. *(Fauci, pp1465-1467.)* The history and physical examination findings suggest mitral stenosis. Dyspnea may be present secondary to pulmonary edema; palpitations are often related to atrial arrhythmias (PACs, SVT, atrial flutter or fibrillation); hemoptysis may occur as a consequence of pulmonary hypertension with rupture of bronchial veins. A diastolic rumbling apical murmur is characteristic. If the patient is in sinus rhythm, a late diastolic accentuation of the murmur occurs because of increased flow across the mitral valve with atrial contraction. A loud first heart sound and early diastolic opening snap may also be present. The etiology of mitral stenosis is usually rheumatic, rarely congenital. Hypertension may cause an S_4 gallop but not a diastolic murmur. Myocardial infarction may cause mitral regurgitation because of papillary muscle dysfunction and anemia may cause a pulmonic flow murmur; both of these are systolic murmurs.

154. The answer is c. *(Fauci, pp1386-1387.)* A holosystolic murmur at the mid–left sternal border is most characteristic of ventricular septal defect. Both the murmur of ventricular septal defect and the murmur of mitral regurgitation are enhanced by exercise and diminished by amyl nitrite. Aortic stenosis causes systolic crescendo-decrescendo murmur heard best at the right upper sterna border. Atrial septal defect may give rise to a systolic murmur at the pulmonic region (pulmonic flow murmur) with a diastolic rumble along the left sternal border (mitral flow murmur). Aortic insufficiency causes a diastolic decrescendo murmur at the mid–left sternal border. A patent ductus arteriosus results in a continuous murmur best heard at the upper left sternal border.

155. The answer is e. *(Fauci, pp1469-1472.)* The patient has severe mitral regurgitation (MR) with resultant pulmonary edema. During systole, blood follows the course of least resistance. Cardiac output is determined by the amount of resistance to flow into the aorta (afterload) and the amount of resistance to flow across the malfunctioning mitral valve. As the resistance to retrograde flow across the leaky mitral valve decreases, a larger proportion of stroke volume flows into the left atrium rather than across the aortic valve. This patient's pulmonary edema is primarily caused by retrograde flow across the MV. To increase antegrade flow (thereby increasing cardiac output and decreasing pulmonary vascular congestion) we should reduce the left ventricular afterload. Lower resistance to flow through the LV outflow tract will increase the proportion of stroke volume that enters systemic circulation. Vasodilators such as ACE inhibitors and hydralazine are frequently used. Nitroprusside is another consideration. This patient will likely benefit from MV replacement, but his perioperative risk will be reduced if he can be stabilized first. An intra-aortic balloon pump will not help and may actually worsen the situation by increasing resistance to flow in the aorta. Beta-blockers do not have a major vasodilator effect and will not be useful in afterload reduction. A second loop diuretic is unlikely to be as beneficial as an intervention that improves the patient's hemodynamics.

156. The answer is e. *(Fauci, p 236.)* Minimally symptomatic PVCs in the absence of structural heart disease are benign and do not require treatment. Antiarrhythmic therapy in this setting has not been shown to reduce sudden cardiac death or overall mortality. A beta-blocker would be the best choice if symptoms begin to interfere with daily activities. Digoxin is not useful in this setting. Type 1 antiarrhythmics (such as quinidine) carry significant risks including an increased incidence of ventricular tachycardia.

157. The answer is e. (*Fauci, pp 1428-1430, 2521-2522.*) Aspirin or other antiplatelet therapy alone would be appropriate for a stroke patient without evidence of cardiogenic embolism. However, in patients with atrial fibrillation and a risk factor (including stroke or TIA, hypertension, LV dysfunction, coronary artery disease, rheumatic mitral valvular disease, prosthetic valve, diabetes, or thyrotoxicosis), the incidence of stroke averages 5% per year (up to 15% per year in those with multiple risk factors). Therapeutic anticoagulation with warfarin (Coumadin) reduces this risk more than antiplatelet agents. The target INR is generally 2.0 to 3.0. Target INR in patients with prosthetic valves is 2.5 to 3.5. In the long run, this patient might be a candidate for medical or electrical cardioversion. Prior to elective cardioversion, however, patients should be anticoagulated for 3 weeks unless fibrillation is clearly of recent (48 hour) onset. Alternatively, a transesophageal echocardiogram (TEE) could be performed to exclude the presence of left atrial thrombus, followed by cardioversion and then maintenance anticoagulation. An AICD/pacemaker would be useful in ventricular, not atrial, fibrillation.

158. The answer is a. (*Fauci, pp 1425, 1431.*) The rhythm strip reveals atrial flutter with 2:1 atrioventricular (AV) block. Management of atrial fibrillation or atrial flutter with rapid ventricular response is determined by the patient's hemodynamic stability. A hemodynamically unstable patient may require emergent cardioversion. In the stable patient, consideration should be given to initially controlling the ventricular response rate. This patient has a normal blood pressure and would probably respond to AV nodal blockade with metoprolol. Adenosine is also a nodal blockade agent, but its extremely short half-life limits its utility to diagnostic maneuvers. Amiodarone can be used to maintain NSR after cardioversion, but immediate management should focus on rate control. Chest compressions are inappropriate given the normal blood pressure.

159. The answer is c. (*Fauci, pp 1564-1565.*) Abdominal aortic aneurysms occur in 1% to 2% of men older than 50 years and to a lesser extent in women. Smoking and hypertension are major risk factors for the development of an AAA. Abdominal aneurysms are commonly asymptomatic, and acute rupture may occur without warning. Some will expand and become painful, with pain as a harbinger of rupture. The risk of rupture increases with the size of the aneurysm. The 5-year risk of rupture is 1% to 2% if the aneurysm is less than 5 cm, but 20% to 40% if the size is greater than 5 cm. Other studies indicate that, in patients with AAAs less than 5.5 cm, there is no difference in mortality rate between those followed with ultrasound and those who undergo elective aneurysmal repair. Therefore, operative repair is typically recommended in asymptomatic individuals when the AAA diameter is greater than 5.5 cm; other indications for surgery are rapid expansion or onset of symptoms. With careful preoperative evaluation and postoperative care, the surgical mortality rate should be less than 1% to 2%. Renal artery involvement increases the complexity of surgical repair but does not increase the risk of rupture. Endovascular stent grafts for infrarenal AAAs are successful in selected patients.

160. The answer is e. (*Fauci, pp 1420-1422.*) AV conduction block is classified as first, second, or third degree. First degree AV block is defined simply as a prolongation of the PR interval (greater than 0.2 seconds). Second degree AV block is divided into two types, also known as Mobitz types. Mobitz type 1 (usually termed Wenckebach phenomenon) is characterized by progressive PR interval prolongation prior to the nonconducted P wave and a "dropped" QRS complex. Mobitz type 2 refers to intermittent nonconducted P wave without prior PR prolongation. In Mobitz type 2, the ECG shows complexes of normal AV conduction with an intermittent "dropped" QRS complex. Third degree AV block refers to a complete dissociation between atrial conduction (the P wave) and ventricular conduction (the QRS complex). This ECG shows Wenckebach second-degree AV block (ie. progressive PR interval prolongation before the blocked atrial impulse). This rhythm generally does not require therapy. It may be seen in normal individuals; other causes include inferior MI and drug intoxications from digoxin, beta-blockers, or calcium-channel blockers. Even in the post-MI setting, Wenckebach second degree AV block is usually stable; it rarely progresses to higher-degree AV block with consequent need for pacemaker.

161. The answer is d. (*Fauci, pp 1436, 1708.*) The standard approach to ventricular fibrillation or hypotensive ventricular tachycardia involves defibrillation (with 200 J, then 300, then 360 if using a monophasic defibrillator; 200 J maximum if using a biphasic defibrillator), followed by epinephrine if needed. Therapy with lidocaine, amiodarone, or procainamide may be warranted if prior interventions fail. Magnesium sulfate may be given in torsades de pointes or when arrhythmia caused by hypomagnesemia is suspected.

162. The answer is d. *(Fauci, pp 1565-1566.)* This patient's presentation strongly suggests aortic dissection. Aortic insufficiency is common with proximal dissection, as is hypertension and evidence of CHF. Hypotension may be present in severe cases. Distal dissection can lead to obstruction of other major arteries with neurological symptoms (carotids), bowel ischemia, or renal compromise. In aortic dissection, the first line of defense is emergent therapy with parenteral beta-blockers. After beta-blockade is established, nitroprusside is commonly used to titrate systolic blood pressure to less than 120. The diagnosis is established with transesophageal echo, MR, or CT angiography. Urgent surgery may be required, especially in proximal (Type A) dissections.

Although endocarditis may cause aortic insufficiency, this patient's sudden onset of symptoms as well as widened mediastinum would be unusual in endocarditis. Myocardial ischemia can cause mitral (but not aortic) insufficiency. Furosemide might help the pulmonary edema but would not address the primary problem; digoxin increases shear force on the aortic wall and could worsen the dissection. Anticoagulation is contraindicated if aortic dissection is suspected, as it may increase the risk of fatal rupture and exsanguinating hemorrhage.

163. The answer is b. *(Fauci, pp 1561-1562.)* Malignant hypertension occurs when diastolic blood pressure above 130 is associated with acute (or ongoing) target organ damage. This patient shows evidence of damage, namely hypertensive encephalopathy (headache, visual disturbance, and altered mental status). Immediate therapy with nitroprusside in the ICU setting is indicated, although renal insufficiency would be a contraindication. Other options include intravenous nitroglycerin, fenoldopam, or enalapril. Intravenous labetalol is often used in hypertensive urgencies but, as a nonselective beta-blocker, is relatively contraindicated in asthma. An oral medication such as clonidine would be slow acting and difficult to administer in a lethargic patient. Sublingual nifedipine is no longer advised because of increased potential for overshoot hypotension with adverse cardiovascular events such as MI, stroke, or ischemic optic neuropathy. Loop diuretics do not lower blood pressure rapidly.

164. The answer is b. *(Fauci, pp 2092-2095.)* This 18-year-old presents with features of rheumatic fever. Rheumatic fever is diagnosed according to the Jones criteria. Evidence of recent streptococcal infection plus two major manifestations or one major and two minor manifestations satisfy the Jones criteria for diagnosis of acute rheumatic fever. Major criteria include carditis, polyarthritis, chorea, erythema marginatum, and subcutaneous nodules. Minor manifestations include fever, polyarthralgia, elevated erythrocyte sedimentation rate, and PR prolongation on ECG. This patient's clinical manifestations include arthritis, fever, and murmur (consistent with mitral regurgitation). The rash suggests erythema marginatum, and a subcutaneous nodule is noted. Rheumatic subcutaneous nodules are pea sized and usually overlie extensor tendons. The rash is usually pink with clear centers and serpiginous margins. Laboratory data include an elevated erythrocyte sedimentation rate. The ECG shows evidence of first-degree AV block. An antistreptolysin O antibody is necessary to document prior streptococcal infection. Endocarditis (for which blood cultures and an echocardiogram would be ordered) might cause fever, joint symptoms and the tender nodule but would not account for the diastolic murmur or the characteristic skin lesion. There is no evidence of lupus or myocardial infarction.

165. The answer is a. (*Fauci, p 1425.*) Adenosine, with its excellent safety profile and extremely short half-life, is the drug of choice for supraventricular tachycardia. The initial dose is 6 mg. A dose of 12 mg can be given a few minutes later if necessary. Verapamil is the next alternative; if the initial dose of 2.5 to 5 mg does not yield conversion, one or two additional boluses 10 minutes apart can be used. Diltiazem and digoxin may be useful in rate control and conversion, but have a slower onset of action. Electrical cardioversion is reserved for hemodynamically unstable patients. Lidocaine is useful in ventricular (not supraventricular) arrhythmias.

166. The answer is b. (*Fauci, pp 1420-1422.*) The ECG shows complete heart block. Although at first glance the P waves and QRS complexes may appear related, on closer inspection they are completely independent of each other (ie, dissociated). Complete heart block in the setting of acute myocardial infarction requires temporary (and often permanent) transvenous pacemaker placement. Atropine may be used as a temporizing measure. You would certainly want to avoid digoxin, beta-blockers, or any other medication that promotes bradycardia. There is no indication on this strip for cardioversion such as for atrial fibrillation/flutter or ventricular tachycardia/fibrillation. Lidocaine is contraindicated because it might suppress the ventricular pacemaker, leading to asystole.

167. The answer is d. *(Anderson et al, pp e16-29, e41-43)* The patient's history suggests acute coronary syndrome (ACS). The combination of elevated troponin and lack of ST segment elevation on ECG is most consistent with non-ST elevation myocardial infarction (NSTEMI). Initial therapy for acute coronary syndrome includes aspirin, nitroglycerin, anticoagulation, and morphine. A cardioselective beta-blocker, such as metoprolol, is frequently given in the immediate management of ACS to decrease myocardial oxygen demand, limit infarct size, reduce pain, and decrease the risk of ventricular arrhythmias. Elevated blood pressure also increases myocardial oxygen demand. Given this patient's increased blood pressure and continued pain, administration of a beta-blocker is the appropriate next step in his management. Administration of intravenous morphine would also be appropriate.

Cardiac catheterization may well be necessary at some point during his evaluation, but there is no mortality benefit for emergent catheterization in NSTEMI. There is no role for thrombolytic therapy in patients with ACS without ST segment elevation. All patients with ACS should be admitted to a monitored cardiac unit with serial cardiac biomarkers to estimate the extent of cardiac damage, but the patient's continued pain demands urgent treatment, not just further observation. Clopidogrel therapy is indicated for patients with ACS who will not be undergoing immediate coronary artery bypass grafting. Clopidogrel therapy, however, will not improve this patient's elevated blood pressure nor decrease myocardial oxygen demand. The correct dose of clopidogrel is a loading dose of 300 to 600 mg, then 75 mg po daily.

168. The answer is c. *(Fauci, pp 89-91, 1393-1394)* The ECG shows ST-segment elevation in inferior leads (II, III, and a VF) with reciprocal ST depression in aVL, diagnostic of an acute inferior MI. An anterior MI would produce ST-segment elevation in the precordial leads. Pericarditis classically produces pleuritic chest pain and diffuse ST segment elevation (except aVR) on ECG. Costochondritis and gastroesophageal reflux are confounding considerations raised by the history. Both can cause substernal chest pain, but not these ECG findings.

169. The answer is a. *(Fauci, p 1561)* The most common cause of refractory hypertension is nonadherence to the medication regimen. A history from the patient is useful, and pill count is the best compliance check. Although Cushing syndrome, coarctation of the aorta, renal artery stenosis, and primary aldosteronism are classic secondary causes of hypertension, there are no clues of these diagnoses on physical examination or laboratory tests. In addition to noncompliance, excessive salt ingestion, alcoholism, and occult sleep apnea are common explanations for persistent hypertension despite appropriate therapy.

170. The answer is c. (*Fauci, pp 1492-1493.*) The patient's pleuritic chest pain that is relieved by sitting up is classic for pericarditis. A pericardial friction rub may initially be present, then disappear, with the heart sounds becoming fainter as an effusion develops. Lung sounds are clear; rales or basilar dullness suggest an alternate diagnosis. An enlarged cardiac silhouette without other chest x-ray findings of heart failure suggests pericardial effusion.

Echocardiography is the most sensitive and specific way of determining whether pericardial fluid is present. The effusion appears as an echo-free space between the moving epicardium and stationary pericardium. Lateral decubitus chest film would show pleural, not pericardial, fluid. It is unnecessary to perform cardiac catheterization for the purpose of evaluating pericardial effusion. A stress test is helpful in coronary artery disease, but not pericarditis. ECG may show diffuse ST segment elevation or PR depression, but an echocardiogram is more sensitive in the diagnosis of pericardial effusion.

171. The answer is c. (*Fauci, pp 1489-1492.*) This patient has developed cardiac tamponade, a condition in which pericardial fluid under increased pressure impedes diastolic filling, resulting in reduced cardiac output and hypotension. Physical examination reveals elevation of jugular venous pressure. An important confirmatory clue to cardiac tamponade is pulsus paradoxus, a greater than normal (10 mm Hg) inspiratory decline in systolic arterial pressure. In contrast to pulmonary edema, the lungs are usually clear. Neither a strong apical beat nor an S_3 gallop would be expected in pericardial tamponade. Epigastric and right upper quadrant tenderness can be seen in either acute right-sided heart failure or in pericardial tamponade (due in both cases to passive congestion of the liver) but would be nonspecific. Immediate echocardiogram and pericardiocentesis may be lifesaving.

172. The answer is e. (*Fauci, pp 1391, 1453-1454.*) Cor pulmonale describes pulmonary hypertension leading to right ventricular enlargement and failure. Its causes include diseases leading to hypoxic vasoconstriction, as in cystic fibrosis; occlusion of the pulmonary vasculature, as in pulmonary thromboembolism; other pulmonary vascular problems, such as the collagen-vascular disease; parenchymal destruction as in sarcoidosis; and COPD. Primary pulmonary hypertension is diagnosed when no cause of right-sided heart failure can be found. With a chronic increase in afterload, the RV hypertrophies, dilates, and fails. The electrocardiographic findings include tall peaked P waves in leads II, III, and aVF (indicating right atrial enlargement), tall R waves in leads V_1 to V_3 and a deep S wave in V_6 with associated ST-T wave changes (indicating right ventricular hypertrophy) and right axis deviation. Right bundle branch block occurs in 15% of patients.

Inferior MI causes ST segment elevation and Q waves in the inferior limb leads (leads II, III, and aVF). Acute pericarditis leads to ST elevation in all limb leads (except for the maverick, aVR) and in the precordial leads, followed by T wave inversion in these leads. The Wolff-Parkinson-White syndrome is associated with a short PR interval (pre-excitation) and slurring in the initial forces of the QRS complex (the delta wave).

173. The answer is c. *(Fauci, p 1431)* The rhythm strip reveals atrial flutter with 4:1 atrioventricular (AV) block. Atrial flutter is characterized by an atrial rate of 250 to 350/minute; the electrocardiogram typically reveals a sawtooth baseline configuration characteristic of flutter waves. In this strip, every fourth atrial depolarization is conducted through the AV node, resulting in a ventricular rate of 75/minute (although 2:1 conduction is more commonly seen). The rapid atrial rate excludes sinus rhythm (where the atrial and ventricular rates are the same) and junctional rhythm. In PAT the atrial rate is around 150, and inverted P waves usually follow the QRS complexes because of retrograde atrial conduction from the impulse which starts in the AV node. Regular atrial depolarizations at a rate of 300/minute (as in this case) would exclude PAT.

174. The answer is a. *(Fauci, pp 1485-1486, 2430-2431.)* The patient's history of sickle cell disease should raise the suspicion of iatrogenic iron overload. Multiple transfusions in a patient whose anemia is not attributed to blood loss lead to tissue iron accumulation and end organ damage just like genetic hemochromatosis. Measures to assess body iron status (transferrin saturation, serum ferritin level) are the initial diagnostic studies. This patient's diabetic status may also be related to iron accumulation. Evidence of cardiomegaly (from physical examination and chest x-ray) together with a low voltage on ECG suggests an infiltrative process affecting the heart. Brain-natriuretic peptide (BNP) is released from the cardiac myocytes in response to ventricular stretch and can be a useful tool in determining whether someone is suffering from heart failure. BNP will not, however, help determine the cause of the heart failure. Holter monitoring and cardiac catheterization are not necessary in patients without evidence of intermittent arrhythmias or coronary ischemia respectively. CT of the chest is used to assess lung nodules or parenchymal abnormalities (such as interstitial lung disease) but would not be useful in this patient with clear lung fields on CXR.

175. The answer is d. (*Wilson et al, pp 1736-1754.*) Recommendations for prophylaxis of infective endocarditis (IE) from transient bacteremia associated with dental, gynecologic, or gastrointestinal procedures has recently undergone major revision. Only patients with history of prior infective endocarditis (IE), patients with prosthetic heart valves, patients with unrepaired congenital cyanotic heart disease, and patients with prosthetic graft material which has not yet endothelialized (typically 6 months from placement of the graft material) are given prophylactic antibiotics. Therefore, the patients with coarctation of the aorta, repaired VSD, mitral valve prolapse, and aortic stenosis do not require pretreatment. A typical adult prophylactic regimen is a single dose of amoxicillin 2 grams orally 30 to 60 minutes prior to the procedure. Any dental procedure that causes bleeding can cause transient bacteremia. Sterile procedures (ie, cardiac catheterization) and procedures with a very low risk of bacteremia (ie, endoscopy without biopsy) do not need preprocedure antibiotics.

176. The answer is e. (*Fauci, pp 1428-1430.*) Most patients with atrial fibrillation tolerate rate control without loss of exercise tolerance, increased morbidity, or increased mortality. "Rate control" means that the heart rate is slowed but the patient remains in atrial fibrillation. Cardioversion (either electrical or mechanical) is reserved for those with symptoms (troubling palpitations, exertional dyspnea) despite rate control alone. If cardioversion is required, the patient is usually treated with an antiarrhythmic agent (type 1 antiarrhythmic or amiodarone), with its own side effects. Many patients who undergo cardioversion are continued on warfarin because of the high risk (up to 70%) of going back in to atrial fibrillation despite antiarrhythmic drug treatment. Cardioversion therefore does not obviate the risks associated with long-term warfarin use. This patient's left atrial enlargement makes it unlikely that she would remain in sinus rhythm after cardioversion. Therefore, rate control with prolonged anticoagulation is appropriate. Indefinite anticoagulation with warfarin is necessary.

177. The answer is d. (*Fauci, pp 1393, 1426, 1434.*) The ECG reveals shortened PR interval and a delta wave causing widening of the QRS. The delta wave is a "slurring" of the upstroke of the R wave caused by the early depolarization of ventricular myocardium. This is consistent with an accessory conduction pathway or WPW. The aberrant conduction tissue bypasses the normal AV node (hence the PR interval of < 0.20 seconds); it leads the electrical impulse directly to the ventricle (bypassing the His-Purkinje fibers and widening the QRS complex). Q waves are not infrequent and can be mistaken for evidence of prior MI. Myocardial infarction, however, does not cause shortened PR interval or delta wave. This patient's QT interval is normal (less than 0.45 seconds). Patients with HOCM usually have voltage criteria for left ventricular hypertrophy and prominent ST/T wave changes but may also have large Q waves owing to hypertrophy of the septum. Rheumatic mitral stenosis would cause left atrial enlargement and perhaps atrial fibrillation, not the changes seen on this ECG.

178. The answer is c. (*Chobonian, pp 2560-2572.*) Hypertension is defined as elevated blood pressure on two or more separate readings. In a patient with stage 1 HTN and no other cardiac risk factors, consideration may be given to a therapeutic trial of diet and lifestyle modification. This patient, however, has diabetes mellitus. Both the American Diabetes Association and JNC-7 recommend a target blood pressure of 130/80 or lower in patients with diabetes. It is unlikely that the patient will be able to reach target blood pressure with diet and lifestyle modification alone, although these interventions will be important adjunct therapies. The JNC-7 recommends a thiazide diuretic as initial therapy for most patients with hypertension. Patients with diabetes and hypertension, however, benefit more from an ACE inhibitor, especially if they have signs of renal damage (elevated creatinine or proteinuria). There is no contraindication to the use of calcium-channel blockers, but their increased expense without increased benefit would prevent answer **d** from being correct. Evidence of end-organ damage, such as left ventricular hypertrophy on an echocardiogram, is unlikely to change your initial management.

179. The answer is b. (*US Preventive Services Task Force, pp 198-202.*) The US Preventive Services Task Force recommends that all males between the ages of 65 and 75 with any history of smoking undergo one-time screening for abdominal aortic aneurysm (AAA). There is no evidence that screening carotid ultrasonography (ie, in the patient without cerebrovascular symptoms or carotid bruits) or treadmill testing are beneficial to the patient. Although lipoprotein(a) and homocysteine levels have some predictive value in assessing CAD risk, their measurement is not recommended by the USPS Task Force.

180. The answer is b. (*Fauci, pp1568-1570.*) This patient has symptomatic peripheral arterial disease (PAD). Initial intervention should focus on lifestyle modification, most notably smoking cessation. Claudication can be improved by a graduated exercise regimen. Cilostazol, a phosphodiesterase inhibitor, improves exercise tolerance. In addition, patients with PAD usually have underlying coronary disease. Aggressive risk factor modification (especially lipid and blood pressure control) may decrease the risk of their chief cause of death, which is coronary artery disease. Calcium-channel blockers have not been shown to improve exercise tolerance, and there is no role for systemic anticoagulation in patients with PAD. Invasive interventions (angioplasty, surgery) are typically reserved for patients who have failed medical therapy or have critical ischemia. Arteriography would likely be needed before invasive intervention is attempted.

181. The answer is e. (*Fauci, pp 283-285, 1395-1396.*) The patient's ECG findings are most consistent with hyperkalemia. Additional ECG findings may include prolongation of the PR interval and QRS interval. Further electrical deterioration may lead to QRS widening and development of a sine wave. Ventricular fibrillation and asystole are potential terminal consequences. The patient's diabetes mellitus and kidney disease are predisposing factors; ACE inhibitors, beta-blockers, and spironolactone can increase the serum potassium.

Hyperkalemia less than 7.5 mEq/L usually does not result in fatal arrhythmias, but evidence of hyperkalemia on an ECG should prompt rapid intervention. Calcium gluconate is commonly administered to decrease membrane excitability. Its effects begin within 5 to 10 minutes and last up to 1 hour. There are no contraindications to calcium in this patient. Insulin causes K^+ to shift into the intracellular space and decreases serum potassium concentration. In euglycemic patients, a combination of insulin and glucose is typically administered concomitantly to decrease the risk of hypoglycemia. In hyperglycemic patients insulin alone should be given. In our patient, however, labs are still pending. It would be prudent to check a blood sugar before administering insulin. Sodium bicarbonate therapy also will shift K^+ into the cells. Patients with severe kidney disease or hypervolemic states, such as CHF, may not tolerate alkalinization or the associated sodium load. Ideally, the serum bicarbonate and creatinine should be checked before intravenous sodium bicarbonate is administered.

Each of the above therapies only shifts K^+ into the cells. Attention must then be given to removing excess K^+ from the body. Sodium polystyrene sulfonate (Kayexalate) is a cation exchange resin that binds K^+ in the GI tract and decreases serum K^+. The delayed onset of action of this drug prevents this from being the best initial intervention. Diuretic therapy (eg, furosemide) or hemodialysis can decrease total body K^+. Depending on the patient's kidney function and volume status, these may be considered, but they too take hours to work and should not take the place of immediate therapy. There is no role for hypertonic saline in the management of hyperkalemia.

182. The answer is b. (*Fauci, p 1381.*) The patient has a prolonged QT interval; her QTc is approximately 520 ms (normal 450 ms or less, although it may be slightly longer in women). As a general rule of thumb, a QT interval less than half of the RR interval should not raise alarm. Her recent thyroid surgery suggests hypocalcemia resulting from parathyroid damage. Besides hypocalcemia, toxins, hypothermia, and many medications may also lead to QT prolongation. Prolonged QT can cause torsades de pointes, a life-threatening ventricular arrhythmia. Magnesium may be used in the therapy of torsades, but this patient has not developed arrhythmia. Subarachnoid hemorrhage may lead to prolongation of the QT interval, and in the correct clinical setting a noncontrast CT scan of the head may be appropriate. This patient has no evidence of intracranial bleeding. There are several congenital QT prolongation syndromes, with Romano-Ward syndrome being most common. Romano-Ward is characterized by prolonged QT and congenital deafness, and there may be a family history of sudden cardiac death. Formal auditory testing would be unlikely to expose congenital deafness not discovered during routine patient interaction. Simple reassurance would not be appropriate, as potential hypocalcemia would remain undiagnosed.

183. The answer is c. (*Fauci, pp 1529-1531.*) The ECG shows acute ST-segment elevation in the anterior precordial leads. The symptoms have persisted for only 1 hour, so the patient is a candidate for primary percutaneous coronary intervention (angioplasty and/or stenting) or thrombolytic therapy, depending on the setting. Aspirin should be given. Nitroglycerin and morphine are indicated for pain control. Beta-blockers reduce pain, limit infarct size, and decrease ventricular arrhythmias. There is no role for calcium-channel blockers in this acute setting (in fact, short-acting dihydropyridines may increase mortality).

184 to 186. The answers are 184-e, 185-b, 186-g. (*Fauci, pp 1563-1564, 2468, 1386-1387, 1479, 1484-1485.*) The first patient displays the classic triad of Marfan syndrome: (1) long, thin extremities, possibly with arachnodactyly or other skeletal changes; (2) reduced vision as a result of lens dislocations;

and (3) aortic root dilatation or aneurysm. The diastolic murmur described is characteristic of aortic regurgitation (insufficiency), accompanied by the peripheral signs of water-hammer pulse and widened pulse pressure. Findings in the second patient suggest tricuspid regurgitation. Recall that inspiration increases right heart volume and therefore augments right-sided murmurs. The symptoms and low-grade fever raise the suspicion of infective endocarditis; the vegetations of IE usually cause regurgitant murmurs. Further history and physical signs of IV drug abuse should be sought. The final vignette suggests hypertrophic cardiomyopathy. The worst-case scenario is sudden cardiac death as the first manifestation of the disease, often occurring with or after physical exertion. Diagnosis is confirmed by echocardiography, which shows left ventricular hypertrophy with preferential hypertrophy of the interventricular septum. Both dynamic ventricular outflow tract obstruction and mitral regurgitation contribute to the harsh systolic crescendo-decrescendo murmur of HOCM. Management includes avoidance of strenuous exertion, good hydration, and beta-blockers. First-degree relatives should be screened with echocardiography.

187 to 189. The answers are 187-b, 188-a, 189-i. (*Fauci, pp 1416, 1435-1436.*) The first patient has sinus bradycardia, a common rhythm disturbance in acute inferior MI. It is usually caused by increased vagal tone and not by destruction of the SA node. When associated with hypotension, atropine should be given. Intravenous chronotropic agents are generally not required. In the second vignette, ventricular tachycardia in the context of cardiac ischemia warrants the use of amiodarone. More than 10 PVCs per minute in association with decreased LV function has been associated with increased mortality. Beta-blockers may also be of benefit, but this patient has already started beta-blocker therapy. Infrequent, sporadic PVCs do not require treatment. The last case illustrates that accelerated idioventricular rhythm ("slow V tach") with rate 60 to 100 develops in 25% of post-MI patients. This is a benign rhythm and rarely degenerates into ventricular tachycardia or other serious arrhythmia; so observation is the appropriate choice.

Endocrinology and Metabolic Disease

Questions

190. A 50-year-old obese female is taking oral hypoglycemic agents. While being treated for an upper respiratory infection, she develops lethargy and is brought to the emergency room. Neurological examination is nonfocal; she does not have neck rigidity. Laboratory results are as follows:

Na: 134 mEq/L
K: 4.0 mEq/L
HCO$_3$: 25 mEq/L
Glucose: 900 mg/dL
BUN: 84 mg/dL
Creatinine: 3.0 mg/dL
HgA1c: 6.8%
BP: 120/80 lying down, 105/65 sitting

Which of the following is the most likely cause of this patient's coma?

a. Diabetic ketoacidosis
b. Hyperosmolar coma
c. Inappropriate ADH
d. Noncompliance with medication
e. Bacterial meningitis

191. A 24-year-old white male presents with a persistent headache for the past few months. The headache has been gradually worsening and not responding to over-the-counter medicines. He reports trouble with his peripheral vision which he noticed while driving. He takes no medications. He denies illicit drug use but has smoked one pack of cigarettes per day since the age of 18. Past history is significant for an episode of kidney stones last year. He tells you no treatment was needed as he passed the stones, and he was told to increase his fluid intake.

Family history is positive for diabetes in his mother and a brother (age 20) who has had kidney stones from too much calcium and a "low sugar problem." His father died of some type of tumor at age 40. Physical examination reveals a deficit in temporal fields of vision and a few subcutaneous lipomas. Laboratory results are as follows:

Calcium: 11.8 mg/dL (normal 8.5-10.5)
Cr: 1.1 mg/dL
Bun: 17 mg/dL
Glucose: 70 mg/dL
Prolactin: 220 μg/L (normal 0-20)
Intact parathormone: 90 pg/mL (normal 8-51)

You suspect a pituitary tumor and order an MRI which reveals a 0.7 cm pituitary mass. Based on this patient's presentation, which of the following is the most probable diagnosis?

a. Tension headache
b. Multiple endocrine neoplasia Type 1 (MEN 1)
c. Primary hyperparathyroidism
d. Multiple endocrine neoplasia Type 2A (MEN 2A)
e. Prolactinoma

192. A 50-year-old female is 5 ft 7 in tall and weighs 185 lb. There is a family history of diabetes mellitus. Fasting blood glucose (FBG) is 160 mg/dL and 155 mg/dL on two occasions. HgA1c is 7.8%. You educate the patient on medical nutrition therapy. She returns for reevaluation in 8 weeks. She states she has followed diet and exercise recommendations but her FBG remains between 130 and 140 and HgA1C is 7.3%. She is asymptomatic, and physical examination shows no abnormalities. Which of the following is the treatment of choice?

a. Thiazolidinediones
b. Encourage compliance with medical nutrition therapy
c. Insulin
d. Metformin
e. Observation with repeat HgA1C in 6 weeks.

193. A 30-year-old female complains of palpitations, fatigue, and insomnia. On physical examination, her extremities are warm and she is tachycardic. There is diffuse thyroid gland enlargement and proptosis. There is thickening of the skin in the pretibial area. Mild clubbing of digits is present. Which of the following laboratory values would you expect in this patient?

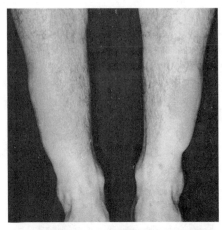

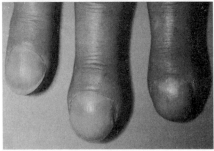

Modified with permission, from Fauci A et al. *Harrison's Principles of Internal Medicine*, 17th ed. New York, NY: McGraw-Hill, 2008.

a. Increased free thyroxine (free T₄), increased TSH
b. Increased free thyroxine, decreased TSH
c. Increased free thyroxine, normal TSH
d. Normal free thyroxine, elevated triiodothyronine (T₃), normal TSH
e. Normal free thyroxine, decreased TSH

194. A 65-year-old black female presents for an annual examination. Physical examination is unremarkable for her age. In completing the appropriate screening tests you order a dual x-ray absorptiometry (DXA) to evaluate whether the patient has osteoporosis. DXA results reveal a T-score of −3.0 at the total hip and −2.7 at the spine, consistent with a diagnosis of osteoporosis. Since her Z-score is −2.0, you proceed with an initial evaluation of secondary osteoporosis. Laboratory evaluation reveals:

Calcium: 9.7 mg/dL
Cr: 1.0 mg/dL
Bun: 19 mg/d
Glucose: 98 mg/dL
25,OH vitamin D: 12 ng/mL (optimal > 25)
WBC: 7700/μL
Hg: 12 g/dL
HCT: 38 g/dL
PLT: 255,000/μL

Based on the above information, additional laboratory would most likely reveal which of the following?

a. Elevated iPTH (intact parathormone), low ionized calcium, normal alkaline phosphatase
b. Normal iPTH, normal ionized calcium, elevated alkaline phosphatase
c. Elevated iPTH, normal ionized calcium, elevated alkaline phosphatase
d. Normal iPTH, low ionized calcium, elevated alkaline phosphatase
e. Elevated iPTH, low ionized calcium, normal alkaline phosphatase

195. You recently evaluated a 28-year-old woman who presented with complaints of shakiness and heat intolerance. The patient plans to have children and is currently using no contraception. On examination you noted tachycardia with an HR of 102, a fine tremor, a diffuse goiter, and proptosis. You now have the laboratory results and note a TSH < 0.001, elevated total T_4 of 17.8, and increased T_3 uptake. Radionuclide uptake by the thyroid gland is elevated. You tell her that she has Graves disease. What is the best treatment plan for this patient?

a. Propylthiouracil
b. Radioactive iodine
c. Propranolol
d. Thyroid surgery
e. Oral corticosteroids

196. A 50-year-old female is evaluated for hypertension. Her blood pressure is 130/98. She complains of polyuria and mild muscle weakness. She is on no blood pressure medication. On physical examination, the PMI is displaced to the sixth intercostal space. There is no sign of congestive heart failure and no edema. Laboratory values are as follows:

Na^+: 147 mEq/dL
K^+: 2.3 mEq/dL
Cl^-: 112 mEq/dL
HCO_3: 27 mEq/dL

The patient denies the use of diuretics or over-the-counter agents to decrease fluid retention or promote weight loss. She does not eat licorice. Which of the following tests is most useful in establishing a diagnosis?

a. 24-hour urine for cortisol
b. Urinary metanephrine
c. Plasma renin activity
d. Renal angiogram
e. Ratio of serum aldosterone to plasma renin activity

197. A 36-year-old female complains of inability to lose weight despite low-calorie diet and daily exercise. She has also noticed that she is cold intolerant. She is wearing a jacket even though it is summer. She also reports constipation and hair loss. These symptoms have been worsening over the past 2 to 3 months. An elevated TSH and low total and free T_4 confirm your suspicion of hypothyroidism. You suspect the etiology of this patient's hypothyroidism to be autoimmune thyroiditis. What is the best test to confirm the diagnosis of autoimmune thyroiditis?

a. Thyroid peroxidase antibody (TPOAb)
b. Antinuclear antibody
c. 24-hour radioactive iodine uptake
d. Thyroid ultrasound
e. Thyroid aspiration

198. A 58-year-old male is referred to your office after evaluation in the emergency room for abdominal pain. The patient was diagnosed with gastritis but a CT scan with contrast performed during the workup of his pain revealed a 2-cm adrenal mass. The patient has no history of malignancy and denies erectile dysfunction. Physical examination reveals a BP of 122/78 with no gynecomastia or evidence of Cushing syndrome. His serum potassium is normal. What is the next step in determining whether this patient's adrenal mass should be resected?

a. Plasma aldosterone/renin ratio.
b. Estradiol level.
c. Plasma metanephrines and dexamethasone-suppressed cortisol level.
d. Testosterone level.
e. Repeat CT scan in 6 months.

199. On routine physical examination, a 28-year-old woman is found to have a thyroid nodule. She denies pain, hoarseness, hemoptysis, or local symptoms. Serum TSH is normal. Which of the following is the best next step in evaluation?

a. Thyroid ultrasonography
b. Thyroid scan
c. Surgical resection
d. Fine needle aspiration of thyroid
e. No further evaluation

200. A 55-year-old type-2 diabetic patient has lost weight and has had good control of his blood glucose on oral metformin, with HgA1c of 6.4%. He has a history of mild hypertension and hyperlipidemia. Which of the following statements is correct regarding routine testing for diabetic patients?

a. Dilated eye examination twice yearly
b. 24-hour urine protein annually
c. Home fasting blood glucose measurement at least once per week
d. Urine microalbumin annually
e. Referral to neurologist for peripheral neuropathy evaluation

201. As part of a review of systems, a 55-year-old male describes an inability to achieve erection. The patient has mild diabetes and is on an ACE inhibitor for hypertension. Which of the following is the most appropriate first step in evaluation?

a. Penile Doppler ultrasound
b. Serum gonadotropin level
c. Information about libido and morning erections
d. Therapeutic trial of sildenafil
e. Nocturnal penile tumescence testing

202. A 90-year-old male complains of hip and back pain. He has also developed headaches, hearing loss, and tinnitus. On physical examination the skull appears enlarged, with prominent superficial veins. There is marked kyphosis, and the bones of the leg appear deformed. Serum alkaline phosphatase is elevated. Calcium and phosphorus levels are normal. Skull x-ray shows sharply demarcated lucencies in the frontal, parietal, and occipital bones. X-rays of the hip show thickening of the pelvic brim. Which of the following is the most likely diagnosis?

a. Multiple myeloma
b. Paget disease
c. Vitamin D intoxication
d. Metastatic bone disease
e. Osteitis fibrosa cystica

203. A 58-year-old postmenopausal female presents to your office on suggestion from a urologist. She has passed 3 kidney stones within the past 3 years. She is taking no medications. Her basic laboratory work shows the following:

Na: 139 mEq/L
K: 4.2 mEq/L
HCO_3: 25 mEq/L
Cl: 101 mEq/L
BUN: 19 mg/dL
Creatinine: 1.1 mg/dL
Ca: 11.2 mg/dL

A repeat calcium level is 11.4 mg/dL; PO_4 is 2.3 mmol/L (normal above 2.5). Which of the following tests will confirm the most likely diagnosis?

a. Serum ionized calcium
b. Thyroid function profile
c. Intact parathormone (iPTH) level
d. Liver function tests
e. 24-hour urine calcium

204. A patient comes to your office for a new-patient visit. He has moved recently to your city due to a job promotion. His last annual examination was 1 month prior to his move. He received a letter from his primary physician stating that laboratory workup had revealed an elevated alkaline phosphatase and that he needed to have this evaluated by a physician in his new location. On questioning, his only complaint is pain below the knee that has not improved with over-the-counter medications. The pain increases with standing. He denies trauma to the area. On examination you note slight warmth just below the knee, no deformity or effusion of the knee joint, and full ROM of the knee without pain. You order an x-ray, which shows cortical thickening of the superior fibula and sclerotic changes. Laboratory evaluation shows an elevated alkaline phosphatase of 297 mg/dL with an otherwise normal metabolic panel. Which of the following is the treatment of choice for this patient?

a. Observation
b. Nonsteroidal anti-inflammatory
c. A bisphosphonate
d. Melphalan and prednisone
e. Ursodeoxycholic acid (UDCA)

205. Your patient is a 48-year-old Hispanic male with a 4-year history of diabetes mellitus type 2. He is currently utilizing NPH insulin/Regular insulin 40/20 units prior to breakfast and 20/10 units prior to supper. His supper time has become variable due to a new job and ranges from 5 to 8 PM. In reviewing his glucose diary you note some very low readings (40-60 mg/dL) during the past few weeks at 3 AM. When he awakens to urinate, he feels sweaty or jittery so has been checking a fingerstick blood glucose. Morning glucose levels following these episodes are always higher (200-250) than his average fasting glucose level (120-150). Which change in his insulin regimen is most likely to resolve this patient's early AM hypoglycemic episodes?

a. Increase morning NPH and decrease evening NPH.
b. Decrease morning NPH and decrease evening regular insulin.
c. Change regimen to glargine at bedtime and continue morning and evening regular insulin.
d. Discontinue both NPH and regular insulin; implement sliding scale regular insulin with meals.
e. Change regimen to glargine at bedtime with lispro prior to each meal.

206. A 40-year-old alcoholic male is being treated for tuberculosis, but he has not been compliant with his medications. He complains of increasing weakness, fatigue, weight loss, and nausea over the preceding three weeks. He appears thin, and his blood pressure is 80/50 mm Hg. There is increased pigmentation over the elbows and in the palmar creases. Cardiac examination is normal. Which of the following is the best next step in evaluation?

a. CBC with iron and iron-binding capacity
b. Erythrocyte sedimentation rate
c. Early morning serum cortisol and cosyntropin stimulation
d. Blood cultures
e. Esophagogastroduodenoscopy (EGD)

207. A 53-year-old woman suffers from long-standing obesity complicated by DJD of the knees, making it difficult for her to exercise. Recently her fasting blood glucose values have been 148 mg/dL and 155 mg/dL; you tell her that she has developed type 2 diabetes. She wonders if diet will allow her to avoid medications. In addition, her daughter also suffers from obesity and has impaired fasting glucose, and the patient wonders about the management of her prediabetes. Which of the following is a correct statement based on the American Diabetes Association 2008 guidelines regarding *nutrition recommendations and interventions for diabetes?*

a. Low-carbohydrate diets such as "South Beach" and "Atkins" should be avoided.
b. Outcomes studies show that medical nutrition therapy (MNT) can produce a 1 to 2 point decrease in hemoglobin A1c in type 2 diabetics.
c. Prediabetic patients should be instructed to lose weight and exercise but a referral to a medical nutritionist is not necessary until full-blown diabetes is diagnosed.
d. Very low-calorie diets (< 800 cal/day) produce weight loss that is usually maintained after the diabetic patient returns to a self-selected diet.
e. Bariatric surgery may be considered for patients with type 2 diabetes and a BMI of > 30 kg/m^2.

208. A 45-year-old G2P2 female presents for annual examination. She reports regular menstrual cycles lasting 3 to 5 days. She exercises 5 times per week and reports no difficulty sleeping. Her weight is stable 140 lbs and she is 5 ft 8 in tall. Physical examination is unremarkable. Laboratory studies are normal with the exception of a TSH value of 6.6 mU/L (normal 0.4-4.0 mU/L). Which of the following represents the best option for management of this patient's elevated TSH?

a. Repeat TSH in 3 months and reassess for signs of hypothyroidism.
b. Begin low dose levothyroxine (25-50 μg/d).
c. Recommend dietary iodide supplementation.
d. Order thyroid uptake scan.
e. Measure thyroid peroxidase antibodies (TPOAb).

209. A family brings their 82-year-old grandmother to the emergency room stating that they cannot care for her anymore. They tell you, "She has just been getting sicker and sicker." Now she stays in bed and won't eat because of stomach pain. She has diarrhea most of the time and can barely make it to the bathroom because of her weakness. Her symptoms have been worsening over the past year, but she has refused to see a doctor. The patient denies symptoms of depression. Blood pressure is 90/54 with the patient supine; it drops to 76/40 when she stands. Heart and lungs are normal. Skin examination reveals a bronze coloring to the elbows and palmar creases. What laboratory abnormality would you expect to find in this patient?

a. Low serum Ca^+
b. Low serum K^+
c. Low serum Na^+
d. Normal serum K^+
e. Microcytic anemia

210. A 60-year-old woman comes to the emergency room in a coma. The patient's temperature is 32.2°C (90°F). She is bradycardic. Her thyroid gland is enlarged. There is diffuse hyporeflexia. BP is 100/60. Which of the following is the best next step in management?

a. Await results of T_4 and TSH.
b. Obtain T_4 and TSH; begin intravenous thyroid hormone and glucocorticoid.
c. Begin rapid rewarming.
d. Obtain CT scan of the head.
e. Begin intravenous fluid resuscitation.

211. A 19-year-old man with insulin-dependent diabetes mellitus is taking 30 units of NPH insulin each morning and 15 units at night. Because of persistent morning glycosuria with some ketonuria, the evening dose is increased to 20 units. This worsens the morning glycosuria, and now moderate ketones are noted in urine. The patient complains of sweats and headaches at night. Which of the following is the most appropriate next step in management?

a. Measure blood glucose levels at bedtime.
b. Increase the evening dose of NPH insulin further.
c. Add regular insulin to NPH at a ratio of 2/3 NPH to 1/3 regular.
d. Obtain blood sugar levels between 2:00 and 5:00 AM
e. Add lispro via a calculated scale to each meal; continue NPH.

212. A 25-year-old woman is admitted for hypertensive crisis. The patient's urine drug screen is negative. In the hospital, blood pressure is labile and responds poorly to antihypertensive therapy. The patient complains of palpitations and apprehension. Her past medical history shows that she developed hypertension during an operation for appendicitis at age 23.

Hct: 49% (37-48)
WBC: 11×10^3 mm (4.3-10.8)
Plasma glucose: 160 mg/dL (75-115)
Plasma calcium: 11 mg/dL (9-10.5)

Which of the following is the most likely diagnosis?

a. Anxiety attack
b. Renal artery stenosis
c. Essential hypertension
d. Type 1 diabetes mellitus
e. Pheochromocytoma

213. The young man pictured below on the left complains of persistent headache. He has noticed gradual increase in his ring size and his shoe size over the years. He has a peculiar deep, hollow-sounding voice. Which of the following is his most likely visual field defect?

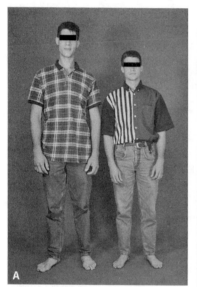
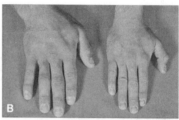
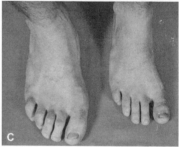

Reproduced, with permission, from Fauci A et al. *Harrison's Principles of Internal Medicine,* 17th ed. New York, NY: McGraw-Hill, 2008.

a. Bitemporal hemianopsia
b. Unilateral blindness
c. Left homonymous hemianopsia
d. Right homonymous hemianopsia
e. Diplopia

214. A patient with small cell carcinoma of the lung develops increasing fatigue but is otherwise alert and oriented. Serum electrolytes show a serum sodium of 118 mg/L. There is no evidence of edema, orthostatic hypotension, or dehydration. Urine is concentrated with an osmolality of 550 mmol/L. Serum BUN, creatinine, and glucose are within normal range. Which of the following is the next appropriate step?

a. Normal saline infusion
b. Diuresis
c. Fluid restriction
d. Demeclocycline
e. Hypertonic saline infusion

215. The 40-year-old woman shown below complains of weakness, amenorrhea, and easy bruisability. She has hypertension and diabetes mellitus. She denies use of any medications other than hydrochlorothiazide and metformin. What is the most likely explanation for her clinical findings?

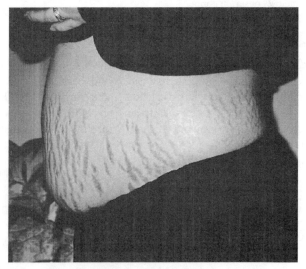

Reproduced, with permission, from Fauci A et al. *Harrison's Principles of Internal Medicine,* 17th ed. New York, NY: McGraw-Hill, 2008.

a. Pituitary tumor
b. Adrenal tumor
c. Ectopic ACTH production
d. Hypothalamic tumor
e. Partner abuse (domestic violence)

216. A 24-year-old male presents with gynecomastia and infertility. On examination, he has small, firm testes and eunuchoid features. He has scant axillary and pubic hair. Which of the following is correct?

a. The patient has Turner syndrome.
b. The patient will have a normal testosterone level.
c. His most likely karyotype is 47 XXY.
d. The patient will have normal sperm count.
e. The patient is likely to have low levels of gonadotropins.

217. A 52-year-old man complains of impotence. On physical examination, he has an elevated jugular venous pressure, S$_3$ gallop, and hepatomegaly. He also appears tanned, with pigmentation along joint folds. His left knee is swollen and tender. The plasma glucose is 250 mg/dL, and liver enzymes are elevated. Which of the following studies will help establish the diagnosis?

a. Detection of nocturnal penile tumescence
b. Determination of iron saturation
c. Determination of serum copper
d. Detection of hepatitis B surface antigen
e. Echocardiography

218. A 30-year-old man is evaluated for a thyroid nodule. The patient reports that his father died from thyroid cancer and that a brother had a history of recurrent renal stones. Blood calcitonin concentration is 2000 pg/mL (normal is less than 100); serum calcium and phosphate levels are normal. The patient is referred to a thyroid surgeon. Which of the following studies should also be obtained?

a. Obtain a liver scan.
b. Measure parathormone level.
c. Measure urinary catecholamines.
d. Administer suppressive doses of thyroxine and measure levels of thyroid-stimulating hormone.
e. Treat the patient with radioactive iodine.

219. A 32-year-old woman has a 3-year history of oligomenorrhea that has progressed to amenorrhea during the past year. She has observed loss of breast fullness, reduced hip measurements, acne, increased body hair, and deepening of her voice. Physical examination reveals frontal balding, clitoral hypertrophy, and a male escutcheon. Urinary free cortisol and dehydroepiandrosterone sulfate (DHEAS) are normal. Her plasma testosterone level is 6 ng/mL (normal is 0.2 to 0.8). Which of the following is the most likely diagnosis?

a. Cushing syndrome
b. Arrhenoblastoma
c. Polycystic ovary syndrome
d. Granulosa-theca cell tumor
e. Ovarian teratoma

220. A 54-year-old man who has had a Billroth II procedure for peptic ulcer disease now presents with abdominal pain and is found to have recurrent ulcer disease. The physician is considering this patient's illness to be secondary either to retained antrum or to gastrinoma. Which of the following tests would best differentiate the two conditions?

a. Random gastrin level
b. Determination of 24-hour acid production
c. Serum calcium level
d. Secretin infusion
e. Insulin-induced hypoglycemia

221. A 55-year-old woman with a history of severe depression and radical mastectomy for carcinoma of the breast 1 year previously develops polyuria, nocturia, and excessive thirst. Laboratory values are as follows:

Serum electrolytes: Na$^+$ 149 mEq/L; K$^+$ 3.6 mEq/L
Serum calcium: 9.5 mg/dL
Blood glucose: 110 mg/dL
Blood urea nitrogen: 30 mg/dL
Urine osmolality: 150 mOsm/kg

Which of the following is the most likely diagnosis?

a. Psychogenic polydipsia
b. Renal glycosuria
c. Hypercalciuria
d. Diabetes insipidus
e. Inappropriate antidiuretic hormone syndrome

222. A 30-year-old nursing student presents with confusion, sweating, hunger, and fatigue. Blood sugar is 40 mg/dL. The patient has no history of diabetes mellitus, although her sister is an insulin-dependent diabetic. The patient has had several similar episodes over the past year, all occurring just prior to reporting for work in the early morning. At the time of hypoglycemia, the patient is found to have a high insulin level and a low C peptide level. Which of the following is the most likely diagnosis?

a. Reactive hypoglycemia
b. Pheochromocytoma
c. Factitious hypoglycemia
d. Insulinoma
e. Sulfonylurea use

223. A 50-year-old female presents with complaints of more than 10 severe hot flashes per day. Her last menstrual period was 13 months ago. She denies fatigue, constipation, or weight gain. Current medical issues include osteopenia diagnosed by central DXA. Family history is positive for hypertension in her father and osteoporosis in her mother. The patient uses no medications other than calcium and vitamin D supplements.

Physical examination reveals weight 145 lbs, height 5ft 6 in, BMI 24, BP 126/64, HR 68. Otherwise the examination is normal.
Screening laboratory studies:
Fasting glucose: 98
Cholesterol: 200 mg/dL
LDL: 100 mg/dL
Triglycerides: 150 mg/dL
HDL: 50 mg/dL
TSH: 1.0 mU/L

The patient requests hormone therapy to decrease hot flashes. Which of the following statements is true regarding hormone replacement therapy?

a. Progesterone therapy alone can alleviate hot flashes.
b. Hormone therapy does not affect bone density.
c. Her symptoms do not warrant systemic HT.
d. Oral estrogen therapy does not affect lipid levels.
e. The risk of breast cancer is directly related to duration of estrogen use.

Questions 224 to 226

Select the most likely disease process for the clinical syndromes described. Each lettered option may be used once, more than once, or not at all.

a. Acromegaly
b. Essential hypertension
c. Empty sella syndrome
d. Cushing disease
e. TSH-secreting adenoma
f. Diabetes insipidus
g. Chronic oral glucocorticoid use
h. Prolactin-secreting adenoma

224. A 30-year-old woman has prominent cervical and dorsal fat pads, purple abdominal striae, unexplained hypokalemia, and diabetes mellitus.

225. A nonpregnant woman has headaches, bitemporal hemianopsia, irregular menses, and galactorrhea.

226. An obese hypertensive woman has chronic headaches, normal visual fields, and normal pituitary function.

Questions 227 to 229

Match each symptom or sign with the appropriate disease. Each lettered option may be used once, more than once, or not at all.

a. Subacute thyroiditis
b. Graves disease
c. Factitious hyperthyroidism
d. Struma ovarii
e. Multinodular goiter
f. Thyroid nodule
g. Iodide deficiency
h. TSH-secreting pituitary adenoma

227. 20-year-old female presents with tachycardia, tremor, and heat intolerance. On physical examination, no thyromegaly is noted, but she does have RLQ fullness on pelvic examination. TSH is < 0.01, and radionuclide scan reveals low uptake in the thyroid gland.

228. A male nursing assistant presents with weakness and tremor. Examination shows no ophthalmopathy or pretibial myxedema. No thyroid tissue is palpable. T_4 is elevated; radioactive iodine uptake is reduced.

229. A 20-year-old presents after recent upper respiratory infection. She complains of neck pain and heat intolerance. The thyroid is tender. Erythrocyte sedimentation rate is elevated; free thyroxine value is modestly elevated.

Endocrinology and Metabolic Disease

Answers

190. The answer is b. *(Fauci, p 2285.)* This obese patient on oral hypoglycemics has developed hyperglycemia and lethargy during an upper respiratory infection. Hyperosmolar nonketotic states typically occur in type 2 diabetes and can be fatal. When hyperglycemia and dehydration cause severe hypertonicity, lethargy or coma occurs. Serum osmolarity is calculated by the formula:

$$\frac{\text{Plasma glucose}}{18} + 2(\text{Na}^+ + \text{K}^+) + \frac{\text{blood urea nitrogen}}{2.8}$$

This patient's serum osmolality is as follows:

$$\frac{900}{18} + 2(134 + 4) + \frac{84}{2.8} = 50 + 276 + 30 = 356$$

Thus the serum osmolarity is greater than 350 mOsm/L. Although the serum sodium is usually the main determinant of osmolarity, extreme hyperglycemia contributes significantly to this patient's hypertonicity. Osmotically active particles in the extracellular fluid space pull water out of the intracellular space. This causes cellular dehydration in the brain and consequently the patient's CNS changes. The serum bicarbonate is too high to be consistent with diabetic ketoacidosis. The hyponatremia is minimal and is related to hyperglycemia. SIADH could not be diagnosed in this clinical setting. Patients with SIADH have an inappropriate production of ADH, leading to water retention and consequent hypotonicity. The patient's diabetes likely went out of control owing to infection.. There is no evidence of noncompliance since the patient's most recent HgA1C is 6.8% (goal < 6.5-7.0%). There is no clinical evidence for meningitis.

191. The answer is b. *(Fauci, p. 2357-2361.)* This young man presents with two obvious serum abnormalities—hypercalcemia and hyperprolactinemia most likely secondary to the pituitary tumor. This, along with his positive family history of a younger sibling with high calcium and low blood sugar and a father who died from an unknown tumor, indicates this family has one of the multiple endocrine neoplasia syndromes. MEN I is associated with parathyroid hyperplasia/adenoma, islet cell hyperplasia/adenoma/carcinoma, pituitary hyperplasia/adenoma, pheochromocytoma, carcinoid and subcutaneous lipomas. Although MEN 2A is associated with parathyroid hyperplasia/adenoma, there is no pituitary abnormality with the MEN 2 syndromes (either MEN 2A or MEN 2B). It would not be prudent to treat the patient's issues as two separate abnormalities (primary hyperparathyroidism and prolactinoma). Tension headache is unlikely in the face of a pituitary tumor and visual field deficit.

192. The answer is d. (*Fauci, pp 2301-2302.*) The classification of diabetes mellitus has changed to emphasize the process that leads to hyperglycemia.

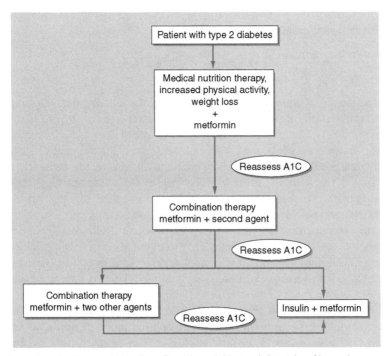

Reproduced, with permission, from Fauci A et al. *Harrison's Principles of Internal Medicine,* 17th ed. New York, NY: McGraw-Hill, 2008.

Type 2 DM is a group of heterogeneous disorders characterized by insulin resistance, impaired secretion of insulin, and increased glucose production. In this type 2 patient, the first intervention, medical nutrition therapy, failed to achieve the goal HgA1c of < 7.0%. *Medical nutrition therapy* (MNT) is a term now used to describe the best possible coordination of calorie intake, weight loss, and exercise. It emphasizes modification of risk factors for hypertension and hyperlipidemia, not just weight loss and calorie restriction. Blood glucose control should be evaluated after 4 to 6 weeks and additional therapy should be added; therefore, continued observation is not the best option. Metformin is considered first-line therapy in that it promotes mild weight loss, has known efficacy and side effect profile, and is available as a generic with very low cost. Thiazolidinediones ("glitazones"), sulfonylureas, and insulin are considered second line or add-on therapy for most patients with type 2 DM.

193. The answer is b. *(Fauci, pp 2233-2235.)* This patient has clinical symptoms consistent with thyrotoxicosis, and her examination is consistent with Graves disease. Most patients with thyrotoxicosis have increases in total and free concentrations of T_3 and T_4 (some may have isolated T_3 elevation). Thyrotoxicosis results in suppression of pituitary TSH secretion, so low TSH levels can confirm the diagnosis. Normal TSH with elevated T_4 usually indicates thyroid hormone resistance syndrome (or very rarely a TSH secreting pituitary tumor). Elevated free T_4 with an elevated TSH would indicate a TSH producing pituitary tumor, which might cause a diffuse goiter but would not cause proptosis or pretibial myxedema (characteristics of Graves disease).

194. The answer is c. *(Fauci, pp 2375-2376.)* This patient has vitamin D deficiency, a common cause of secondary osteoporosis, as diagnosed by the suboptimal serum 25,OH vitamin D level. Vitamin D deficiency at less than 15 ng/mL can lead to low bone density. Vitamin D deficiency leads to impaired intestinal absorption of calcium and lower serum calcium levels. The low serum calcium causes elevated iPTH. In order to maintain serum calcium homeostasis, calcium is sacrificed from the skeleton leading to low bone density. With increasing bone turnover alkaline phosphatase levels can be increased. With significant vitamin D deficiency the following pattern is characteristic: elevated iPTH, normal ionized calcium, and elevated alkaline phosphatase. The patient with uncomplicated postmenopausal osteoporosis (ie, primary osteoporosis) has normal iPTH, ionized calcium, and alkaline phosphatase levels.

195. The answer is a. *(Fauci, p 2236.)* Antithyroid drugs are the treatment of choice in a patient with Graves disease who may become pregnant. Iodine 131 has been used successfully in Graves disease and is a reasonable option if the patient is willing to practice secure contraception for at least 6 months.. However, it often causes permanent hypothyroidism and may worsen ophthalmopathy in some patients. The treatment of choice is the oral agent propylthiouracil. Propylthiouracil is chosen in cases such as this owing to low transplacental transfer. Methimazole is preferred in men and non–childbearing women because it can be given once daily. Propranolol relieves the adrenergic symptoms resulting from Graves disease but will not treat the underlying disease. Subtotal thyroidectomy is reserved for thyrotoxic pregnant women who have had severe side effects to medication. Surgical complications include hypoparathyroidism and recurrent laryngeal nerve injury. Corticosteroids are used in thyroid storm but not in the stable patient with Graves disease.

196. The answer is e. (*Fauci, p 2260.*) The patient has diastolic hypertension with unprovoked hypokalemia. She is not taking diuretics. There is no edema on physical examination. Inappropriate aldosterone overproduction is a prime consideration in hypertension with hypokalemia. Hypersecretion of aldosterone increases distal tubular exchange of sodium for potassium with progressive depletion of body potassium. The hypertension is caused by increased sodium absorption. Interestingly, peripheral edema does not occur despite the sodium retention.

Elevated aldosterone level and low plasma renin activity suggest the diagnosis of primary hyperaldosteronism. The plasma aldosterone to renin ratio is a useful screening test. A high ratio of > 30 strongly suggests aldosterone oversecretion. Lack of suppression of aldosterone (ie, autonomous overproduction), however, is necessary to definitively diagnose primary hyperaldosteronism. High aldosterone levels that are not suppressed by a 2 L saline load prove the diagnosis. CT scan of the adrenal glands is then ordered to distinguish an aldosterone producing tumor from bilateral adrenal hyperplasia. Renin levels alone lack specificity. Suppressed renin activity occurs in about 25% of hypertensive patients with essential hypertension. Twenty-four-hour urine for free cortisol would be used in the workup of a patient with Cushing syndrome. Urinary metanephrine is a screening test for pheochromocytoma. Renal angiography is a test for renal artery stenosis.

197. The answer is a. (*Fauci, pp 2230-2232.*) Once hypothyroidism is diagnosed (clinical features, a low free T_4 and elevated TSH), the etiology can be confirmed by measuring the presence of autoantibody—particularly thyroid peroxidase (TPOAb), which is present in 90% to 95% of patients with autoimmune hypothyroidism. Ultrasound can be used to decide if a thyroid nodule is solid or cystic but will not help determine the pathogenesis of hypothyroidism. The thyroid uptake scan is useful in the diagnosis of hyperthyroidism, not in hypothyroidism.. Antinuclear antibodies are normal in immune-mediated endocrine disorders. Biopsy by fine needle aspirate is used to evaluate thyroid nodules, not autoimmume thyroiditis.

198. The answer is c. *(Fauci, pp 2257-2259.)* This patient has what is commonly referred to as an adrenal incidentaloma. If the mass is > 1 cm the first step is to determine whether it is a functioning or nonfunctioning tumor via measurement of serum metanephrines (pheochromocytoma) and dexamethasone suppressed cortisol (Cushing syndrome) levels. As the patient has no history of malignancy, a CT-guided fine-needle aspiration is not required. The patient has normal BP and potassium; therefore, plasma aldosterone/plasma renin level to evaluate primary hyperaldosteronism is not required. There are no signs of feminization or erectile dysfunction, so sex-steroid measurement is not indicated. Unenhanced CT would be required after appropriate serum workup to determine true size and characteristics (Hounsfield units). Malignant indicators include large size (>4-6 cm), irregular margins, soft tissue calcifications, tumor inhomogeneity, or high unenhanced CT attenuation values > 10 HU. CT scans should be performed in 6 months and again in 1 year to ensure stability of the adrenal mass, but only after a functioning tumor has been excluded.

199. The answer is d. *(Fauci, p 2247.)* Palpable thyroid nodules are common, occurring in about 5% of all adults. Thyroid fine needle biopsy now plays a central role in the differential diagnosis of thyroid nodules. If the TSH is normal, as it is in this patient, then fine needle aspirate biopsy is indicated and will distinguish cysts from benign lesions or neoplasms. In about 14% of such cases, biopsy will be suspicious or diagnostic for malignancy and surgery will be necessary. Thyroid scan can show a "hot" nodule, which is almost always benign, but the TSH is suppressed in most autonomously overactive nodules. Thyroid sonography by itself cannot rule out malignancy in palpable nodules. Thyroid cancer can present even in a young, asymptomatic patient like this; so option e would not be appropriate.

200. The answer is d. *(Fauci, p 2302.)* Guidelines for ongoing medical care in diabetic patients recommend that the following screenings or interventions be performed annually: dilated eye examination, lipid profile, and medical nutrition therapy and education. Annual screening for diabetic nephropathy begins with dipstick assessment of urine protein and, if negative, testing of a single voided specimen for albumin/creatinine ratio. Twenty-four-hour urine testing is not recommended. A foot examination should be performed yearly by the physician and daily by the patient. Peripheral neuropathy is first suggested by distal loss of sensation on clinical exam. HgA1c testing should be performed 2 to 4 times a year depending on patient's diabetes control (if patient HgA1c at goal, twice yearly is adequate). Blood pressure should be measured quarterly. Home glucose measurements are usually performed once daily in well-controlled type 2 diabetics.

201. The answer is c. (*Fauci, pp 297-298.*) The first step in the evaluation of erectile dysfunction is a complete and detailed history, including onset, libido, interpersonal relationship issues, and ability to attain spontaneous erection unrelated to sexual intercourse. Most men will obtain erection during REM sleep and will wake with at least a partial if not full erection. Loss of all erectile function including spontaneous morning erections suggests vascular, neuropathic, or other organic cause for the disease. Erectile dysfunction will often occur in the wake of an extramarital relationship; therefore, evaluation of interpersonal relationship issues is crucial. Diabetes may cause impotence because of its effect on penile blood supply or parasympathetic nervous system function. Serum testosterone and prolactin should be measured after psychogenic ED is ruled out. If testosterone level is low, serum gonadotropins should be measured. Specialized imaging/testing (eg, penile Doppler, nocturnal penile tumescence testing) can be performed at the discretion of the clinician, but cost and invasiveness limit its use. Physicians should not institute sildenafil or other phosphodiesterase inhibitors without considering the potential etiology of the impotence, as important diseases (pituitary tumor, peripheral arterial disease, diabetes) can be missed.

202. The answer is b. (*Fauci, p 1764, pp 2409-2410.*) This patient has widespread Paget disease of bone. Excessive resorption of bone is followed by replacement with dense, trabecular, disorganized bone. Hearing loss and tinnitus result from direct involvement of the ossicles of the inner ear. Neither myeloma, metastatic bone disease, nor osteitis fibrosa cystica would result in bony changes such as skull enlargement or long bone deformity. Serum alkaline phosphatase levels indicate increased bone turnover and are always elevated in Paget disease. The alkaline phosphatase level is normal in purely tic processes such as multiple myeloma. Hypervitaminosis D causes hypercalcemia owing to excess intestinal absorption of calcium and would not cause these bony changes.

203. The answer is c. *(Fauci pp 2380)* Hypercalcemia must first be confirmed since misleading laboratory values can be caused by hemoconcentration of the serum sample. Ninety percent of hypercalcemia is attributed either to hyperparathyroidism or to malignancy. Almost all patients with malignancy-associated hypercalcemia have previously diagnosed cancer or symptoms (weight loss, anorexia, cough, hemoptysis) to suggest this diagnosis. In this otherwise healthy patient, confirmed hypercalcemia should lead to measurement of intact parathyroid hormone (iPTH). Other causes of hypercalcemia include familial hypocalciuric hypercalcemia, Vitamin D intoxication, sarcoidosis and other granulomatous diseases, hyperthyroidism, prolonged immobilization, and milk-alkali syndrome. Thyroid studies and liver enzymes (to evaluate for granulomatous hepatitis) might be ordered if the iPTH level is suppressed. Urine calcium excretion is assessed before parathyroidectomy to rule out familial hypocalciuric hypercalcemia, which can otherwise mimic hyperparathyroidism. Urine calcium determination, however, would not be the first test obtained in the assessment of hypercalcemia. Osteoporosis should be considered in this postmenopausal woman with hyperparathyroidism and appropriate screening for osteoporosis performed with central dual x-ray absorptiometry (DXA).

204. The answer is c. *(Fauci, pp 2410-2411.)* The radiographs and elevated alkaline phosphatase suggest Paget disease of the bone. Most patients with Paget disease do not require treatment, as they are asymptomatic. Bone pain, hearing loss, bony deformity, congestive heart failure, hypercalcemia, and repeated fractures are all indications for specific therapy beyond just symptomatic treatment for pain. Bisphosphonates bind to hydroxyapatite crystals to decrease bone turnover; they are now recommended as the treatment of choice for symptomatic Paget disease. Newer bisphosphonates such as alendronate and risedronate have replaced editronate because they are more potent and do not produce mineralization defects. The recommended dose in Paget disease is higher than the bisphosphonate dose used to treat osteoporosis. Subcutaneous injectable calcitonin is still used in patients who cannot tolerate the GI side effects of bisphosphonates. Melphalan and prednisone can be used to treat multiple myeloma, but myeloma causes osteolytic (rather than sclerotic) changes and does not cause elevation of the serum alkaline phosphatase. Ursodeoxycholic acid (UDCA) is utilized in the treatment of primary biliary cirrhosis (which can also present with elevated alkaline phosphatase) but has no effect on bone mineralization.

205. The answer is e. *(Fauci, pp 2297-2298.)* To recognize the best insulin regimen, you must first understand the pharmacokinetics of different insulin preparation—namely the peak time of onset of action and effective duration. The following describes the insulin preparations from shortest to longest duration. Lispro has a peak onset of 0.5 to 1.5 hours and effective duration of 3 to 4 hours. Regular insulin has a peak onset of 2 to 3 hours and effective duration of 4 to 6 hours. NPH has a peak onset of 6 to 10 hours and effective duration of 10 to 16 hours. Glargine provides basal insulin with an effective duration of 24 hours and no peak effect. This patient is experiencing early morning hypoglycemia resulting from his erratic supper time; in addition his fasting blood glucose levels (120 to 150 mg/dL) are not adequately controlled. The most appropriate insulin regimen for this patient is a long-acting insulin such as glargine at bedtime along with a short-acting insulin such as lispro before each meal. This will allow better regulation of basal glucose levels while providing coverage at mealtime and will address the issue of variable mealtimes. Twice daily regimens with NPH and regular insulin have fallen out of favor as they rarely provide sufficient coverage for either basal or meal-associated glucose production. Although premeal regular insulin is cheaper, lispro more closely matches the meal-associated glucose surge and provides better overall control. .

206. The answer is c. *(Fauci, pp 2263-2264.)* This patient's symptoms of weakness, fatigue, and weight loss in combination with hypotension and extensor hyperpigmentation are all consistent with Addison disease (adrenal insufficiency). Tuberculosis can involve the adrenal glands and result in adrenal insufficiency. Measurement of serum cortisol baseline and then stimulation with ACTH will confirm the clinical suspicion. The ACTH stimulation test is used to determine the adrenal reserve capacity for steroid production. Cortisol response is measured 60 minutes after cosyntropin is given intramuscularly or intravenously; a value of 18 μg/dL or above effectively excludes adrenal insufficiency. Hemochromatosis can cause hyperpigmentation but not the weight loss and hypotension. Bacteremia would not cause the gradually increasing symptoms or the hyperpigmentation. In some patients with weight loss and nausea, an EGD may be warranted; however, the clinical features of adrenal insufficiency in conjunction with poorly treated tuberculosis would first direct attention toward adrenal status.

207. The answer is b. *(ADA, pp S61-S78)* The 2008 ADA *Guidelines for Nutrition Recommendations and Diabetes* is a position statement based on evidence-based information. Medical nutrition therapy has been shown to reduce the HgA1c in type 2 diabetics by 1 to 2 points. The guidelines state that both low carbohydrate AND low-fat diets can produce beneficial weight loss in diabetes. However, if a low-carbohydrate diet is utilized, renal function, lipid profile and protein intake should be monitored (especially in patients with nephropathy). This is because low carbohydrate diets are high in animal protein. Referral to a medical nutritionist is recommended for both prediabetics and diabetics. Although very low-calorie diets (< 800 calories) produce beneficial weight loss, weight gain is usually occurs after self-selecting diet resumes. Bariatric surgery is an option for diabetic patients with a BMI of >35 kg/m² NOT 30 kg/m².

208. The answer is a. *(Fauci, p 2233)* In this patient with a TSH below 10 mU/L and no symptoms of hypothyroidism, the diagnosis is subclinical hypothyroidism. Recommendations include checking a free thyroxine level (it should be normal in subclinical hypothyroidism) and repeating the TSH in 3 months to monitor for progression toward overt hypothyroidism. The patient should be informed about the symptoms of hypothyroidism. Thyroxine therapy is not currently recommended for asymptomatic patients in whom the TSH level is below 10 mU/L.

Although an abnormal TPOAb increases the risk of progression to overt hypothyroidism, it does not affect your present management. Thyroid uptake scan may be useful in the diagnosis of hyperthyroidism, but not in possible hypothyroidism. Iodide deficiency is not seen in the United States because of dietary iodide supplementation.

209. The answer is c. *(Fauci, pp 2263-2264.)* This patient's presentation suggests adrenal insufficiency (Addison disease). Hyponatremia is caused by loss of sodium in the urine (aldosterone deficiency) and free-water retention. Sodium loss causes volume depletion and orthostatic hypotension. Hyperkalemia is caused by aldosterone deficiency, impaired glomerular filtration, and acidosis. Ten to twenty percent of patients with adrenal insufficiency will have mild hypercalcemia; hypocalcemia is not expected. Complete blood count can reveal a normocytic anemia, relative lymphocytosis, and a moderate eosinophilia. Microcytic anemia would suggest an iron disorder or thalassemia. The hyperpigmentation results from the release of pro-opiomelanocortin which has melanocyte stimulating activity.

Hyperpigmentation is not seen if pituitary dysfunction is causing the adrenal insufficiency (ie, in secondary hypoadrenalism).

210. The answer is b. *(Fauci, pp 2233.)* The clinical picture strongly suggests myxedema coma. Unprovoked hypothermia is a particularly important sign. Myxedema coma constitutes a medical emergency; treatment should be started immediately. Should laboratory results fail to support the diagnosis, treatment can be stopped. An intravenous bolus of levothyroxine is given (500 mcg loading dose), followed by daily intravenous doses (50 to 100 mcg). Impaired adrenal reserve may accompany myxedema coma; so parenteral hydrocortisone is given concomitantly. Intravenous fluids are also needed but are less important than thyroxine and glucocorticoids; rewarming should be accompanied slowly, so as not to precipitate cardiac arrhythmias. If alveolar ventilation is compromised, then intubation may also be necessary. Hyponatremia and an elevated PCO_2 are laboratory markers of severe myxedema. CT of the head would not be the first choice, since a structural brain lesion would not explain the hypothermia, diffuse goiter, or hyporeflexia seen in this case.

211. The answer is d. *(Fauci, pp 2296-2305)* Episodic hypoglycemia at night is followed by rebound hyperglycemia. This condition, called the Somogyi effect, develops in response to excessive insulin administration. An adrenergic response to hypoglycemia results in increased glycogenolysis, gluconeogenesis, and diminished glucose uptake by peripheral tissues; hence the prebreakfast blood sugars are often elevated. Checking the blood sugars at 2 and 5 AM will demonstrate the hypoglycemia and allow the proper treatment changes— less long-acting insulin at bedtime, not more—to be made. Nocturnal hypoglycemia is a common problem with intermediate-acting insulins such as NPH and lente. The nearly peakless long-acting insulins glargine and detimir infrequently lead to the Somogyi effect.

212. The answer is e. *(Fauci, pp 2269-2270.)* Hypertensive crisis in this young woman suggests a secondary cause of hypertension. In the setting of palpitations, apprehension, and hyperglycemia, pheochromocytoma should be considered. Pheochromocytomas are derived from the adrenal medulla. They are capable of producing and secreting catecholamines. Unexplained hypertension associated with surgery or trauma may also suggest the disease. Clinical symptoms are the result of catecholamine secretion. For example, the patient's hyperglycemia is a result of a catecholamine effect of insulin suppression and stimulation of hepatic glucose output. Hypercalcemia has been attributed to ectopic secretion of parathormone-related protein. Renal artery stenosis can cause severe hypertension but would not explain the systemic symptoms or laboratory abnormalities in this case. An anxiety attack can produce palpitations, apprehension and mild to moderate elevation in blood pressure but would not produce hypercalcemia nor elevated blood pressure poorly responsive to treatment. Essential hypertension can occur in a 25-year-old but again would not account for the laboratory changes. Diabetes mellitus does not cause hypertension unless renal insufficiency has already developed; her hyperglycemia will likely resolve when the pheochromocytoma is removed. Once pheochromocytoma is suspected, a 24-hour urine specimen for metanephrines or fractionated catecholamines is the commonly used diagnostic study. After biochemical evidence of catecholamine overproduction is found, imaging studies (CT scan, radionuclide imaging) will localize the problem for curative surgery.

213. The answer is a. *(Fauci, p 2203 and p 2210.)* The patient shows excessive growth of soft tissue that has resulted in coarsening of facial features, prognathism, and frontal bossing—all characteristic of acromegaly. This growth hormone–secreting pituitary tumor will result in bitemporal hemianopsia when the tumor impinges on the optic chiasm, which lies just above the sella turcica. Growth hormone secreting tumors are the second commonest functioning pituitary tumors (second to prolactinomas). Serum IGF-1 (insulin-like growth factor-1) level will be elevated and is usually the first diagnostic test. Growth hormone secretion is pulsatile and a single GH level is often equivocal; the GH level must be suppressed (usually with glucose) to diagnose autonomous overproduction. Unilateral blindness would be caused by optic neuritis or occlusion of the ophthalmic artery, as in temporal arteritis. Homonymous hemianopsia occurs with disease posterior to the optic chiasm—in the optic radiation or the occipital lobe. A right-sided lesion would cause left homonymous hemianopsia and vice versa. Diplopia usually implies an abnormality in cranial nerve three, four, or six, or else an eye muscle imbalance (as in Graves disease or myasthenia gravis).

214. The answer is c. *(Fauci, pp 2222-2223.)* The patient described has hyponatremia, normovolemia, and concentrated urine. These features are sufficient to make a diagnosis of inappropriate antidiuretic hormone secretion. If ADH were responding normally to the patient's hypotonic state, the urine would be dilute and the excess water load would be excreted. Treatment necessitates restriction of fluid (free water) intake. Insensible and urinary water loss results in a rise in serum Na$^+$ and serum osmolality and symptom improvement. If the patient has CNS symptoms such as confusion, obtundation, or seizures, hypertonic saline is cautiously administered to raise the serum sodium out of the danger zone (usually a rise of 4-8 mEq/L). Normal saline would treat volume depletion, but this patient is euvolemic. Isotonic saline would not address the free water excess. Loop diuretics lead to modest free water loss in the urine but would be less important than fluid restriction. The tetracycline derivative demeclocycline decreases renal response to ADH and can be used in cases where the hyponatremia does not respond to fluid restriction. SIADH can occur as a side effect of many drugs or from carcinoma (especially small cell carcinoma of the lung), CNS disorders (head trauma, CNS infection) or benign lung diseases (especially lung abscesses or other chronic infections).

215. The answer is a. (*Fauci, pp 2255-2256.*) The clinical findings all suggest an excess production of cortisol by the adrenal gland. Hypertension, truncal obesity, and dark abdominal striae are common physical findings; patients often have ecchymoses at points of trauma (especially legs and forearms) because of increased capillary fragility. The process responsible for hypercortisolism is most often an ACTH-producing pituitary microadenoma. An adrenal adenoma that directly produces cortisol is the next most likely option. Most ectopic ACTH-producing neoplasms (usually small cell carcinoma of the lung) progress too rapidly for the full Cushing syndrome to develop. These patients usually present with muscle weakness due to profound hypokalemia. The initial test to diagnose endogenous cortisol overproduction is either the overnight dexamethasone suppression test (in normals, the AM cortisol should suppress to less than 2 micrograms/dL after a midnight dose of 1 mg dexamethasone) or 24-hour urine collection for free cortisol. More extensive testing is then required to determine the source. Hypothalamic tumors can affect ADH production and eating behavior but do not produce cortisol or ACTH. Unexpected bruising should prompt questions about domestic violence, but partner abuse would not account for the constellation of this patient's findings.

216. The answer is c. (*Fauci, pp 2341-2342.*) The picture of infertility, gynecomastia, and tall stature (arms and legs longer than expected for truncal size) is consistent with Klinefelter syndrome and an XXY karyotype. The patient has abnormal gonadal development with hyalinized testes that result in low testosterone levels. Pituitary function in Klinefelter syndrome is normal, so gonadotropin levels are elevated in response to underproduction of testosterone. Although Klinefelter patients may have sexual function, they do not produce sperm and are infertile. Turner syndrome refers to the 45 XO karyotype that results in abnormal sexual development in a female.

217. The answer is b. *(Fauci, pp 2430-2431.)* Iron overload should be considered among patients who present with any one or a combination of the following: hepatomegaly, weakness, hyperpigmentation, atypical arthritis, diabetes, impotence, unexplained chronic abdominal pain, or cardiomyopathy. Diagnostic suspicion should be particularly high when the family history is positive for similar clinical findings. The most frequent cause of iron overload is the common genetic disorder (idiopathic) hemochromatosis. Secondary iron storage problems can occur after multiple transfusions in a variety of anemias. The most practical screening test is the determination of serum iron, transferrin saturation, and ferritin. Transferrin saturation greater than 50% in males or 45% in females suggests increased iron stores. Substantially elevated serum ferritin levels confirm total body iron overload. Genetic screening is now used to assess which patients are at risk for severe fibrosis of the liver. Definitive diagnosis can be established by liver biopsy. Determination of serum copper is needed when Wilson disease is the probable cause of hepatic abnormalities. Wilson disease does not cause hypogonadism, heart failure, diabetes, or arthropathy. Chronic liver disease caused by hepatitis B would not account for the heart failure, hyperpigmentation, or diabetes. Nocturnal penile tumescence and echocardiogram can confirm clinical findings but will not establish the underlying diagnosis.

218. The answer is c. *(Fauci pp 2361-2362.)* For the patient described, the markedly increased calcitonin level indicates the diagnosis of medullary carcinoma of the thyroid. In view of the family history, the patient most likely has multiple endocrine neoplasia (MEN) type IIA, which includes medullary carcinoma of the thyroid gland, pheochromocytoma, and parathyroid hyperplasia. Pheochromocytoma may exist without sustained hypertension, as indicated by excessive urinary catecholamines. Before thyroid surgery is performed on this patient, a pheochromocytoma must be ruled out through urinary catecholamine determinations; the presence of such a tumor might expose him to a hypertensive crisis during surgery. The serum calcium serves as a screening test for hyperparathyroidism. At surgery, the entire thyroid gland must be removed because foci of parafollicular cell hyperplasia, a premalignant lesion, may be scattered throughout the gland. Successful removal of the medullary carcinoma can be monitored with serum calcitonin levels. Medullary carcinoma of the thyroid rarely metastases to the liver; so a liver scan would be unnecessary if liver enzymes are normal. Thyroxine will be needed after surgery, but MEN type II is not associated with hypothyroidism. Radioactive iodine can be used to treat malignancies that arise from the follicular cells of the thyroid; parafollicular cells, however, do not take up iodine and do not respond to radioactive iodine. Hyperparathyroidism, while unlikely in this eucalcemic patient, is probably present in his brother.

219. The answer is b. *(Fauci, p 301, p 606, p 2195.)* The symptoms of masculinization (eg, alopecia, deepening of voice, clitoral hypertrophy) in this patient are characteristic of an active androgen-producing tumor. Such extreme virilization is very rarely observed in polycystic ovary syndrome or in Cushing syndrome; moreover, the presence of normal cortisol and adrenal androgens (DHEA-S) plus markedly elevated plasma testosterone levels indicates an ovarian rather than adrenal cause of the findings. Arrhenoblastomas are the most common androgen-producing ovarian tumors. Their incidence is highest during the reproductive years. Composed of varying proportions of Leydig and Sertoli cells, they are generally benign. In contrast to arrhenoblastomas, granulosa-theca cell tumors produce feminization, not virilization. Dermoid cysts (benign teratomas) do not produce gonadotropins but cause symptoms by enlargement or ovarian torsion (pain) or rupture with contents spilling into the peritoneal cavity.

220. The answer is d. *(Fauci, p 2354, p 2359.)* The diagnosis of gastrinoma should be considered in all patients with recurrent ulcers after surgical correction for peptic ulcer disease, ulcers in the distal duodenum or jejunum, ulcer disease associated with diarrhea, or evidence suggestive of the multiple endocrine neoplasia (MEN) type I (familial association of pituitary, parathyroid, and pancreatic tumors) in ulcer patients. Because basal serum gastrin and basal acid production may both be normal or only slightly elevated in patients with gastrinomas, provocative tests may be needed for diagnosis. Both the secretin and calcium infusion tests are used; a paradoxical increase in serum gastrin concentration is seen in response to both infusions in patients with gastrinomas. In contrast, other conditions associated with hypergastrinemia, such as duodenal ulcers, retained antrum, gastric outlet obstruction, antral G cell hyperplasia, and pernicious anemia, will respond with either no change or a decrease in serum gastrin. Serum calcium level should be obtained to rule out concomitant hyperparathyroidism but would not help in the assessment of gastrinoma per se. Insulin-induced hypoglycemia is used as a provocative test for adrenal insufficiency, not for the evaluation of acid hypersecretory states.

221. The answer is d. *(Fauci, pp 2218-2219.)* Metastatic tumors rarely cause diabetes insipidus, but of the tumors that cause it, carcinoma of the breast is by far the most common. In this patient, the diagnosis of diabetes insipidus is suggested by hypernatremia and low urine osmolality. To distinguish between central (ADH deficiency) and nephrogenic (peripheral resistance to ADH action) diabetes insipidus, vasopressin (ADH by another name) is administered. If the urine osmolality rises and the urine output falls, the diagnosis is central DI. There will be little response to vasopressin in nephrogenic DI.

Psychogenic polydipsia is an unlikely diagnosis since serum sodium is usually mildly reduced in this condition. Renal glycosuria would be expected to induce higher urine osmolality than this patient has because of the osmotic effect of glucose. While nephrocalcinosis secondary to hypercalcemia may produce polyuria, hypercalciuria does not. Finally, the findings of inappropriate antidiuretic hormone syndrome are the opposite of those observed in diabetes insipidus and thus are incompatible with the clinical picture in this patient.

222. The answer is c. *(Fauci, p 2299, p 2309.)* This clinical picture and laboratory results suggest factitious hypoglycemia caused by self-administration of insulin. The diagnosis should be suspected in healthcare workers, patients or family members with diabetes, and others who have a history of malingering. Patients present with symptoms of hypoglycemia and low plasma glucose levels. Insulin levels will be high, but C peptide will be undetectable. Endogenous hyperinsulinism, such as would be seen with an insulinoma, would result in elevated plasma insulin concentrations (> 36 pmol/L) and elevated C peptide levels (> 0.2 mmol/L). C peptide is derived from the breakdown of proinsulin, which is produced endogenously; thus C peptide will not rise in the patient who develops hypoglycemia from exogenous insulin. Reactive hypoglycemia occurs after meals and is self-limited. A rapid postprandial rise in glucose may induce a brisk insulin response that causes transient hypoglycemia hours later. It may be associated with gastric or intestinal surgery. Pheochromocytoma causes hyperglycemia due to the insulin counter-regulatory effect of catecholamines. Sulfonylurea, an insulin secretagogue, would increase natural insulin secretion resulting in elevated insulin and elevated C peptide levels.

223. The answer is e. (*Fauci, pp 2335-2336.*) Estrogen is the most effective medication for decreasing vasomotor symptoms related to menopause. Hormone therapy (HT) favorably affects the lipid panel by decreasing LDL and increasing HDL, but HT also increases triglyceride levels. HT has an antiresorptive effect on bone, thus stabilizing or increasing bone density. In the Women's Health Initiative Study, HT was shown to decrease the incidence of hip fractures. Hormone therapy should be implemented in women with moderate to severe hot flashes who lack contraindications to use (endometrial cancer, history of venous thromboembolism, breast cancer, or gallbladder disease). This patient has a low risk for cardiovascular disease and has no direct contraindications for HT. The risk of breast cancer with HT use is directly related to the length of use. Five or more years is considered long-term use and is the cut-off where most research studies and meta-analyses found increasing risk of breast cancer. Progestational agents alone do not improve vasomotor symptoms.

224 to 226. The answers are 224-d, 225-h, 226-c. (*Fauci, pp 2255, 2205-2206, 2199.*) Cushing disease produces hypercortisolism secondary to excessive secretion of pituitary ACTH. It often affects women in their childbearing years. Prominent cervical fat pads, purple striae, hirsutism, and glucose intolerance are characteristic features, as well as muscle wasting, easy bruising, amenorrhea, and psychiatric disturbances. Diabetes mellitus can result from chronic hypercortisolism. Exogenous glucocorticoid use will not produce hirsutism but will produce cervical fat pad, purple striae, muscle wasting, easy bruising and secondary diabetes mellitus. Prolactinoma, or prolactin-secreting adenoma, may cause bitemporal hemianopsia—as can all pituitary tumors. Galactorrhea (lactation not associated with pregnancy) and irregular menses or amenorrhea are the clinical clues. Serum prolactin levels are usually over 250 ng/mL, higher than usually seen in other causes of hyperprolactinemia such as medications or renal failure. Empty sella syndrome is enlargement of the sella turcica from CSF pressure compressing the pituitary gland. It is most common in obese, hypertensive women. There are no focal findings. Some patients have chronic headaches; others are asymptomatic. MRI will distinguish this syndrome from a pituitary tumor. These patients have normal pituitary function, the rim of pituitary tissue being fully functional.

227 to 229. The answers are 227-d, 228-c, 229-a. (*Fauci, pp 2233-2238.*) In a young female with hyperthyroidism, low or absent radioiodine uptake in the thyroid and a coexisting pelvic mass, you should consider struma ovarii (ectopic thyroid tissue in a teratoma of the ovary). Whole body radionuclide scanning can demonstrate ectopic thyroid tissue. Surreptitious use of thyroid supplements (factitious hyperthyroidism) can occur in healthcare workers who have access to thyroid hormone. Classic symptoms of hyperthyroidism occur and the serum T_4 is elevated. Radioactive iodine uptake would show subnormal values, as there is no thyroid hormone production in the gland itself. The thyroid gland is not palpable. A tender thyroid gland and elevated ESR make subacute thyroiditis a likely diagnosis. Hyperthyroid symptoms are common early in the illness. The condition is self-limited (usually lasting 6-8 weeks); so antithyroid drugs are not used. Beta-blockers can alleviate symptoms until the inflammation resolves.

Gastroenterology

Questions

230. A 35-year-old alcoholic man is admitted with nausea, vomiting, and abdominal pain that radiates to the back. He has had several previous episodes of pancreatitis presenting with the same symptoms. Which of the following laboratory values suggests a poor prognosis in this patient?

a. Elevated serum lipase
b. Elevated serum amylase
c. Leukocytosis of 20,000/μm
d. Diastolic blood pressure greater than 90 mm Hg
e. Heart rate of 100 beats/minute

231. A 60-year-old woman with depression and poorly controlled type 2 diabetes mellitus complains of episodic vomiting over the last three months. She has constant nausea and early satiety. She vomits once or twice almost every day. In addition, she reports several months of mild abdominal discomfort that is localized to the upper abdomen and that sometimes awakens her at night. She has lost 5 lb of weight. Her diabetes has been poorly controlled (glycosylated hemoglobin recently was 9.5). Current medications are glyburide, metformin, and amitriptyline.

Her physical examination is normal except for mild abdominal distention and evidence of a peripheral sensory neuropathy. Complete blood count, serum electrolytes, BUN, creatinine, and liver function tests are all normal. Gallbladder sonogram is negative for gallstones. Upper GI series and CT scan of the abdomen are normal.

What is the best next step in the evaluation of this patient's symptoms?

a. Barium esophagram
b. Scintigraphic gastric emptying study
c. Colonoscopy
d. Liver biopsy
e. Small bowel biopsy

232. A 56-year-old woman becomes the chief financial officer of a large company and, several months thereafter, develops upper abdominal pain that she ascribes to stress. She takes an over-the-counter antacid with temporary benefit. She uses no other medications. One night she awakens with nausea and vomits a large volume of coffee grounds-like material; she becomes weak and diaphoretic. Upon hospitalization, she is found to have an actively bleeding duodenal ulcer. Which of the following statements is true?

a.   The most likely etiology is adenocarcinoma of the duodenum.
b.   The etiology of duodenal ulcer is different in women than in men.
c.   The likelihood that she harbors *Helicobacter pylori* is greater than 50%.
d.   Lifetime residence in the United States makes *H pylori* unlikely as an etiologic agent.
e.   Organisms consistent with *H pylori* are rarely seen on biopsy in patients with duodenal ulcer.

233. A 40-year-old man with long-standing alcohol abuse complains of abdominal swelling, which has been progressive over several months. He has a history of gastrointestinal bleeding. On physical examination, there are spider angiomas and palmar erythema. Abdominal collateral vessels are seen around the umbilicus. There is shifting dullness, and bulging flanks are noted. Which of the following is the most important first step in the patient's evaluation?

a.   Diagnostic paracentesis
b.   Upper GI series
c.   Ethanol level
d.   CT scan of the abdomen
e.   Examination of peripheral blood smear

234. A 70-year-old man presents with a complaint of fatigue. There is no history of alcohol abuse or liver disease; the patient is taking no medications. Scleral icterus is noted on physical examination; the liver and spleen are nonpalpable. The patient has a normocytic, normochromic anemia. Urinalysis shows bilirubinuria with absent urine urobilinogen. Serum bilirubin is 12 mg/dL, AST and ALT are normal, and alkaline phosphatase is 300 U/L (three times normal). Which of the following is the best next step in evaluation?

a.   Ultrasound or CT scan of the abdomen
b.   Viral hepatitis profile
c.   Reticulocyte count
d.   Serum ferritin
e.   Antimitochondrial antibodies

235. A 58-year-old white man complains of intermittent rectal bleeding and, at the time of colonoscopy, is found to have internal hemorrhoids and the lesion shown at the splenic flexure. Pathology shows tubulovillous changes. Repeat colonoscopy should be recommended at what interval?

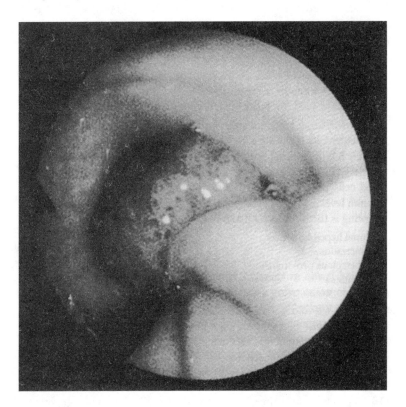

a. In 1 to 2 months
b. In 1 year
c. In 3 years
d. In 10 years
e. Repeat colonoscopy is not necessary

236. A 36-year-old man presents for a well-patient examination. He gives a history that, over the past 20 years, he has had three episodes of abdominal pain and hematemesis, the most recent of which occurred several years ago. He was told that an ulcer was seen on a barium upper GI radiograph. You obtain a serum assay for H pylori IgG, which is positive. What is the most effective regimen to eradicate this organism?

a. Omeprazole 20 mg orally once daily for 6 weeks
b. Ranitidine 300 mg orally once daily at bedtime for 6 weeks
c. Omeprazole 20 mg twice daily, amoxicillin 1000 mg twice daily, and clarithromycin 500 mg twice daily for 14 days
d. Pepto-Bismol and metronidazole twice daily for 7 days
e. Benzathine penicillin, 1.2 million units intramuscularly weekly for three doses

237. A 60-year-old woman complains of fever and constant left lower quadrant pain of 2 days duration. She has not had vomiting or rectal bleeding. She has a history of hypertension but is otherwise healthy. She has never had similar abdominal pain, and has had no previous surgeries. Her only regular medication is lisinopril.

On examination blood pressure is 150/80, pulse 110, and temperature 38.9°C (102°F). She has normal bowel sounds and left lower quadrant abdominal tenderness with rebound. A complete blood count reveals WBC = 28,000. Serum electrolytes, BUN, creatinine and liver function tests are normal. What is the next best step in evaluating this patient's problem?

a. Colonoscopy
b. Barium enema
c. Exploratory laparotomy
d. Ultrasound of the abdomen
e. CT scan of the abdomen and pelvis

238. A 63-year-old woman with cirrhosis caused by chronic hepatitis C is hospitalized because of confusion. She has guaiac-positive stools and a low-grade fever. She has received lorazepam for sleep disturbance. On physical examination, the patient is confused. She has no meningeal signs and no focal neurologic findings. There is hyperreflexia and a nonrhythmic flapping tremor of the wrists. Which of the following is the most likely explanation for this patient's mental status change?

a. Tuberculous meningitis
b. Subdural hematoma
c. Alcohol withdrawal seizure
d. Hepatic encephalopathy
e. Central nervous system vasculitis from cryoglobulinemia

239. A 50-year-old man with a history of alcohol and tobacco abuse has complained of difficulty swallowing solid food for the past 2 months. More recently, swallowing fluids has also become a problem. He has noted black, tarry stools on occasion. The patient has lost 10 lb. Which of the following statements is correct?

a. A CT scan of the abdomen and pelvis is the best next test.
b. Barium contrast esophagram will likely establish a diagnosis.
c. The most likely diagnosis is peptic ulcer disease.
d. The patient has achalasia.
e. Herpes simplex virus infection of the esophagus is likely.

240. A 34-year-old man presents with substernal discomfort. The symptoms are worse after meals, particularly a heavy evening meal, and are sometimes associated with hot/sour fluid in the back of the throat and nocturnal awakening. The patient denies difficulty swallowing, pain on swallowing, or weight loss. The symptoms have been present for 6 weeks; the patient has gained 20 lb in the past 2 years. Which of the following is the most appropriate initial approach?

a. Therapeutic trial of ranitidine
b. Exercise test with thallium imaging
c. Esophagogastroduodenoscopy
d. CT scan of the chest
e. Coronary angiography

241. A 48-year-old woman presents with a change in bowel habit and 10-lb weight loss over the past 2 months despite preservation of appetite. She notices increased abdominal gas, particularly after fatty meals. The stools are malodorous and occur 2 to 3 times per day; no rectal bleeding is noticed. The symptoms are less prominent when she follows a clear liquid diet. Which of the following is the most likely histological abnormality associated with this patient's symptoms?

a. Signet ring cells on gastric biopsy
b. Mucosal inflammation and crypt abscesses on sigmoidoscopy
c. Villous atrophy and increased lymphocytes in the lamina propria on small bowel biopsy
d. Small, curved gram-negative bacteria in areas of intestinal metaplasia on gastric biopsy
e. Periportal inflammation on liver biopsy

242. An otherwise healthy 40-year-old woman sees you because of recurrent abdominal pain. In the past month she has had four episodes of colicky epigastric pain. Each of these episodes has lasted about 30 minutes and has occurred within an hour of eating. Two of the episodes have been associated with sweating and vomiting. None of the episodes have been associated with fever or shortness of breath. She has not lost weight. She does not drink alcohol or take any prescription or over-the-counter medications. Other than three previous uneventful vaginal deliveries, she has never been hospitalized.

Her examination is negative except for mild obesity (BMI = 32). A complete blood count and multichannel chemistry profile that includes liver function test is normal. A gallbladder sonogram reveals multiple gallstones.

What is the next best step in the treatment of this patient?

a. Omeprazole, 20 mg daily for eight weeks.
b. Ursodeoxycholic acid
c. Observation without specific therapy
d. Laparoscopic cholecystectomy
e. Weight reduction

243. A 56-year-old chronic alcoholic has a 1 year history of ascites. He is admitted with a 2-day history of diffuse abdominal pain and fever. Examination reveals scleral icterus, spider angiomas, a distended abdomen with shifting dullness, and diffuse abdominal tenderness. Paracentesis reveals slightly cloudy ascitic fluid with an ascitic fluid PMN cell count of 1000/μL. Which of the following statements about treatment is true?

a. Antibiotic therapy is unnecessary if the ascitic fluid culture is negative for bacteria.
b. The addition of albumin to antibiotic therapy improves survival.
c. Repeated paracenteses are required to assess the response to antibiotic treatment.
d. After treatment of this acute episode, a recurrent episode of spontaneous bacterial peritonitis would be unlikely.
e. Treatment with multiple antibiotics is required because polymicrobial infection is common.

244. A 60-year-old man with known hepatitis C and a previous liver biopsy showing cirrhosis requests evaluation for possible liver transplantation. He has never received treatment for hepatitis C. Though previously a heavy user of alcohol, he has been abstinent for over 2 years. He has had 2 episodes of bleeding esophageal varices. He was hospitalized 6 months ago with acute hepatic encephalopathy. He has a 1 year history of ascites that has required repeated paracentesis despite treatment with diuretics.

Medications are aldactone 100 mg daily and lactulose 30 cc 3 times daily.

On examination he appears thin, with obvious scleral icterus, spider angiomas, palmar erythema, gynecomastia, a large amount ascites, and small testicles. There is no asterixis.

Recent laboratory testing revealed the following: hemoglobin = 12.0 mg/dL (normal 13.5-15.0), MCV = 103 fL (normal 80-100), creatinine = 2.0 mg/dL (normal 0.7-1.2), bilirubin = 6.5 mg/dL (normal 0.1-1.2), AST = 25 U/L (normal < 40), ALT = 45 U/L (normal < 40), INR = 3.0 (normal 0.8-1.2).

What is the next best step?

a. Repeat liver biopsy.
b. Start treatment with interferon and ribavirin.
c. Refer the patient for hospice care.
d. Continue to optimize medical treatment for his ascites and hepatic encephalopathy and tell the patient he is not eligible for liver transplantation because of his previous history of alcohol abuse.
e. Refer the patient to a liver transplantation center.

245. A 40-year-old white male complains of weakness, weight loss, and abdominal pain. On examination, the patient has diffuse hyperpigmentation and a palpable liver edge. Polyarthritis of the wrists and hips is also noted. Fasting blood sugar is 185 mg/dL. Which of the following is the most likely diagnosis?

a. Insulin-dependent diabetes mellitus
b. Pancreatic carcinoma
c. Addison disease
d. Hemochromatosis
e. Metabolic syndrome

246. A 32-year-old white woman complains of abdominal pain off and on since the age of 17. She notices abdominal bloating relieved by defecation as well as alternating diarrhea and constipation. She has no weight loss, GI bleeding, or nocturnal diarrhea. On examination, she has slight LLQ tenderness and gaseous abdominal distension. Laboratory studies, including CBC, are normal. Which of the following is the most appropriate initial approach?

a. Recommend increased dietary fiber, antispasmodics as needed, and follow-up examination in 2 months.
b. Refer to gastroenterologist for colonoscopy.
c. Obtain antiendomysial antibodies.
d. Order UGI series with small bowel follow-through.
e. Order small bowel biopsy.

247. A 55-year-old white woman has had recurrent episodes of alcohol-induced pancreatitis. Despite abstinence, the patient develops postprandial abdominal pain, bloating, weight loss despite good appetite, and bulky, foul-smelling stools. KUB shows pancreatic calcifications. In this patient, you should expect to find which of the following?

a. Diabetes mellitus
b. Malabsorption of fat-soluble vitamins D and K
c. Guaiac-positive stool
d. Courvoisier sign
e. Markedly elevated amylase

248. A 34-year-old white woman is treated for a UTI with amoxicillin. Initially she improves, but 5 days after beginning treatment, she develops recurrent fever, abdominal bloating, and diarrhea with six to eight loose stools per day. What is the best diagnostic test to confirm your diagnosis?

a. Identification of *Clostridium difficile* toxin in the stool
b. Isolation of *C difficile* in stool culture
c. Stool positive for white blood cells (fecal leukocytes)
d. Detection of IgG antibodies against *C difficile* in the serum
e. Visualization of clue cells on microscopic examination of stool

249. A 27-year-old female is found to have a positive hepatitis C antibody at the time of plasma donation. Physical examination is normal. Liver enzymes reveal ALT of 62 U/L (normal < 40), AST 65 U/L (normal < 40), bilirubin 1.2 mg/dL (normal), and alkaline phosphatase normal. Hepatitis C viral RNA is 100,000 copies/mL. Hepatitis B surface antigen and HIV antibody are negative. Which of the following statements is true?

a. Liver biopsy is necessary to confirm the diagnosis of hepatitis C.
b. Most patients with hepatitis C eventually resolve their infection without permanent sequelae.
c. This patient should not receive vaccinations against other viral forms of hepatitis.
d. Serum ALT levels are a good predictor of prognosis.
e. Patients with hepatitis C genotype 2 or 3 are more likely to have a favorable response to treatment with interferon and ribavirin.

250. A 72-year-old woman notices progressive dysphagia to solids and liquids. There is no history of alcohol or tobacco use, and the patient takes no medications. She denies heartburn, but occasionally notices the regurgitation of undigested food from meals eaten several hours before. Her barium swallow is shown. Which of the following is the cause of this condition?

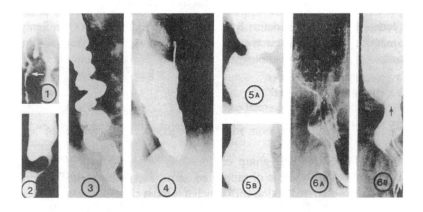

a. Growth of malignant squamous cells into the muscularis mucosa
b. Scarring caused by silent gastroesophageal reflux
c. Spasm of the lower esophageal sphincter
d. Loss of intramural neurons in the esophagus
e. Psychiatric disease

251. A 37-year-old woman presents for evaluation of abnormal liver chemistries. She has long-standing obesity (current BMI 38) and has previously taken anorectic medications but not for the past several years. She takes no other medications and has not used parenteral drugs or had high-risk sexual exposure. On examination, her liver span is 13 cm; she has no spider angiomas or splenomegaly. Several sets of liver enzymes have shown transaminases two to three times normal. Bilirubin and alkaline phosphatase are normal. Hepatitis B surface antigen and hepatitis C antibody are normal, as are serum iron and total iron-binding capacity. Which of the following is the likely pathology on liver biopsy?

a. Macrovesicular fatty liver
b. Microvesicular fatty liver
c. Portal triaditis with piecemeal necrosis
d. Cirrhosis
e. Copper deposition

Questions 252 to 254

Match the patient described with the most likely diagnosis. Each lettered option may be used once, more than once, or not at all.

a. Acute diverticulitis
b. Acute pancreatitis
c. Acute cholecystitis
d. Intestinal obstruction
e. Irritable bowel syndrome
f. Mesenteric ischemia

252. A 45-year-old diabetic woman presents with two days of severe upper abdominal pain that radiates into the back and has been associated with nausea and vomiting. She takes insulin but has been noncompliant for several weeks. She denies alcohol consumption. Her serum is lipemic.

253. A 78-year-old white man with coronary artery disease presents with several months of postprandial generalized abdominal pain that typically lasts 30-60 minutes. He has become fearful of eating and has lost 15 lb of weight.

254. A 68-year-old woman who has had a previous hysterectomy presents with an 8-hour history of cramping periumbilical pain. Each episode of pain lasts 3 to 5 minutes and then abates. Over several hours she develops nausea, vomiting, and abdominal distension. She has been unable to pass stool or flatus for the past 4 hours.

Questions 255 to 256

Match the clinical description with the most likely disease process. Each lettered option may be used once, more than once, or not at all.

a. Primary biliary cirrhosis
b. Sclerosing cholangitis
c. Anaerobic liver abscess
d. Hepatocellular carcinoma
e. Hepatitis C
f. Hepatitis D
g. Hemochromatosis

255. A 40-year-old white female complains of pruritus. Physical examination reveals xanthelasma and mild splenomegaly. She has an elevated alkaline phosphatase, but her transaminases are normal. The antimitochondrial antibody test is positive.

256. A 58-year-old male with long-standing cirrhosis resulting from hepatitis C develops vague right upper quadrant pain and weight loss. A right upper quadrant mass is palpable. Serum alkaline phosphatase is elevated.

Questions 257 to 259

Match the clinical description with the most likely disease process. Each lettered option may be used once, more than once, or not at all.

a. Hemolysis secondary to G6PD deficiency
b. Pancreatic carcinoma
c. Acute viral hepatitis
d. Crigler-Najjar syndrome
e. Gilbert syndrome
f. Cirrhosis of liver

257. An African American male develops mild jaundice while being treated for a urinary tract infection. Urine bilirubin is negative. Serum bilirubin is 3 mg/dL, mostly unconjugated. Hemoglobin is 7 g/dL.

258. A 60-year-old male is noted to have mild jaundice and 15-lb weight loss. The patient has noted pruritus and pale, clay-colored stools. On examination, the gallbladder is palpable. Alkaline phosphatase is very elevated.

259. A young woman complains of one week of fatigue, change in skin color, and dark brown urine. She has right upper quadrant tenderness and ALT of 1035 U/L (normal <40).

Questions 260 to 262

For each case scenario, select the most likely diagnosis. Each lettered option may be used once, more than once, or not at all.

a. Gastric ulcer
b. Aortoenteric fistula
c. Mallory-Weiss tear
d. Esophageal varices
e. Hereditary hemorrhagic telangiectasia (HHT)
f. Colon polyp
g. Adenocarcinoma of the colon

260. An 88-year-old white woman with osteoarthritis has noticed mild epigastric discomfort for several weeks. Naproxen has helped her joint symptoms. She suddenly develops hematemesis and hypotension.

261. A 76-year-old white man presents with painless hematemesis and hypotension. He has no previous GI symptoms but did have resection of an abdominal aortic aneurysm 12 years previously. EGD shows no bleeding source in the stomach or duodenum.

262. A 39-year-old alcoholic presents with massive hematemesis and hypotension. Examination reveals hemorrhoids and ascites.

Questions 263 to 265

For each case scenario, select the most likely diagnosis. Each lettered option may be used once, more than once, or not at all.

a. Ulcerative colitis
b. Crohn disease
c. Ischemic colitis
d. Diverticulitis
e. Amebic colitis
f. Tuberculoma of the colon

263. A 35-year-old white man presents with diarrhea, weight loss, and RLQ pain. On examination, a tender mass is noted in the RLQ; the stool is guaiac-positive. Colonoscopy shows segmental areas of inflammation. Barium small bowel series shows nodular thickening of the terminal ileum.

264. A 75-year-old African American woman, previously healthy, presents with low-grade fever, diarrhea, and rectal bleeding. Colonoscopy shows continuous erythema from rectum to mid-transverse colon. The cecum is normal.

265. A 70-year-old white woman presents with LLQ abdominal pain, low-grade fever, and mild rectal bleeding. Examination shows LLQ tenderness. Unprepped sigmoidoscopy reveals segmental inflammation beginning in the distal sigmoid colon through the mid-descending colon. The rest of the examination is negative.

Questions 266 to 268

For each of the following case scenarios, select the most likely pathogen. Each lettered option may be used once, more than once, or not at all.

a. *Staphylococcus aureus*
b. *Shigella dysenteriae*
c. *Entamoeba histolytica*
d. *Escherichia coli O157H7*
e. *Salmonella* species
f. *Giardia lamblia*

266. A 21-year-old male develops bloody diarrhea and fever. He owns and operates an exotic pet store, which specializes in reptile sales.

267. Two hours after ingesting potato salad at a picnic, a 50-year-old white woman develops severe nausea and vomiting. She has no diarrhea, fever, or chills. On examination, she appears hypovolemic, but the abdomen is benign.

268. Last week a 30-year-old woman received treatment with trimethoprim-sulfamethoxazole for bloody diarrhea. She now presents with a creatinine of 6.0 mg/dL (normal 0.5-1.0) and a hemoglobin of 7.2 g/dL (normal 12.5-14.0).

Gastroenterology

Answers

230. The answer is c. (*Fauci, pp 2006-2010.*) The Ranson criteria are used to determine prognosis in acute pancreatitis. Factors that adversely affect survival include age greater than 55 years, leukocytosis greater than 16, 000/μm, glucose greater than 200 mg/dL, LDH greater than 400 U/L, and AST greater than 250 U/L. After the initial 48 hours, a decrease in hematocrit, hypocalcemia, hypoxemia, an increase in BUN, and hypoalbuminemia predict a poor prognosis. Hypotension with systolic BP less than 90 mm Hg is also a poor prognostic sign; diastolic hypertension is not correlated with prognosis. Although serum amylase and lipase elevations are important in the diagnosis of pancreatitis, the degree of elevation is not prognostic. Tachycardia is frequently associated with the pain of pancreatitis but is not a risk factor in the Ranson criteria.

231. The answer is b. (*Fauci, pp 241-242.*) Delayed gastric emptying (gastroparesis) is a common cause of recurrent vomiting, nausea, early satiety, and weight loss in poorly controlled diabetics. Abdominal discomfort is often nonspecific, but may be localized to the upper abdomen and often awakens the patient at night. Drugs with anticholinergic properties may aggravate the problem. The best diagnostic test is a scintigraphic gastric emptying study, which will show delay in gastric emptying. Treatment includes withdrawal of aggravating drugs such as opiates and those that have anticholinergic properties, good diabetes control, and drug therapy with metoclopropamide or erythromycin. The patient's symptoms are not those of esophageal disease (dysphagia, odynophagia), so a barium esophagram would not be useful. Her symptoms also do not suggest colonic pathology; in the absence of iron deficiency, colonoscopy would not be indicated. You would not order a liver biopsy in a patient with normal liver enzymes and CT scan of the abdomen. Small bowel biopsy would be indicated if her symptoms suggest intestinal malabsorption.

232. The answer is c. (*Fauci, pp 1857-1858.*) Duodenal ulcer is more common in men than women, but *H pylori* is present in 70% of patients (men and women) who have a duodenal ulcer not associated with NSAID ingestion. In gastric ulcer disease, the incidence of H pylori is 30 to 60%. H pylori is more common in developing countries but is often seen in the United States. It is more common in patients with low socioeconomic status, in particular those with unsanitary living conditions, which suggests that H pylori is transmitted by fecal-oral or oral-oral routes. In patients with duodenal ulcer, organisms consistent with H pylori are frequently seen on biopsy. Before the discovery of H pylori, most duodenal ulcers would reoccur. Adenocarcinoma of the duodenum is a rare cause of upper gastrointestinal bleeding.

233. The answer is a. *(Fauci, pp 267-268, 1978-1979.)* Paracentesis is required to evaluate new-onset ascites. While cirrhosis and portal hypertension are most likely in this patient, complicating diseases such as tuberculous peritonitis and hepatoma are ruled out by analysis of ascitic fluid. An ultrasound or CT scan can be used to demonstrate ascitic fluid in equivocal cases. A serum albumin minus ascitic fluid albumin greater than 1.1 suggests portal hypertension alone as a cause for ascites. Tuberculosis, pancreatitis, and malignancy would cause inflammation and increased capillary permeability, causing protein to leak into the ascitic fluid. This would result in a gradient between the serum and ascitic fluid of less than 1.1. Upper GI radiographs are less useful than endoscopy in demonstrating the esophageal varices that may be associated with cirrhosis. Neither serum ethanol level nor an evaluation of the peripheral blood smear for evidence of folate deficiency would specifically address the ascites.

234. The answer is a. *(Fauci, pp 1927-1931.)* Patients with jaundice should be characterized as having unconjugated (indirect reacting) or conjugated (direct) hyperbilirubinemia. Causes of unconjugated hyperbilirubinemia include hemolysis, ineffective erythropoiesis, or enzyme deficiencies (the commonest in adults being Gilbert syndrome). The patient, however, has conjugated hyperbilirubinemia, which almost always indicates significant liver dysfunction, either hepatocellular or cholestatic (obstructive); this patient's predominant elevation of alkaline phosphatase suggests a cholestatic pattern. Normal transaminases rule out hepatocellular damage (such as viral or alcoholic hepatitis). Instead, a disease of bile ducts or a cause of impaired bile excretion should be considered. Ultrasound or CT scan will evaluate the patient for an obstructing cancer or stone disease versus intrahepatic cholestasis. Ferritin values would evaluate for hemochromatosis, but this disease typically causes transaminase elevation and hepatomegaly. Primary biliary cirrhosis (evaluated by the antimitochondrial antibody test) might be considered if imaging studies show a nondilated biliary system (suggesting intrahepatic cholestasis), but PBC is usually seen in middle-aged women.

235. The answer is c. *(Fauci, pp 573-575.)* It is likely that most colon cancers start out as adenomatous polyps; this explains the rationale for using colonoscopy as a preventative test for colon cancer, despite the fact that proof is lacking. Larger polyps, sessile polyps, and those that contain villous elements are more likely to harbor malignancies. Patients who have had one adenomatous polyp removed have a 30% to 50% chance of developing another polyp, but the regrowth is slow (taking at least 3 years to become clinically significant). Repeat colonoscopy is, therefore, recommended 3 years after the adenoma has been removed.

236. The answer is c. *(Fauci, pp 1862-1867.)* Although acid suppression therapy leads to 80% healing rates after 4 weeks of treatment, acid reduction with omeprazole or ranitidine alone does not eradicate H pylori. Three-or four-drug therapy, including bismuth or (most often) proton pump inhibitor, combined with two antibiotics effective against H pylori, will be necessary to eradicate the organism. Longer duration of therapy (ie, 14 days) leads to a greater healing rate. This regimen will eradicate H pylori in more than 90% of patients. Patients whose H pylori has been eradicated have only a 5% chance of ulcer recurrence (compared to 60 to 70% of patients not treated for H pylori). Follow-up tests to prove H pylori eradication are not recommended in the usual patient who becomes asymptomatic. If the peptic ulcer should recur (again, this happens infrequently), either direct testing of a biopsy specimen or a test for urease activity in the stomach (ie, the C 13 breath test) is necessary, as the serological studies remain positive for many years. Benzathine penicillin is commonly used to treat syphilis but not Helicobacter.

237. The answer is e. *(Fauci, pp 1903-1906.)* The most likely diagnosis in this patient is acute diverticulitis. Diverticulitis results from obstruction of a preexisting colon diverticulum. Colonic diverticulosis is very common in Western societies, and over half of Americans over age 60 have diverticula. Diverticulosis is asymptomatic. However, obstruction of a diverticulum can result in a microscopic perforation contained by the mesentery, or frank perforation and development of a peridiverticular abscess. Diverticulitis is classically associated with abdominal pain and fever. The pain is typically located in the left lower quadrant because the sigmoid is the most common region of the colon to be affected by diverticulosis. The marked leukocytosis in this patient combined with rebound tenderness suggests the possibility of a peridiverticular abscess. Diverticulitis can usually be diagnosed by CT scan of the abdomen and pelvis, which can also detect an associated diverticular abscess. Abdominal ultrasound is rarely useful in assessing colon pathology. Diverticulitis should be treated with antibiotics that are effective against coliforms and anaerobes. A typical choice is ciprofloxacin and metronidazole. Diverticular abscesses frequently require drainage which can often be done percutaneously. Immediate surgery is reserved for cases refractory to antibiotics and percutaneous drainage. Because of the increased risk of colon perforation, colonoscopy and barium enema are usually deferred for 4 to 6 weeks in patients with acute diverticulitis.

238. The answer is d. *(Fauci, pp 1920-1921, 1979.)* Hepatic encephalopathy presents as a change of consciousness, behavior, and neuromuscular function associated with liver disease. Hyperreflexia and asterixis (flapping tremor) are clinical manifestations of toxins in the systemic circulation as a result of impaired hepatic clearance. Fever, gastrointestinal bleeding, and sedation are all potential precipitating factors in a patient with liver disease. Meningitis, subdural hematoma, and postictal state can occur in the alcoholic patient but would not cause asterixis. In difficult cases, these may need to be distinguished from encephalopathy by additional tests such as lumbar puncture, CT scan, or EEG. Cryoglobulinemia can be associated with hepatitis C but does not cause CNS symptoms.

239. The answer is b. *(Fauci, pp 570-571.)* The most likely diagnosis in this patient is esophageal carcinoma. Dysphagia is progressive, first for solids and then liquids. There is blood in the stool and a history of weight loss. Alcohol use and cigarette smoking are risk factors. Prognosis is not good in this patient. Difficulty swallowing suggests significant esophageal narrowing, and usually this means that the disease is incurable. A barium contrast study should demonstrate an esophageal carcinoma with marked narrowing and an irregular, ragged mucosal pattern. Formerly, squamous cell carcinoma accounted for 90% of esophageal cancer, but its incidence is decreasing. Now more than 50% are adenocarcinomas, most often associated with Barrett esophagus. CT scan of the abdomen and pelvis is not helpful in demonstrating esophageal pathology. Peptic ulcer disease does not cause dysphagia. Achalasia would not cause guaiac-positive stools or progressive symptoms. Herpes simplex virus can cause an acute esophagitis in immunocompromised patients. It is characterized by odynophagia, not progressive dysphagia.

240. The answer is a. (*Fauci, pp 1851-1852.*) In the absence of alarm symptoms (such as dysphagia, odynophagia, weight loss, or gastrointestinal bleeding), a therapeutic trial of acid reduction therapy is reasonable. Mild to moderate GERD symptoms often respond to H_2 blockers. More severe disease, including erosive esophagitis, usually requires proton pump inhibitor therapy for 8 weeks to ensure healing. If the patient has recurrent symptoms or has had symptomatic GERD for over 5 years, endoscopy may be indicated to rule out Barrett esophagus (intestinal metaplasia of the lower esophagus). Barrett esophagus is a premalignant condition, and most patients receive surveillance EGD every 2 to 3 years, although evidence of mortality benefit from this approach is not available. In the absence of alarm symptoms, a therapeutic trial is generally favored over more expensive diagnostic studies (endoscopy, CT scan). Classic symptoms of GERD do not mandate an evaluation for coronary artery disease unless other features suggest this diagnosis.

241. The answer is c. (*Fauci, pp 1877-1885.*) The patient's history suggests malabsorption. Weight loss despite increased appetite goes with either a hypermetabolic state (such as hyperthyroidism) or nutrient malabsorption. The gastrointestinal symptoms support the diagnosis of malabsorption. Patients may notice greasy malodorous stools, increase in stool frequency, stools that are tenacious and difficult to flush, as well as changes in bowel habit according to the fat content of the diet. In the United States, celiac sprue (gluten-sensitive enteropathy) and chronic pancreatic insufficiency are the commonest causes of malabsorption. The histological pattern described in option c is associated with celiac sprue. IgA antiendomysial antibodies and antibodies against tissue transglutaminase provide supporting evidence. Signet ring cells are seen with gastric cancer. This lesion can cause weight loss through anorexia or early satiety but would not cause malabsorption. The changes described in option b are associated with ulcerative colitis; since this disease affects only the colon, small bowel absorption is not affected. *Helicobacter pylori* (which can be seen as curved gram-negative rods on gastric biopsy) is not associated with malabsorption. Periportal inflammation is seen in chronic hepatitis but does not cause malabsorption.

242. The answer is d. (*Fauci, pp 1992-1995.*) Cholelithiasis (gallstone disease) is very common. Risk factors for the development of gallstones include advancing age, female gender, obesity, prior pregnancies, native American or Mexican American ancestry, and rapid weight loss. Many patients are asymptomatic but some develop biliary colic. About half of symptomatic patients will have recurrent episodes, and 1% to 2% will develop complications annually. The treatment of choice is cholecystectomy, which can usually be performed laparoscopically. This woman's symptoms are classic for biliary colic; acid reducers such as omeprazole would not be useful. Although ursodeoxycholic acid can dissolve gallstones, they usually recur, and this drug is no longer considered appropriate therapy unless surgery is contraindicated. Weight reduction does not dissolve gallstones, and rapid weight loss can precipitate symptoms. In order to prevent complications, symptomatic patients with low operative risk are usually managed with surgery rather than with observation. Asymptomatic gallstone disease is followed and treated surgically if symptoms develop.

243. The answer is b. (*Fauci pp 808, 1978-1979.*) Spontaneous bacterial peritonitis is the occurrence of a bacterial infection in preexisting ascitic fluid without bowel wall perforation. It is almost always caused by a single species; isolation of multiple species would suggest a bowel wall perforation. The typical patient has preexisting cirrhosis and ascites, and presents with fever and abdominal pain. Acute deterioration of liver function and hepatic encephalopathy are common. An ascitic fluid PMN cell count of greater than $250/\mu L$ confirms the diagnosis, even if the culture is negative. Standard antibiotic therapy is a fluoroquinolone or third-generation cephalosporin for 7 to 10 days. Response to therapy can be judged clinically and repeated paracentesis is not usually necessary. The addition of albumin to antibiotic therapy has been shown to improve survival. Recurrence rates are high, and long-term prophylactic therapy with a fluoroquinolone is recommended.

244. The answer is e. (*Fauci, pp 1983-1990.*) Cirrhosis caused by hepatitis C is the most common cause for liver transplantation in the United States. A previous history of alcoholism is not a contraindication to transplantation, although most transplant centers require abstinence from alcohol for 6 months before transplantation is considered. Three-year survival rate after transplantation in most centers now exceeds 80%. The model for end-stage liver disease (MELD) scoring system is used in the United States to allocate cadaveric livers to potential donors. Patients with complications of cirrhosis (esophageal variceal bleeding, hepatic encephalopathy, and uncontrolled ascites) or who have significantly elevated bilirubin, INR, and serum creatinine are usually made eligible for transplantation. Repeat liver biopsy would be unnecessary and potentially risky due to the patient's coagulopathy. Patients with end-stage cirrhosis from hepatitis C do not benefit from interferon and ribavirin therapy.

245. The answer is d. (*Fauci, pp 2429-2433.*) Hemochromatosis is a disorder of iron storage that results in deposition of iron in parenchymal cells. The liver is usually enlarged, and excessive skin pigmentation is present in 90% of symptomatic patients at the time of diagnosis. Diabetes occurs secondary to direct damage of the pancreas by iron deposition. Arthropathy develops in 25% to 50% of cases. Other diagnoses listed could not explain all the manifestations of this patient's disease process. Diabetes and pancreatic cancer would not account for the hyperpigmentation or joint symptoms. Addison disease can cause weight loss and hyperpigmentation but does not affect the liver or joints; it is associated with hypoglycemia rather than diabetes mellitus. Metabolic syndrome is not associated with weight loss, hyperpigmentation, or joint symptoms.

246. The answer is a. (*Fauci, pp 1899-1902.*) This patient meets the Rome II criteria for irritable bowel syndrome. The major criterion is abdominal pain relieved with defecation and associated with change in stool frequency or consistency. In addition, these patients often complain of difficult stool passage, a feeling of incomplete evacuation, and mucus in the stool. In this young patient with long-standing symptoms and no evidence of organic disease on physical and laboratory studies, further evaluation (ie, colonoscopy or small bowel studies for sprue) is unnecessary. Irritable bowel syndrome is a motility disorder associated with altered sensitivity to abdominal pain and distension. It is the commonest cause of chronic GI symptoms and is three times more common in women than in men. Associated lactose intolerance may cause similar symptoms and should be considered in all cases. Patients older than 40 years with new symptoms, weight loss, or positive family history of colon cancer should have further workup, usually with colonoscopy.

247. The answer is a. (*Fauci, pp 2001-2017.*) Chronic pancreatitis is caused by pancreatic damage from repeated attacks of acute pancreatitis.

The classic triad is abdominal pain, malabsorption, and diabetes mellitus. Twenty-five percent of cases are idiopathic. Vitamins D and K are absorbed intact from the intestine without digestion by lipase and are therefore absorbed normally in pancreatic insufficiency. Forty percent of patients, however, develop B$_{12}$ deficiency. Treatment of the malabsorption with pancreatic enzyme replacement will lead to weight gain, but the pain can be difficult to treat. Courvoisier sign is a palpable, nontender gall-bladder in a jaundiced patient. This finding suggests the presence of a malignancy, usually pancreatic cancer. Chronic pancreatitis per se does not produce guaiac-positive stools. Amylase is usually normal in patients with chronic pancreatitis.

248. The answer is a. *(Fauci, pp 818-821.)* *Clostridium difficile* is an important cause of diarrhea in patients who receive antibiotic therapy. *C difficile* proliferates in the gastrointestinal tract when the normal enteric bacteria are altered by antibiotics. Commonly implicated antibiotics include ampicillin, penicillin, clindamycin, cephalosporins, and trimethoprim-sulfamethoxazole. The diarrhea is usually mild to moderate, but can be profound. Other clinical findings include fever, abdominal pain, abdominal tenderness, leukocytosis, and serum electrolyte abnormalities. The diagnosis is made by demonstration at sigmoidoscopy of yellowish plaques (pseudomembranes) that cover the colonic mucosa or by detection of *C difficile* toxin in the stool. The pseudomembranes consist of a tenacious fibrinopurulent mucosal exudate that contains extruded leukocytes, mucin, and sloughed mucosa. Isolation of *C difficile* from stool cultures is nonspecific because of asymptomatic carriage, particularly in infants. Testing for fecal leukocytes is also nonspecific and may be negative in *C difficile* colitis. Serological tests are not clinically useful for diagnosing this infection. Pseudomembranous colitis demands discontinuation of the offending antibiotic. Antibiotic therapy for moderate or severe disease includes oral metronidazole or vancomycin. Cholestyramine can be used therapeutically to bind the diarrheogenic toxin. Clue cells are bacteria-coated vaginal epithelial cells, used to diagnose bacterial vaginosis. They are not seen in stool.

249. The answer is e. *(Fauci, pp 1962-1966.)* This patient has chronic hepatitis C. A positive test for hepatitis C viral RNA confirms the diagnosis. Liver biopsy is not necessary for confirmation, but may be useful in predicting candidacy for treatment. Chronic hepatitis C rarely resolves spontaneously. Untreated, about 15% of patients with hepatitis C will eventually develop cirrhosis. The levels of ALT and viral RNA correlate poorly with histologic disease and eventual prognosis. Treatment with pegylated interferon and ribavirin is aimed at preventing cirrhosis. Females, patients under age 40, patients with minimal or no cirrhosis, and those infected with genotypes 2 and 3 are more likely to respond to treatment. All patients with chronic hepatitis C should receive vaccination against hepatitis A and B, which can cause fulminate hepatic failure in patients with preexisting hepatitis C.

250. The answer is d. *(Fauci, pp 1847-1851.)* The barium swallow shows the dilated baglike proximal esophagus and tapered distal esophageal ring characteristic of achalasia. This is a motor disorder of the esophagus and classically produces dysphagia to both solids and liquids. Structural disorders such as cancer and stricture usually cause trouble swallowing solids as the first manifestation. In achalasia, manometry shows elevated pressure and poor relaxation of the lower esophageal sphincter. In classic achalasia the contractions of the esophagus are weak, although a variant called *vigorous achalasia* is associated with large-amplitude prolonged contractions. Medications (nitrates, calcium channel blockers, botox injections into the LES) or physical procedures (balloon dilatation or surgical myotomy) that decrease LES pressure are the recommended treatments. Squamous cell carcinoma would not cause esophageal dilation and would be associated with ratty rather than smooth tapering of the esophagus. Achalasia is not associated with gastroesophageal reflux disease. Although anxiety can cause dysphagia and a globus-like sensation in the cricoid region, it would not cause the anatomical changes seen on this barium swallow.

251. The answer is a. *(Fauci, pp 1980-1983.)* This woman likely has non-alcoholic fatty liver (NAFL), which is associated with macrovesicular accumulation of fat in the liver. If hepatocellular necrosis is present, the condition is termed *nonalcoholic steatohepatitis* (NASH). This condition is histologically similar to alcoholic hepatitis, and increasing evidence suggests that it too is a precirrhotic condition. With the increasing incidence of obesity in Western societies, NASH may become the commonest cause of cirrhosis and end-stage liver disease. Microvesicular fat is seen in the acute life-threatening conditions of acute fatty liver of pregnancy and Reye syndrome. Portal triaditis and piecemeal necrosis of cells in the hepatic lobule are associated with several disorders, including autoimmune and chronic viral hepatitis. Cirrhosis, characterized by bands of fibrous tissue, regenerating nodules, and disruption of the hepatic architecture, is the final common pathway of various chronic insults to the liver. Copper deposition is seen in Wilson disease.

252 to 254. The answers are 252-b, 253-f, 254-d. *(Fauci, pp 2007-2009, 1910-1914.)* Pancreatitis typically causes severe abdominal pain that radiates into the back. It is almost always associated with nausea and vomiting. The most common etiology is heavy alcohol use. Other etiologies include gallstones, hyperlipidemia, certain medications (such as azathioprine and hydrochlorothiazide), trauma, and after ERCP. Serum amylase and lipase are typically elevated. Mild elevation of the amylase can also occur in renal failure, appendicitis, and mumps.

Intermittent mesenteric ischemia occurs from atherosclerotic obstruction of visceral arteries. Patients typically present with postprandial abdominal pain and weight loss ("intestinal angina"). Men are more commonly affected than women and usually have atherosclerotic disease elsewhere. Cigarette smoking is a risk factor. Diagnosis is usually made by Doppler ultrasound of the mesenteric vessels and confirmed by contrast angiography. Treatment is usually surgical.

Acute intestinal obstruction is most often associated with adhesive bands from previous surgery. Hysterectomy and appendectomy are the most common preceding surgeries, although any operation associated with entry into the peritoneum can cause adhesions. The patient usually has the classic colicky pain associated with several pain-free minutes before the pain again builds up to maximum intensity. This kind of pain is much more commonly associated with intestinal obstruction than biliary or renal disease (so-called biliary and renal colic are often constant pains).

255 to 256. The answers are 255-a, 256-d. *(Fauci, pp 580-585, 1974-1976.)* Primary biliary cirrhosis usually occurs in women between the ages of 35 and 60. The earliest symptom is pruritus, often accompanied by fatigue. Serum alkaline phosphatase is elevated two- to fivefold, and a positive antimitochondrial antibody test greater than 1:40 is both sensitive and specific.

Hepatocellular carcinoma is more common in men than women and has a peak incidence between 40 and 60 years of age. A major risk factor is cirrhosis. Hepatitis B and hepatitis C are independent risk factors. The typical patient has preexisting cirrhosis and presents with right upper quadrant pain and a palpable mass. Serum alkaline phosphatase and alpha-fetoprotein are elevated. Diagnosis is confirmed by biopsy. Surgical resection offers the only chance for cure, but most patients do not have resectable disease at presentation.

257 to 259. The answers are 257-a, 258-b, 259-c. *(Fauci, pp 261-265.)* The young African American male with mild jaundice has unconjugated hyperbilirubinemia and an anemia. Unconjugated bilirubin is bound to albumin in the circulation and is not excreted in the urine; hence the urine bilirubin level is negative. His jaundice may be secondary to G6PD deficiency with hemolysis precipitated by an offending antibiotic (sulfonamide or trimethoprim-sulfamethoxazole). These patients are unable to maintain an adequate level of reduced glutathione in their red blood cells when an antibiotic or other toxin causes oxidative stress to the red cells. The 60-year-old male with jaundice has an obstructive process, as his pale stools suggest the lack of bilirubin in the stool. A high alkaline phosphatase also indicates that there is an obstructive jaundice. Pancreatic carcinoma would be the most likely cause of obstructive jaundice in this patient. The young woman's case is most consistent with acute hepatitis—srtikingly elevated hepatocellular enzymes and conjugated hyperbilirubinemia. Tenderness of the liver on palpation is common in acute hepatitis.

260 to 262. The answers are 260-a, 261-b, 262-d. *(Fauci, pp 257-260.)* Nonsteroidal anti-inflammatory drugs, even over-the-counter brands, are common causes of GI bleeding. Preceding symptoms may be mild before the bleeding occurs. Cotreatment with misoprostol decreases GI bleeding but is quite expensive. Selective COX-2 inhibitors decrease the incidence of GI bleeding, but have recently been shown to increase cardiovascular events and to carry the same risk of renal dysfunction, edema, and blood pressure elevation as nonselective NSAIDs.

Erosion of the proximal end of a woven aortic graft into the distal duodenum or proximal jejunum can occur many years after surgery for abdominal aortic aneurysm. Often, the patient will have a smaller herald bleed, which is then followed by catastrophic bleeding. A high index of suspicion is necessary, as timely surgery can be lifesaving.

Cirrhosis is often associated with portal hypertension, esophageal varices, and hemorrhoids. Acute bleeding from esophageal varices frequently causes massive hematemesis and can be fatal. Endoscopic band ligation is the treatment of choice. Patients with large varices are less likely to hemorrhage if they receive prophylactic treatment with beta-blockers such as propranolol.

263 to 265. The answers are 263-b, 264-a, 265-c. *(Fauci, pp 1886-1899.)* Crohn disease can affect the entire GI tract from mouth to anus. Right lower quadrant pain, tenderness, and an inflammatory mass would suggest involvement of the terminal ileum. As opposed to ulcerative colitis (a pure mucosal disease), full-thickness involvement of the gut wall can lead to fistula and abscess formation. Skip lesions (ie, segmental involvement) can also help distinguish Crohn disease from UC; granuloma formation on biopsies would also support the diagnosis of Crohn disease.

Although thought of as a disease of young adults, ulcerative colitis has a second peak of incidence in the 60- to 80-year age group and should be considered in the differential diagnosis of diarrhea at any age. Colonic involvement starts in the rectum and proceeds toward the cecum in a continuous fashion (ie, no skip lesions). Inflammation is limited to the mucosa; so fistulas, abscesses, and granulomas are not seen.

Ischemic colitis usually occurs in the older age group. The ischemia is usually confined to the mucosa, so perforation is unusual. Pain is a prominent complaint and may mimic acute diverticulitis. The finding of segmental inflammation in watershed areas in the vascular distribution of the colon is characteristic. Most patients improve without surgical intervention.

266 to 268. The answers are 266-e, 267-a, 268-d. *(Fauci, pp 247-249, 813-818.)* Infection with *Salmonella* usually occurs by ingesting contaminated poultry or eggs, but has also been associated with handling turtles, lizards, and other reptiles. *Salmonella* gastroenteritis is often associated with fever and bloody diarrhea. Unless the patient is severely ill, antibiotic therapy is withheld because it can be associated with prolonged excretion of the organism in the stool.

Food-borne illness (food poisoning) is a very common cause of acute GI symptoms. This patient's short incubation period (indicating preformed toxin rather than bacterial proliferation in the body) as well as the prominent upper GI symptoms are characteristic of staphylococcal food poisoning.

Infection with certain enterotoxigenic *E coli* can cause bloody diarrhea and fever. A particular strain (O157H7) has been associated with the hemolytic uremic syndrome. This occurs more commonly in patients who have been treated with antibiotics.

Nephrology

Questions

269. A 76-year-old male presents to the emergency room. He had influenza and now presents with diffuse muscle pain and weakness. His past medical history is remarkable for osteoarthritis for which he takes ibuprofen, and hypercholesterolemia for which he takes lovastatin. Physical examination reveals blood pressure of 130/90 with no orthostatic change. The only other finding is diffuse muscle tenderness. Laboratory data include

BUN: 30 mg/dL
Creatinine: 6 mg/dL
K: 6.0 mEq/L
Uric acid: 18 mg/dL
Ca: 6.5 mg/dL
PO_4: 7.5 mg/dL
UA: large blood, 2+ protein. Microscopic study shows muddy brown casts and 0 to 2 RBC/HPF (red blood cells/high power field).

Which of the following is the most likely diagnosis?

a. Nonsteroidal anti-inflammatory drug-induced acute renal failure (ARF)
b. Volume depletion
c. Rhabdomyolysis-induced ARF
d. Urinary tract obstruction
e. Hypertensive nephrosclerosis

270. A 20-year-old male presents with obtundation. Past medical history is unobtainable. Blood pressure is 120/70 without orthostatic change, and he is well perfused peripherally. The neurological examination is nonfocal. His laboratory values are as follows:

Na: 138 mEq/L
K: 4.2 mEq/L
HCO_3: 5 mEq/L
Cl: 104 mEq/L
Creatinine: 1.0 mg/dL
BUN: 14 mg/dL
Ca: 10 mg/dL
Arterial blood gas on room air: Po_2 96, Pco_2 15, pH 7.02
Blood glucose: 90 mg/dL
Urinalysis: normal, without blood, protein, or crystals

Which of the following is the most likely acid-base disorder?

a. Pure normal anion-gap metabolic acidosis
b. Respiratory acidosis
c. Pure high anion-gap metabolic acidosis
d. Combined high anion-gap metabolic acidosis and respiratory alkalosis
e. Combined high anion-gap metabolic acidosis and respiratory acidosis

271. An 83-year-old woman presents for follow-up of hypertension, type 2 diabetes mellitus, and depression. She complains of fatigue and mild dependent edema. Her medications include hydrochlorothiazide 25 mg/d, atenolol 50 mg/d, glyburide 5 mg bid., and paroxetine 20 mg/d. Physical examination shows BP 152/88, weight 42 kg, clear lung fields, normal liver and spleen, and 1+ peripheral edema. She appears mildly pale. CBC shows Hb 9.6 with an MCV of 87 and normal WBC and platelets. Chem profile shows Na 136, K 4.9, CO_2 18, Cl 108, creat 1.5, and glucose 178 mg/dL. Liver enzymes are normal. What is the most likely cause of her anemia?

a. Anemia of chronic kidney disease (CKD)
b. Anemia of chronic disease caused by diabetes
c. Depression with nutritional folate deficiency
d. Occult colon cancer
e. Medication-induced bone marrow suppression

272. A 53-year-old male with septic shock develops acute renal failure with a serum creatinine of 6.4 mg/dL. Which of the following is a specific indication to initiate dialysis?

a. BUN rises to 75 mg/dL.
b. Urine output falls to < 10 mL/h.
c. Pericardial friction rub develops.
d. Hematocrit falls to < 30%.
e. Continued hypotension

273. A 68-year-old woman with stable coronary artery disease undergoes an aortogram with lower extremity run-off studies for symptomatic peripheral vascular disease. The patient is on warfarin (for recurrent deep vein thrombosis), aspirin, lisinopril, metoprolol, and atorvastatin. She received a course of dicloxacillin for cellulitis 1 week ago. Three weeks after angiography the patient is evaluated for general malaise. Physical examination reveals a petechial rash and livedo reticularis on both lower extremities. Laboratory evaluation reveals that her creatinine has risen from 1.5 to 3.7 mg/dL. Other laboratory abnormalities include an ESR of 96 mm/h, leukocytosis, eosinophilia, and a reduced third component of complement (C3). Urine sodium is 40 mEq/L. Urinalysis reveals 5 to 10 eosinophils/HPF, 10 to 20 WBC/HPF, 5 to 10 RBC/HPF, no casts, and 1+ dipstick proteinuria. Which of the following is the most likely diagnosis?

a. Prerenal azotemia
b. Radiocontrast-induced acute renal failure
c. Drug-induced acute interstitial nephritis
d. Acute glomerulonephritis
e. Atheroembolic renal failure

274. A 47-year-old HIV positive man is brought to the emergency room because of weakness. The patient has HIV nephropathy and adrenal insufficiency. He takes trimethoprim-sulfamethoxazole for PCP prophylaxis and is on triple agent antiretroviral treatment. He was recently started on spironolactone for ascites due to alcoholic liver disease. Physical examination reveals normal vital signs, but his muscles are diffusely weak. Frequent extrasystoles are noted. He has mild ascites and 1+ peripheral edema. Laboratory studies show a serum creatinine of 2.5 with a potassium value of 7.3 mEq/L. An EKG shows peaking of the T waves and QRS duration of 0.14. What is the most important immediate treatment?

a. Sodium polystyrene sulfonate (Kayexalate)
b. Acute hemodialysis
c. IV normal saline
d. IV calcium gluconate
e. IV furosemide 80 mg stat

275. A 30-year-old male is brought to the emergency room from prison, where he works in the paint shop. He is barely arousable but has no focal abnormalities. He has no past medical history. CT scan of the head is normal. Urine toxicology screen is negative. Ethanol and acetaminophen are not detectable. Laboratory data is as follows:

Na: 140 mEq/L
K: 5.1 mEq/L
Cl: 100 mEq/L
HCO_3 10 mEq/L
Creatinine 1.2 mg/dL
Blood ethanol: nondetectable
Blood glucose: 110 mg/dL
Arterial blood gases: PO_2 88, PCO_2 23, pH 7.21

Which of the following tests will provide the key to correct diagnosis?

a. Serum ketones
b. Serum lactate
c. Serum creatine kinase
d. Measured plasma osmolality
e. Magnetic resonance scan of the head

276. A 73-year-old male undergoes abdominal aortic aneurysm repair. Postoperatively, his blood pressure is 110/70, heart rate is 110, surgical wound is clean, and a Foley catheter is in place. His urine output drops to 40 cc/h, and creatinine rises from 1.5 to 2.2 mg/dL. Hemoglobin and hematocrit are stable, K 4.6, uric acid 8.2. Which initial diagnostic test is most useful for this patient?

a. Urine sodium/creatinine ratio
b. Urinalysis
c. Renal ultrasound
d. Urine uric acid/creatinine ratio
e. CT renal arteriogram

277. A 25-year-old man is referred to you because of hematuria. He noticed brief reddening of the urine with a recent respiratory infection. The gross hematuria resolved, but his physician found microscopic hematuria on two subsequent first-voided morning urine specimens. The patient is otherwise healthy; he does not smoke. His blood pressure is 114/72 and the physical examination is normal. The urinalysis shows 2+ protein and 10 to 15 RBC/HPF, with some dysmorphic erythrocytes. No WBC or casts are seen. What is the most likely cause of his hematuria?

a. Kidney stone
b. Renal cell carcinoma
c. Acute poststreptococcal glomerulonephritis
d. Chronic prostatitis
e. IgA nephropathy (Berger disease)

278. A 17-year-old male is brought to the emergency room with confusion and incoordination. He is uncooperative and refuses to provide further history. Physical examination reveals an RR of 30; the vital signs are otherwise normal as is the general physical examination. Laboratory values are as follows:

Na: 135 mEq/L
K: 2.7 mEq/L
HCO_3: 15 mEq/L
Cl: 110 mEq/L
Arterial blood gases: Po_2 92, Pco_2 30, pH 7.28
Urine: pH 7.5, glucose—negative
Ca: 9.7 mg/dL
PO_4: 4.0 mg/dL

Which of the following is the most likely cause of the acid base disorder?

a. GI loss owing to diarrhea
b. Proximal renal tubular acidosis
c. Disorder of the renin-angiotensin system
d. Distal renal tubular acidosis
e. Respiratory acidosis

279. A 56-year-old man presents with hypertension and peripheral edema. He is otherwise healthy and takes no medications. Family history reveals that his father and a brother have kidney disease. His father was on hemodialysis before his death at age 68 of a stroke. Physical examination reveals BP 174/96 and AV nicking on funduscopic examination. He has a soft S_4 gallop. Bilateral flank masses measuring 16 cm in length are palpable. Urinalysis shows 15 to 20 RBC/HPF and trace protein but is otherwise normal; his serum creatinine is 2.4 mg/dL.

Which is the most likely long-term complication of his condition?

a. End-stage renal disease requiring dialysis or transplantation
b. Malignancy
c. Ruptured cerebral aneurysm
d. Biliary obstruction owing to cystic disease of the pancreas
e. Dementia

280. A 73-year-old female with arthritis presents with confusion. Neurologic examination is nonfocal, and CT of the head is normal. Laboratory data include

Na: 140 mEq/L
K: 3.0 mEq/L
Cl: 107 mEq/L
HCO_3: 12 mEq/L
Arterial blood gases: PO_2 62, PCO_2 24, pH 7.40

What is the acid-base disturbance?

a. Respiratory alkalosis with appropriate metabolic compensation
b. High anion-gap metabolic acidosis with appropriate respiratory compensation
c. Combined metabolic acidosis and respiratory alkalosis
d. No acid-base disorder
e. Hyperchloremic (normal anion gap) metabolic acidosis with appropriate respiratory compensation

281. A 17-year-old woman presents with peripheral and periorbital edema. She has previously been healthy and takes no medications. Her blood pressure is 146/92; she is afebrile. The patient has mild basilar dullness on lung examination; her cardiac examination is normal. She has periorbital edema and soft doughy 3+ edema in her legs. Her serum creatinine is 0.6 mg/dL and her serum albumin is 2.1 g/L. Urinalysis shows 3+ protein, no RBC or WBC, and some oval fat bodies. What is the most important initial diagnostic test?

a. Serum and urine protein electrophoresis
b. Serum cholesterol and triglyceride measurement
c. Plasma aldosterone and renin activity
d. Quantitation of urine albumin excretion
e. Renal biopsy

282. A 63-year-old male alcoholic with a 50-pack-year history of smoking presents to the emergency room with fatigue and confusion. Physical examination reveals a blood pressure of 110/70 with no orthostatic change. Heart, lung, and abdominal examination are normal and there is no pedal edema. Laboratory data is as follows:

Na: 110 mEq/L
K: 3.7 mEq/L
Cl: 82 mEq/L
HCO_3: 20 mEq/L
Glucose: 100 mg/dL
BUN: 5 mg/dL
Creatinine: 0.7 mg/dL
Urinalysis: normal. Specific gravity: 1.016.

Which of the following is the most likely diagnosis?

a. Volume depletion
b. Inappropriate secretion of antidiuretic hormone
c. Psychogenic polydipsia
d. Cirrhosis
e. Congestive heart failure

283. A 65-year-old diabetic male with a creatinine of 1.6 was started on an angiotensin-converting enzyme inhibitor for hypertension and presents to the emergency room with weakness. His other medications include atorvastatin for hypercholesterolemia, metoprolol and spironolactone for congestive heart failure, insulin for diabetes, and aspirin. Laboratory studies include

K: 7.2 mEq/L
Creatinine: 1.8 mg/dL
Glucose: 250 mg/dL
CK: 400 IU/L

Which of the following is the most likely cause of hyperkalemia in this patient?

a. Worsening renal function
b. Uncontrolled diabetes
c. Statin-induced rhabdomyolysis
d. Drug-induced effect on the renin-angiotensin-aldosterone system
e. High potassium diet

284. A 27-year-old alcoholic presents with the following electrolytes: calcium 6.9 mg/dL, albumin 3.5 g/dL, magnesium 0.7 mg/dL, phosphorus 2.0 mg/dL. Which of the following is the most likely cause of the hypocalcemia?

a. Poor dietary intake
b. Hypoalbuminemia
c. Decreased parathyroid hormone release because of hypomagnesemia
d. Decreased end-organ response to parathyroid hormone because of hypomagnesemia
e. Osteoporosis caused by hypogonadism

285. A 27-year-old female presents to the emergency room with a panic attack. She appears healthy except for tachycardia and a respiratory rate of 30. Electrolytes include calcium 10.0 mg/dL, albumin 4.0 g/dL, phosphorus 0.8 mg/dL, and magnesium 1.5 mg/dL. Arterial blood gases include pH of 7.56, P_{CO_2} 21 mm Hg, P_{O_2} 99 mm Hg. Which of the following is the most important cause of the hypophosphatemia?

a. Hypomagnesemia
b. Hyperparathyroidism
c. Respiratory alkalosis with intracellular shift
d. Poor dietary intake
e. Vitamin D deficiency

286. A diabetic male presents with hypertension. His blood pressure is 146/92. He has no peripheral edema but does note sensory loss to the midcalves bilaterally. A spot urine specimen shows 150 micrograms of albumin per mg creatinine (microalbuminuria present if this value is 30-300 mcg/mg). Which of the following is the most appropriate antihypertensive drug to prevent progression of renal failure?

a. Clonidine
b. Beta-blocker
c. Thiazide diuretic
d. Angiotensin-converting enzyme inhibitor
e. Short-acting dihydropyridine calcium channel blocker (nifedipine)

287. A 29-year-old male with HIV, on indinavir, zidovudine, and stavudine, presents with severe edema and a serum creatinine of 2.0 mg/dL. He has had bone pain for 5 years and takes large amounts of acetaminophen with codeine, aspirin, and ibuprofen. He is on prophylactic trimethoprim-sulfamethoxazole. Blood pressure is 170/110; urinalysis shows 4+ protein, 5 to 10 RBC, 0 WBC; 24-hour urine protein is 6.2 g. The serum albumin is 1.9 g/L (normal above 3.7).Which of the following is the most likely cause of his renal disease?

a. Indinavir toxicity
b. Analgesic nephropathy
c. Trimethoprim-sulfamethoxazole–induced interstitial nephritis
d. Focal glomerulosclerosis
e. Renal artery stenosis

288. A 60-year-old male is brought in by ambulance and is unable to speak. The EMS personnel tell you that a neighbor informed them he has had a stroke in the past. There are no family members present. His serum sodium is 118 mEq/L. Which of the following is the most helpful first step in the assessment of this patient's hyponatremia?

a. Order a chest x-ray
b. Place a Foley catheter to measure 24 hour urine protein
c. Clinical assessment of extracellular fluid volume status
d. CT scan of head
e. Serum AVP (arginine vasopressin) level

289. A 39-year-old woman is admitted to the gynecology service for hysterectomy for symptomatic uterine fibroids. Postoperatively the patient develops an ileus accompanied by severe nausea and vomiting; ondansetron is piggybacked into an IV of D5 $^1/_2$ normal saline running at 125 cc/hr. On the second postoperative day the patient becomes drowsy and displays a few myoclonic jerks. Stat labs reveal Na 118, K 3.2, Cl 88 HCO$_3$ 22, BUN 3, creatinine 0.9. Urine studies for Na and osmolality are sent to the lab. What is the most appropriate next step?

a. Change the IV fluid to 0.9% (normal) saline and restrict free-water intake to 600 cc/d
b. Change the odansetron to promethazine, change the IV fluid to lactated Ringer solution and recheck the Na in 4 hours.
c. Start 3% (hypertonic) saline, make the patient NPO and transfer to the ICU
d. Change the IV fluid to normal saline and give furosemide 40mg IV stat.
e. Make the patient NPO and send for stat CT scan of the head to look for cerebral edema.

290. You evaluate a 48-year-old man for chronic renal insufficiency. He has a history of hypertension, osteoarthritis, and gout. He currently has no complaints. His medical regimen includes lisinopril 40 mg daily, hydrochlorothiazide 25 mg daily, allopurinol 300 mg daily, and acetaminophen for his joint pains. He does not smoke but drinks 8 oz of wine on a daily basis. Examination shows BP 146/86, pulse 76, a soft S_4 gallop and mild peripheral edema. There is no abdominal bruit. His UA reveals 1+ proteinuria and no cellular elements. Serum creatinine is 2.2 mg/dL and his estimated GFR from the MDRD formula is 42 ml/min. What is the most important element is preventing progression of his renal disease?

a. Discontinuing all alcohol consumption
b. Discontinuing acetaminophen
c. Adding a calcium channel blocker to improve blood pressure control
d. Obtaining a CT renal arteriogram to exclude renal artery stenosis
e. Changing the lisinopril to losartan

Questions 291 to 293

Match the clinical presentation with the likely cause of the patient's renal failure. Each lettered option may be used once, more than once, or not at all.

a. Prerenal azotemia because of intravascular volume depletion
b. Ischemia-induced acute tubular necrosis
c. Nephrotoxin-induced acute tubular necrosis
d. Acute interstitial nephritis
e. Postrenal azotemia because of obstructive uropathy
f. Postinfectious glomerulonephritis
g. Acute cortical necrosis

291. A patient is admitted to the hospital with a nursing-home acquired pneumonia. His blood pressure is normal and the extremities well-perfused. Admission creatinine is 1.2 mg/dL. UA is clear. The patient is treated on the floor with piperacillin/tazobactam and improves clinically. On the fourth hospital day, the patient notes a nonpruritic rash over the abdomen. The creatinine has risen to 2.2 mg/dL. The urinalysis shows 2+ protein, 10 to 15 WBC/HPF, and no casts or RBCs.

292. A 62-year-old man is admitted with pneumonia and severe sepsis. Vasopressors are required to maintain peripheral perfusion, and mechanical ventilation is needed because of ARDS. Admission creatinine is 1.0 mg/dL but rises by the second hospital day to 2.2 mg/dL. Urine output is 300 cc/24 hours. UA shows renal tubular epithelial cells and some muddy brown casts. The fractional excretion of sodium is 3.45.

293. A 76-year-old man is admitted with pneumonia. He has a history of diabetes mellitus. Admission creatinine is 1.2 mg/dL. He responds to ceftriaxone and azithromycin. He develops occasional urinary incontinence treated with anticholinergics, but his overall status improves and he is ready for discharge by the fifth hospital day. On that morning, however, he develops urinary hesitancy and slight suprapubic tenderness. The creatinine is found to be 3.0 mg/dL; UA is clear with no RBCs, WBCs or protein.

Questions 294 and 295

Match the clinical and microscopic presentation with the correct primary glomerular disease. Each lettered option may be used once, more than once, or not at all.

a. Minimal change disease
b. IgA nephropathy
c. Focal and segmental glomerulosclerosis
d. Thin basement membrane disease
e. Membranous nephropathy
f. Membranoproliferative glomerulonephritis

294. A 50-year-old white male presents with mild hypertension, nephrotic syndrome, microscopic hematuria, and venous thromboses (including renal vein thrombosis). Renal biopsy reveals a thickened glomerular basement membrane with subepithelial immunoglobulin deposition.

295. A 19-year-old white male presents with hypertension, nephrotic syndrome, mild renal insufficiency, RBC casts in urine, and depressed third component of complement (C3). Renal biopsy shows thickened basement membranes and increased cellular elements. Electron microscopy shows dense deposits within the basement membrane.

Questions 296 and 297

Match the presentation with the most likely systemic disease. Each lettered option may be used once, more than once, or not at all.

a. Macroscopic (classic) polyarteritis nodosa
b. Microscopic polyangiitis
c. Wegener granulomatosis
d. Goodpasture syndrome
e. Churg-Strauss syndrome
f. Essential mixed cryoglobulinemia
g. Systemic lupus erythematosus
h. Behçet disease

296. A 66-year-old male presents with severe hypertension and abdominal pain. He has low grade fever and livedo reticularis over the lower extremities. Neurological examination shows a right peroneal neuropathy and sensory loss in the left radial nerve distribution, consistent with mononeuritis multiplex. UA reveals 1+ proteinuria and 15 to 20 RBC/HPF.

297. A 75-year-old male presents with a 6 month history of nasal congestion, mild epistaxis and sinus tenderness. He develops a cough and peripheral edema. CT scan of the sinuses shows evidence of chronic sinusitis, and the chest x-ray reveals several nodular densities, one with early cavitation. His serum creatinine has risen from 1.1 mg/dL to 2.7 mg/dL over the past 3 weeks. The UA shows 2+ protein and moderate hematuria.

Questions 298 and 299

Match the type of stone with the clinical situation in which it occurs. Each lettered option may be used once, more than once, or not at all.

a. Calcium phosphate
b. Calcium oxalate
c. Cystine
d. Struvite
e. Uric acid
f. Xanthine
g. Bilirubin

298. A 50-year-old man has recurrent stones that cannot be seen on plain film of the abdomen but are readily apparent on CT scan (renal stone protocol). The urinalysis is clear but the urine pH is 4.88 on a 24-hour urine specimen.

299. A 40-year-old paraplegic with an indwelling urinary catheter has recurrent infections. The UA always shows leukocytes and the urine pH is 8. KUB shows the presence of staghorn calculi.

Nephrology

Answers

269. The answer is c. (*Fauci, pp 801-803, 1752-1761.*) Rhabdomyolysis-induced ARF is characterized by hyperkalemia, hyperphosphatemia, and hyperuricemia, all caused by release of intracellular muscle products. The high phosphorus level causes hypocalcemia. The BUN/creatinine ratio, normally 10/1, is reduced because of release of muscle creatine, which is converted to creatinine. The load of creatinine to be excreted by the failing kidney therefore exceeds the urea load, which is little changed. The presence of "blood" on the dipstick determination is caused by myoglobinuria. The dipstick registers red blood cells, hemoglobin (for instance, from intravascular hemolysis) and myoglobin as "blood." Trauma, medications (especially statins), infectious processes (influenza, sepsis), extreme muscular exertion (seizures, exertional heat stroke) are common causes.

All nonsteroidal agents may cause decreased renal function. Usually this is attributed to decreased blood flow—less commonly, to drug-induced interstitial nephritis. The laboratory abnormalities in this case do not suggest decreased blood flow or interstitial nephritis. However, stopping the ibuprofen would be prudent. The absence of orthostatic hypotension makes the diagnosis of volume depletion very unlikely. Nothing on history, physical examination, or electrolyte abnormalities suggests obstruction. However, in a 76-year-old man, a renal sonogram to rule out occult obstruction would be reasonable. Hypertensive nephrosclerosis causes chronic rather than acute renal insufficiency and would not account for the electrolyte abnormalities.

270. The answer is c. (*Fauci, pp 287-296.*) The first step in analyzing an acid-base disturbance is simply to look at the pH. This patient has an acidosis. Then look at the HCO_3 and the P_{CO_2} to determine the primary disturbance, ie, is it a metabolic acidosis or a respiratory acidosis? The serum HCO_3 has decreased from 24 to 5 mEq/L, so this must be a metabolic acidosis. The P_{CO_2} is below the normal value of 40 mm, so this CANNOT be a respiratory acidosis (the P_{CO_2} would be above 40 in a respiratory acidosis). The first two steps are straightforward and unambiguous.

The third (and most difficult) step is to assess the compensatory response. This patient has a metabolic acidosis, so you need to assess the respiratory compensation, that is, has the P_{CO_2} decreased appropriately to compensate for the metabolic acidosis? The normal compensatory response in metabolic acidosis is for the P_{CO_2} to decrease by 1 to 1.5 mm Hg for each 1-mEq decrease in HCO_3. So, this patient's 19 mEq/L drop in bicarbonate is matched by a 25 mm drop in the P_{CO_2}. Hence, this is a compensated metabolic acidosis. Another method of assessing compensation in a metabolic acidosis is to use the Winters formula, which says that the appropriate P_{CO_2} equals 1.5 $(HCO_3) + 8$. This would give an appropriate P_{CO_2} of 15.5, very close to the measured P_{CO_2}. Again, the compensatory response is appropriate for the degree of acidosis; the patient does not have a respiratory acid-base disorder.

The fourth step is to calculate the anion gap. The normal anion gap $(Na - [Cl + HCO_3])$ is 8 to 12 mEq/L; in this case the value is 29 mEq/L. Therefore, this is an anion-gap metabolic acidosis with appropriate respiratory compensation. A brief differential of anion-gap metabolic acidosis is as follows:

Diabetic ketoacidosis
Lactic acidosis
Alcoholic ketoacidosis
Toxic alcohol (methanol, ethylene glycol) ingestion
Salicylate intoxication
Renal failure

271. The answer is a. (*Fauci, pp 1761-1771.*) Although this woman's serum creatinine level is at the upper end of the traditional "normal" level, her GFR is only 19 mL/min, consistent with Stage 4 chronic kidney disease. The serum creatinine is an imprecise indicator of GFR, particularly when the muscle mass is diminished, as in this thin elderly woman. The most accurate way to determine GFR is by an estimation formula, either the Cockroft-Gault equation or the MDRD formula. The Cockroft-Gault formula is easy to remember: $(140 - age)$(lean weight in kilograms)/(serum creatinine)(72). The value is multiplied by 0.85 in women, since a smaller percentage of a woman's body mass is made up of muscle.

A mild hyperchloremic acidosis, indicated by the low serum bicarbonate, and edema are commonly seen in Stage 4 CKD. (ie, GFR between 15 and 30 mL/min). Anemia caused by erythropoietin underproduction usually occurs with this degree of kidney dysfunction. The anemia of CKD is normocytic.

Folic-acid deficiency causes a macrocytic anemia, and iron deficiency resulting from colon cancer would typically cause a microcytic anemia. Diabetes is not an inflammatory or neoplastic disease and does not cause the anemia of chronic disease. Bone marrow suppression usually causes a decrease in all cellular elements on the CBC (ie, leukocytes and platelets in addition to erythrocytes).

272. The answer is c. *(Fauci, pp 1767, 1772-1776.)* Pericarditis in renal failure (acute or chronic) is an indication to initiate hemodialysis, because untreated uremic pericarditis may progress to pericardial tamponade. Other indications include encephalopathy, volume overload, and intractable hyperkalemia. There is no absolute BUN number to initiate dialysis, although 100 mg/dL has been suggested. No degree of oliguria is a specific indication for dialysis, although this situation must be closely watched for volume overload. Bone marrow depression, mainly because of reduced erythropoietin combined with mildly reduced red cell half-life, causes hematocrit to fall almost universally in renal failure (acute and chronic). This does not determine need for dialysis. Hypotension in septic shock makes dialysis MORE difficult, and would be an indication for vasopressors, not for dialysis.

273. The answer is e. *(Fauci, pp 1752-1761, 1812-1813.)* Atheroembolic renal failure is a poorly understood syndrome of subacute renal failure in patients with severe vascular disease who undergo angiography. For unknown reasons, warfarin appears to be a risk factor. Clinical features include the dermatologic findings in this patient, refractile plaques in the retinal arteries (Hollenhorst plaques), and digital cyanosis. Although atheroembolic renal failure was once felt to lead inevitably to end-stage renal disease, it is now recognized that a significant percentage of patients have some recovery of renal function. Volume depletion is not associated with the physical findings and diverse laboratory abnormalities seen in this patient. In addition, a urine sodium less than 20 mEq/L would be expected if the patient is hypovolemic. Radiocontrast-induced acute renal failure occurs immediately after contrast studies and does not cause livedo reticularis, eosinophiluria, or hypocomplementemia. Dicloxacillin may cause drug-induced acute interstitial nephritis, which is characterized by fever, diffuse erythematous rash, white blood cell casts in the urine, and eosinophiluria, but interstitial nephritis does not cause a decreased complement level. Acute glomerulonephritis can cause hypocomplementemia but should be associated with erythrocyte casts in the urine. In addition, glomerulonephritis would be rare in this setting.

274. The answer is d. (*Fauci, pp 283-285.*) This patient has life-threatening hyperkalemia as suggested by the ECG changes in association with documented hyperkalemia. Death can occur within minutes as a result of ventricular fibrillation, and immediate treatment is mandatory. Intravenous calcium is given to combat the membrane effects of the hyperkalemia, and measures to shift potassium acutely into the cells must be instituted as well. IV regular insulin 10 units and (unless the patient is already hyperglycemic) IV glucose (usually 25 grams) can lower the serum potassium level by 0.5 to 1.0 mEq/L. Nebulized albuterol is often used and is probably more effective than IV sodium bicarbonate. It is crucial to remember that measures to promote potassium loss from the body (Kayexalate, furosemide, or dialysis), although important in the long run, take hours to work. These measures will not promptly counteract the membrane irritability of hyperkalemia. IV normal saline will not lower the serum potassium level.

This patient's hyperkalemia is a result of the combination of CKD and several medications (trimethoprim, spironolactone), which can cause hyperkalemia. Adrenal insufficiency could be playing a role as well. An important aspect of the management of CKD is avoiding drugs that can worsen kidney function or the metabolic effects (hyperkalemia, hyperphosphatemia, metabolic acidosis) of renal failure.

275. The answer is d. (*Fauci, pp 287-295.*) This patient appears intoxicated and has a severe anion gap acidosis (AG = 30 mEq/L). This scenario suggests toxic alcohol ingestion, and the osmolar gap should be calculated. The estimated plasma osmolality is calculated as follows: $2 \times Na + BUN/2.8 + glucose/18 + blood\ ethanol/4.6$ (denominators are a function of molecular weight of each substance). Here the calculated osmolality is 288 mOsm/L ($2 \times 138 + 14/2.8 + 90/18 + 0/4.6$). This patient is found to have a measured plasma osmolality of 320 mOsm/L. The measured osmolality of 320 mOsm/L minus the calculated osmolality of 288 mOsm/L gives an osmolar gap of 32 (normal less than 10) due either to methanol or ethylene glycol. In this case, methanol, used in paint thinners, is likely. Ethylene glycol, used in antifreeze, is frequently associated with hypocalcemia, renal failure, and crystalluria. Serum ketones should be checked, but diabetic ketoacidosis is unlikely with a blood sugar of 110 mg/dL, and alcoholic ketoacidosis rarely, if ever, causes acidosis of this severity. Serum lactate should be checked, but in an afebrile patient with normal blood pressure, lactic acidosis is unlikely to be the primary cause. Rhabdomyolysis does not cause a wide anion gap metabolic acidosis; so a CK level would not be helpful.

A primary CNS event would not account for this patient's wide anion gap metabolic acidosis.

276. The answer is b. *(Fauci, pp 1752-1761.)* Urinalysis would be the best test because it is likely to show muddy brown granular casts, suggesting acute tubular necrosis. In oliguric acute renal failure (less than 20 mL urine per hour), a urine sodium less than 10 mEq/L (and a fractional excretion of sodium < 1) suggest prerenal azotemia, whereas a value > 20 mEq/L (FENa > 2) suggests acute tubular necrosis. However, the urine sodium is less useful in nonoliguric ARF. Obstructive uropathy is unlikely since a functioning urinary catheter is in place; a normal urinalysis would raise the index of suspicion both for obstruction and for hypovolemia. Despite the high serum uric acid, acute uric acid nephropathy occurs with chemotherapy of aggressive tumors (eg, Burkitt lymphoma) and rarely in the postoperative setting. A urine uric acid—creatinine ratio > 1 is helpful in diagnosing uric acid nephropathy in the appropriate setting. Any diagnostic study that uses IV radiocontrast agents should be avoided if possible in the setting of acute renal insufficiency.

277. The answer is e. *(Fauci, pp 272-273, 1782-1797.)* Dysmorphic erythrocytes and proteinuria suggest a glomerular source of hematuria. The commonest causes of glomerular hematuria in this population are IgA nephropathy (Berger disease) and thin basement membrane disease. Berger disease can cause hypertension or even renal insufficiency; thin basement membrane disease is a benign condition. Berger disease is associated with IgA deposits in the mesangium. Patients with IgA nephropathy often have an exacerbation of their hematuria with intercurrent respiratory illnesses.

Acute glomerulonephritis usually occurs a week or two AFTER the sore throat (ie, to give enough time for vigorous antibody production against the Streptococcal antigens). Acute glomerulonephritis is usually symptomatic (hypertension, periorbital edema) and is associated with red blood cell casts and an active urinary sediment. Poststreptococcal GN is now a rare condition in the adult population of developed nations. Although urological cancers, kidney stones, and prostatitis are important causes of hematuria (especially in an older or symptomatic patient), they would not cause dysmorphic erythrocytes or protein in the urine.

278. The answer is d. *(Fauci, pp 289-292.)* The patient has a metabolic acidosis. Respiratory compensation is appropriate, and the anion gap is normal. Therefore, he has a hyperchloremic (normal anion gap) metabolic acidosis. Common causes include renal tubular acidosis, bicarbonate loss owing to diarrhea, and mineralocorticoid deficiency.

In a metabolic acidosis, the urine pH should be low (ie, the patient should be trying to excrete the excess acid). This patient's high urine pH is therefore diagnostic of renal tubular acidosis (RTA). Proximal RTA is associated with glycosuria, phosphaturia, and aminoaciduria (Fanconi syndrome). Since the serum phosphorus is normal and glycosuria is absent, proximal RTA is unlikely. GI Loss of bicarbonate caused by diarrhea would be associated with an appropriately acidic urine (pH less than 5.5). Disorders of the renin-angiotensin-aldosterone system are associated with hyperkalemia, not hypokalemia. The low P_{CO_2} excludes respiratory acidosis. So, this patient has a distal RTA, probably because of toluene inhalation (glue sniffing). Toluene can lead to life-threatening metabolic acidosis and hypokalemia.

279. The answer is a. (*Fauci, pp 1797-1799.*) This patient has adult polycystic kidney disease (APCKD), an autosomal dominant condition. It is the commonest genetic renal disease causing ESRD and often presents with hypertension, hematuria, and large palpable kidneys. Imaging studies would confirm the diagnosis by showing numerous bilateral renal cortical cysts. Cysts are often seen in the liver and pancreas but rarely cause symptoms. Most patients progress to end-stage renal disease despite meticulous blood pressure control with ACE inhibitors or angiotensin receptor blockers.

About 10% of patients with adult PCK disease harbor berry aneurysms in the circle of Willis; a ruptured berry aneurysm may have accounted for his father's stroke. APCKD patients also have an increased incidence of abdominal and thoracic aneurysms as well as diverticulosis. The abnormal gene, on chromosome 16 in 85% of patients, appears to encode a structural protein that helps keep the renal tubules open and unobstructed. This same protein provides strength to the walls of arteries and other epithelial structures (pancreatic ductules, bile ductules, colon). Malignancy and dementia are not seen with increased incidence in APCKD patients.

280. The answer is c. (*Fauci, p 287-296.*) This patient's normal pH would initially suggest a normal acid-base status. However, the P_{CO_2} is significantly low, indicating a respiratory alkalosis. If the pH is normal, there must be a superimposed metabolic acidosis, ie, metabolic compensation would NOT return the pH all the way back to 7.4. Indeed the serum bicarbonate is too low for a compensatory response (metabolic compensation for respiratory alkalosis rarely drops the HCO_3 below 17 mEq/L) and the anion gap is elevated at 21. The only cause of a substantially elevated anion gap is metabolic acidosis (the AG can be elevated to 16 or 17 in alkalosis). Therefore, this patient has a combined (mixed) disturbance, ie, combined respiratory alkalosis AND metabolic acidosis.

This is the classic acid-base disturbance associated with salicylate intoxication. Aspirin stimulates central respiratory drive; in addition, several metabolic substances (salicylic acid and lactic acid due to suppression of oxidative phosphorylation, among others) build up to widen the anion gap. Choices a, b, and e are wrong because compensation never normalizes the pH.

281. The answer is d. (*Fauci, pp 1790-1793.*) This patient almost surely has the nephrotic syndrome, which is characterized by sufficient albuminuria to cause hypoalbuminemia and its complications (edema, hyperlipidemia, and hypertension). The degree of albuminuria required to cause the clinical syndrome is 3.5 g per 24 hours or greater. The urine dipstick shows 3+ (300 mg/dL) or 4+ (1000 mg/dL) proteinuria. Proteinuria can be quantified on a spot urine specimen by measuring the urine albumin/creatinine ratio (> 3.5 mg/g). The occasional patient with this degree of proteinuria but without the clinical manifestations of the nephrotic syndrome is said to have nephrotic-range proteinuria. Remember that other proteins (eg, Bence-Jones proteins, myoglobin) can cause severe proteinuria but, since they do not cause albumin loss in the urine, do not cause the nephrotic syndrome. These proteins often do not show up on the urine dipstick, which is relatively albumin specific.

Once the diagnosis of the nephrotic syndrome is made, an underlying cause should be sought. In the absence of diabetes (overwhelmingly the most common cause of nephrotic range proteinuria in adults), most cases will be associated with primary glomerular diseases. Systemic lupus, amyloidosis, and several infectious diseases can cause the nephrotic syndrome but are usually associated with systemic manifestations that point to the proper diagnosis. Kidney biopsy is usually carried out in adults, but in children and adolescents, where minimal change disease is the commonest cause, a trial of corticosteroids usually precedes renal biopsy. Serum and urine protein electrophoresis would help diagnose multiple myeloma, but this would be a very rare condition in a young patient. Measuring serum lipids should be done but would be less important than diagnosing the nephrotic syndrome. Plasma aldosterone and renin levels are useful in ruling out hyperaldosteronism as a cause of hypertension but play no role in the evaluation of proteinuria or the nephrotic syndrome.

282. The answer is b. *(Fauci, pp 274-285, 2217-2224.)* Inappropriate secretion of antidiuretic hormone is suggested in a patient without clinical evidence of volume depletion or an edematous (ie, salt-retaining) condition. This syndrome may be idiopathic, associated with certain pulmonary and intracranial pathologies, resulting from endocrine disorders (eg, hypothyroidism), or drug-induced (eg, many psychotropic agents). Volume depletion is unlikely in the absence of orthostatic hypotension. Psychogenic polydipsia requires the ingestion of huge quantities of water to overcome the kidneys' ability to excrete a free-water load and would be associated with a very dilute urine (ie, urine specific gravity of 1.001 or 1.002). Cirrhosis is unlikely in the absence of ascites and edema. Congestive heart failure can cause hyponatremia but would be associated with edema and evidence of venous congestion.

283. The answer is d. *(Fauci, pp 2262-2268.)* The syndrome of hyporeninemic hypoaldosteronism occurs in older diabetic patients, particularly males with congestive heart failure. The syndrome often presents when aggravating drugs are added. Beta-blockers impair renin secretion; ACE inhibitors decrease aldosterone levels; and spironolactone competes for the aldosterone receptor. Combined with diabetes and mild renal insufficiency, the result may be life-threatening hyperkalemia. Moderate renal insufficiency per se is unlikely to cause such severe hyperkalemia. Hypertonicity caused by hyperglycemia could aggravate hyperkalemia, but a blood glucose of 250 mg/dL should not cause severe hyperkalemia. Statin drugs may cause muscle injury and rhabdomyolysis, but a CK of 400 IU/L is a modest elevation (probably caused by the renal insufficiency) and would not cause severe hyperkalemia. A high potassium diet may contribute modestly to hyperkalemia but is rarely a major factor by itself.

284. The answer is d. *(Fauci, pp 2372-2377.)* The major effect of hypomagnesemia on parathyroid hormone is decreased end-organ response, including bone resistance and reduced renal synthesis of 1, 25(OH)2D. A less important effect is impaired parathormone release. Hypoalbuminemia decreases the serum calcium by 0.8 mg Ca/g albumin below normal; this patient's mild hypoalbuminemia is a minimal factor. Dietary intake is usually a minor factor, as there are huge supplies of mobilizable calcium in the skeletal system. Osteoporosis does not cause hypocalcemia.

285. The answer is c. *(Fauci, p 295.)* Respiratory alkalosis is one of the commonest causes of hypophosphatemia; it results from shift of phosphate from the extracellular to the intracellular space. Hypomagnesemia alone would increase phosphorus by decreasing parathormone effect. Hyper-parathyroidism can decrease phosphorus, but not to this degree; also, cal-cium is not elevated. Severe hypophosphatemia is seen with malnutrition, especially during the refeeding stage when carbohydrate intake causes phos-phate to shift into the intracellular space. Such patients have clear clinical evidence of malnutrition. In addition, malnutrition almost always causes hypoalbuminemia. Vitamin D deficiency is uncommon in this age group and would be associated with hypocalcemia.

286. The answer is d. *(Fauci, pp 1770-1771.)* By a variety of mechanisms, angiotensin-converting enzyme inhibitors help to preserve renal function in diabetes. Angiotensin receptor blockers can be used as well. Be sure to monitor serum potassium and serum creatinine after initiation of therapy. Clonidine has not been shown to slow the progression of diabetic renal dis-ease, and often causes orthostatic hypotension, constipation, and erectile dysfunction. Although many diabetic patients receive beta-blockers because of coronary disease, these are not first-line drugs for preventing progression of renal failure. Beta-blockers may blunt the symptoms and physiologic response to hypoglycemia, but this is primarily a problem in brittle insulin-treated diabetics. Because of low cost and proven efficacy, thiazide diuretics remain a good choice for the general population, but do not have a specific effect on progression of renal disease. Short-acting dihydropyridine cal-cium-channel blockers (eg, nifedipine) may increase the incidence of stroke and myocardial infarction, and have no role in the treatment of hyperten-sion in any patient.

287. The answer is d. *(Fauci, pp 1177, 1709-1791, 1796.)* Although many glomerular lesions occur in association with HIV, focal glomerulosclerosis is by far the commonest etiology of this patient's nephrotic syndrome. While focal sclerosis is more common in intravenous drug users with HIV, the lesion is different from so-called heroin nephropathy. Indinavir toxicity may cause tubular obstruction by crystals and is a cause of renal stones, but does not cause nephrotic syndrome. Analgesic nephropathy is a frequently unrecognized cause of occult renal failure. This entity requires at least 10 years of high-level analgesic use and may cause renal colic owing to papillary necrosis. Analgesic abuse nephropathy, however, is an interstitial disease and does not cause nephrotic range proteinuria. Trimethoprim-sulfamethoxa-zole may cause acute interstitial nephritis, but the patient does not have fever, rash, WBC casts, or eosinophils in the urinalysis. Again, interstitial diseases do not cause high-level proteinuria. Bilateral renal artery stenosis would be rare at this age and is associated with a normal urinalysis.

288. The answer is c. *(Fauci, pp 274-279.)* The first step in the clinical assessment of hyponatremia is a thorough history and physical examination, including assessment of extracellular fluid status. Increased ECF in the setting of hyponatremia may be caused by heart failure, hepatic cirrhosis, nephrotic syndrome, or renal insufficiency. A normal ECF in the same setting would indicate a disorder such as SIADH, whereas a decreased ECF would prompt a search for the cause of the hypovolemia (GI or renal losses being the most common). In hypovolemic states, ADH release is stimulated by the decreased ECF volume status and leads to free-water retention. Remember that, even when ECF volume is decreased, hyponatremia almost always indicates free-water EXCESS (hypotonicity).

Determination of plasma osmolality is helpful in the setting of hyponatremia to confirm the presence of hypotonicity. Most patients with hyponatremia will have a low plasma osmolality. A high plasma osmolality usually indicates hyperglycemia, and a normal plasma osmolality can indicate "pseudohyponatremia" caused by disorders such as hyperproteinemia and hyperlipidemia. In this case, determination of ECF status from the physical examination (history would be limited owing to patient's inability to communicate) would be the best first step. You would not wait for the plasma osmolality before beginning assessment and development of an initial differential diagnosis. Helpful laboratory assessment in the face of hyponatremia includes plasma osmolality, urine osmolality, and urine K and Na concentration. The plasma AVP assay is difficult to perform, and the result would not be available in time to help the patient. Proteinuria does not cause hyponatremia unless overt nephrotic syndrome is present. Chest x-ray and CT scan of the head are indicated if the patient is found to have SIADH (euvolemic hyponatremia), but SIADH cannot be diagnosed until the volume status is determined.

289. The answer is c. *(Fauci, pp 274-279.)* The patient has acute symptomatic hyponatremia, a life-threatening condition. Although some controversy persists as to whether chronic hyponatremia should be rapidly corrected, acute symptomatic hyponatremia should be rapidly treated with hypertonic saline. This patient it is at high risk of seizure and respiratory arrest, the main cause of permanent CNS damage in hyponatremia. ICU care, with frequent monitoring of the serum sodium level and CNS status, is critical. Once the Na has risen 4 to 8 mEq/L and the symptoms have improved, the rate of hypertonic saline infusion can be decreased. Less aggressive methods of treating her free-water overload, such as fluid restriction alone or in combination with furosemide, are not appropriate for this acute emergency. Isotonic fluids such as normal saline and lactated Ringer solution are useful in volume depletion but will NOT treat this patient's free-water excess. Postoperative hyponatremia is particularly common in premenopausal women. The nausea and pain sometimes associated with surgery are very potent stimulators of vasopressin (ADH) release by the neurohypophysis. If hypotonic fluids are used at all in this setting, the serum sodium level should be closely monitored, and isotonic fluids used if there is any trend toward free-water retention (ie, hyponatremia).

290. The answer is c. *(Fauci, pp 1761-1771).* This patient has Stage III chronic kidney disease (estimated GFR 30-60 mL/min). At this stage it is crucial for the internist to prevent progression to end-stage renal disease. Blood pressure control, with a target blood pressure of < 130 systolic and < 80 diastolic, is a critical element in his management. If the patient has proteinuria greater than 1 g/ 24 h, even tighter control is necessary. Other important management issues include avoiding nephrotoxins (such as NSAIDs and IV contrast agents) if possible, modest dietary protein restriction, and atherosclerotic risk factor management. If the patient progresses to Stage IV CKD (estimated GFR 15-30 mL/min), he should be referred to a nephrologist.

Modest ethanol consumption is not a renal or cardiovascular risk factor and need not be modified unless you believe the patient is consuming much more alcohol than he admits. Acetaminophen in usual therapeutic doses is the safest agent to control DJD pain and certainly is preferable to nonsteroidals. Although ARBs are sometimes added to ACEIs in patients with significant proteinuria (with caution to avoid hyperkalemia), there is no reason to discontinue the ACEI at this time. The critical element is tighter blood pressure control.

291 to 293. The answers are 291-d, 292-b, 293-e. *(Fauci, pp 1752-1761.)* Acute renal failure in adults usually occurs during hospitalization for other illness. The history (in particular, exposure to nephrotoxins including intravenous contrast agents), physical examination (in particular, assessment of volume status and search for allergic manifestations such as skin rash), and urine studies will usually establish the diagnosis. The fractional excretion of sodium may demonstrate renal underperfusion if this is not clear from the clinical setting. If the kidneys are underperfused from volume depletion, third space losses or poor cardiac output, the kidneys will retain salt and water, and the fractional excretion of sodium (FENa) will be low. In the cases presented here, the clinical setting suggests the diagnosis.

Interstitial nephritis typically occurs as an allergic reaction to antibiotics, particularly beta-lactams and sulfa derivatives. So-called tubular proteinuria is modest (< 1 g/24 h), albuminuria is minimal and the nephrotic syndrome does not occur. Pyuria and eosinophiluria are usually present. The commonest cause of acute renal failure is acute tubular necrosis. The FENa is usually above two and muddy brown cases may be present on the urinalysis. Ischemia (often owing to sepsis) and nephrotoxins are the usual causes. Obstructive uropathy can occur acutely, particularly in the setting of bladder outlet obstruction (BPH) or neurogenic bladder (as can occur in diabetes). The patient will often have difficulty voiding and the urinalysis will be unremarkable. Complete anuria or fluctuations from oliguria to polyuria also suggest the diagnosis. Bladder catheterization or renal sonography are diagnostic.

294 and 295. The answers are 294-e, 295-f. (*Fauci, pp 1782-1797.*) Glomerular diseases present with proteinuria and sometimes an active urinary sediment (dysmorphic red cells, white blood cells, and red cell casts). Many patients have the nephrotic syndrome. Patients who present with an active sediment, hypertension, and worsening renal function without nephrotic-range proteinuria and hypoalbuminemia are said to have the nephritic syndrome. Finally, some patients (eg, the usual patient with IgA nephropathy) will have asymptomatic proteinuria or hematuria. Serological studies, complement levels and, often, renal biopsy will be necessary to establish a definite diagnosis and to adequately plan treatment.

Membranous nephropathy is the commonest cause of idiopathic nephrotic syndrome in adults. One-third of cases improve spontaneously, one-third remain stable, and one-third progress to end-stage renal disease if untreated. The condition is fairly responsive to corticosteroid and cytotoxic therapy. Membranoproliferative glomerulonephritis is the rarest cause of idiopathic nephrotic syndrome in adults. Depressed C3 is caused by an autoantibody that directly activates the third component of complement. A progressive clinical course and erratic response to therapy are typical.

296 and 297. The answers are 296-a, 297-c. (*Fauci, pp 2119-2131.*) Renal involvement in systemic vasculitis is common and can lead to serious morbidity including end-stage renal disease. The pattern of renal disease can be diagnostically useful. Macroscopic polyarteritis nodosa is a vasculitis of medium-sized blood vessels that causes renal artery aneurysms (severe hypertension), abdominal aneurysms (abdominal pain), and ischemic damage to skin and peripheral nerves. Patients are most commonly older males and anyone who is hepatitis B surface antigen—positive. Microscopic polyangiitis is a different disease entirely. It is often associated with lung involvement and alveolar hemorrhage (pulmonary involvement is rare in classic PAN) and small-vessel (ie, glomerular) renal involvement rather than the arcuate artery aneurysms that are seen on angiography in classic PAN. Wegener granulomatosis is one of the most common of the vasculitides. It usually occurs in older males and typically starts with chronic sinusitis. Pulmonary and renal involvement then develop. A positive c-ANCA (cytoplasmic antineutrophil cytoplasmic antibody) test, associated with antibodies against proteinase 3, is an important diagnostic clue. Perinuclear or p-ANCA positivity is caused by antibodies to myeloperoxidase and can be seen in other vasculitic syndromes.

298 and 299. The answers are 298-e, 299-d. *(Fauci, pp 1815-1820.)* Uric acid stones are associated with low urine pH, owing to decreased NH_3 production by the kidney. Uric acid is underexcreted in an acid urine. These stones are commonly radiolucent on plain film or IVP but are easily visualized on CT. They often dissolve within weeks if the urine is alkalinized (eg, with potassium citrate). Struvite stones are found if the urine is infected with organisms (especially *Proteus* species) that produce the enzyme urease. Urease splits urea to CO_2 and ammonium; the latter produces the characteristic alkaline urine (urine pH usually 8). The ammonium combines with urinary magnesium and phosphate to form the insoluble struvite (magnesium ammonium phosphate). These stones are opaque and are often large, filling the collecting system (staghorn calculi). Calcium containing stones cause over 70% of kidney stones and are radiopaque. Hypercalciuria and hyperoxaluria (as can be seen in intestinal malabsorption) are contributing factors. Hexagonal urinary crystals are found in cystinuria, an uncommon hereditary disease that starts early in life and if untreated progresses to end-stage renal disease. These stones may be lucent or opaque. Xanthine stones are rare. The pigment calcium bilirubinate causes gallstones, not kidney stones.

Hematology and Oncology

Questions

300. A 55-year-old male is being evaluated for constipation. There is no history of prior gastrectomy or of upper GI symptoms. Hemoglobin is 10 g/dL, mean corpuscular volume (MCV) is 72 fL, serum iron is 4 μg/dL (normal is 50-150 μg/dL), iron-binding capacity is 450 μg/dL (normal is 250-370 μg/dL), saturation is 1% (normal is 20%-45%), and ferritin is 10 μg/L (normal is 15-400 μg/L). Which of the following is the best next step in the evaluation of this patient's anemia?

a. Red blood cell folate
b. Serum lead level
c. Colonoscopy
d. Bone marrow examination
e. Hemoglobin electrophoresis with A2 and F levels

301. A 50-year-old woman complains of pain and swelling in her proximal interphalangeal joints, both wrists, and both knees. She complains of morning stiffness. She had a hysterectomy 10 years ago. Physical examination shows swelling and thickening of the PIP joints. Hemoglobin is 10.3 g/dL, MCV is 80 fL, serum iron is 28 μg/dL, iron-binding capacity is 200 μg/dL (normal is 250-370 μg/dL), and saturation is 14%. Which of the following is the most likely explanation for this woman's anemia?

a. Occult blood loss
b. Vitamin deficiency
c. Anemia of chronic disease
d. Sideroblastic anemia
e. Occult renal disease

302. A 35-year-old female who is recovering from *Mycoplasma* pneumonia develops increasing weakness. Her Hgb is 9.0 g/dL and her MCV is 110. Which of the following is the best test to determine whether the patient has a hemolytic anemia?

a. Serum bilirubin
b. Reticulocyte count and blood smear
c. *Mycoplasma* antigen
d. Glucose phosphate dehydrogenase level
e. Liver spleen scan

303. A 70-year-old male complains of 2 months of low back pain and fatigue. He has developed fever with purulent sputum production. On physical examination, he has pain over several vertebrae and rales at the left base. Laboratory results are as follows:

Hemoglobin: 7 g/dL
MCV: 89 fL (normal 86 to 98)
WBC: 12,000/mL
BUN: 44 mg/dL
Creatinine: 3.2 mg/dL
Ca: 11.5 mg/dL
Chest x-ray: LLL infiltrate
Reticulocyte count: 1%

The definitive diagnosis is best made by which of the following?

a. 24-hour urine protein
b. Bone scan
c. Renal biopsy
d. Rouleaux formation on blood smear
e. Greater than 30% plasma cells in the bone marrow

304. A 64-year-old man complains of cough, increasing shortness of breath, and headache for the past 3 weeks. He has mild hypertension for which he takes hydrochlorothiazide; he has smoked one pack of cigarettes a day for 40 years. On examination you notice facial plethora and jugular venous distension to the angle of the jaw. He has prominent veins over the anterior chest and a firm to hard right supraclavicular lymph node. Cardiac examination is normal and lungs are without rales. Peripheral edema is absent. What is the most likely cause of his condition?

a. Long-standing hypertension
b. Gastric carcinoma
c. Emphysema
d. Lung cancer
e. Nephrotic syndrome

305. A 38-year-old woman presents with a 3-day history of fever and confusion. She was previously healthy and is taking no medications. She has not had diarrhea or rectal bleeding. She has a temperature of 38°C (100.4°F) and a blood pressure of 145/85. Splenomegaly is absent. She has no petechiae but does have evidence of early digital gangrene of the right second finger. Except for confusion the neurological examination is normal. Her laboratory studies reveal the following:

Hemoglobin: 8.7
Platelet count: 25,000
Peripheral smear: numerous fragmented RBCs, few platelets
LDH 562 (normal <180)
Creatinine: 2.7
Liver enzymes: normal
Prothrombin time/PTT/fibrinogen level: normal

What is the most likely pathogenesis of her condition?

a. Disseminated intravascular coagulation
b. Antiplatelet antibodies
c. Failure to cleave von Willebrand factor multimers
d. Verotoxin-induced endothelial damage
e. Cirrhosis with sequestration of erythrocytes and platelets in the spleen

306. After undergoing surgical resection for carcinoma of the stomach, a 60-year-old male develops numbness in his feet. On examination, he has lost proprioception in the lower extremities and has a wide-based gait and positive Romberg sign. Peripheral blood smear shows macrocytosis and hypersegmented polymorphonuclear leukocytes. The neurologic dysfunction is secondary to a deficiency of which vitamin?

a. Folic acid
b. Thiamine
c. Vitamin K
d. Vitamin B_{12}
e. Riboflavin

307. A 60-year-old asymptomatic man is found to have leukocytosis on a preoperative CBC. Physical examination shows the spleen tip to be palpable 2 cm below the left costal margin. Rubbery, nontender lymph nodes up to 1.5 cm in size are present in the axillae and inguinal regions. Laboratory data include the following:

Hgb: 13.3 g/dL (normal 14 to 18)
Leukocytes: 40,000/μL (normal 4300 to 10,800)
Platelet count: 238,000 (normal 150,000 to 400,000)
His peripheral blood smear is shown in the accompanying photo.

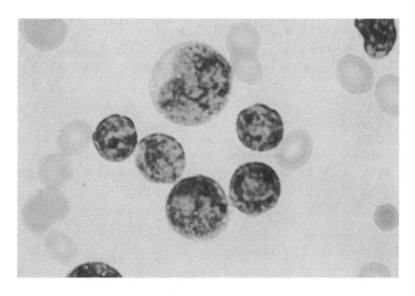

Which of the following is the most likely diagnosis?

a. Acute monocytic leukemia
b. Chronic myelogenous leukemia
c. Chronic lymphocytic leukemia
d. Tuberculosis
e. Infectious mononucleosis

308. A 25-year-old woman complains of persistent bleeding for 5 days after a dental extraction. She has noticed easy bruisability since childhood, and was given a blood transfusion at age 17 because of prolonged bleeding after an apparently minor cut. She denies ecchymoses or bleeding into joints. Her father has noticed similar symptoms but has not sought medical care. Physical examination is normal except for mild oozing from the dental site. She does not have splenomegaly or enlarged lymph nodes. Her CBC is normal, with a platelet count of 230,000. Her prothrombin time is normal but the partial thromboplastin time is mildly prolonged. The bleeding time is 12 minutes (normal 3-9 minutes). What is most appropriate way to control her bleeding?

a. Factor VIII concentrate
b. Fresh frozen plasma
c. Desmopressin (DDAVP)
d. Whole blood transfusion
e. Single donor platelets

309. A 67-year-old male presents with hemoptysis 1 week in duration. He has smoked 1—2 packs of cigarettes per day for 50 years and has been unable to quit smoking despite nicotine replacement therapy and bupropion. He has mild COPD for which he uses an ipratropium inhaler. Chest x-ray reveals a 3-cm right perihilar mass. Which of the following is the most likely cause of this patient's hemoptysis?

a. Adenocarcinoma of the lung
b. Squamous cell carcinoma of the lung
c. Bronchoalveolar cell carcinoma
d. Bronchial adenoma
e. Sarcoidosis

310. A 38-year-old female presents with repeated episodes of sore throat. She is on no medications, does not use ethanol, and has no history of renal disease. Physical examination is normal. On CBC the Hgb is 9.0 g/dL, MCV is 85 fL (normal), white blood cell count is 2,000/μL, and platelet count is 30,000/μL. Which of the following is the best approach to diagnosis?

a. Erythropoietin level
b. Serum B_{12}
c. Bone marrow biopsy
d. Liver spleen scan
e. Therapeutic trial of corticosteroids

311. A 50-year-old female complains of vague abdominal pain, constipation, and a sense of fullness in the lower abdomen. The abdomen is nontender, but there is shifting dullness to percussion. Which of the following is the best next step in evaluation?

a. Abdominal ultrasound
b. Therapeutic trial of diuretics
c. CA-125 cancer antigen
d. Sigmoidoscopy
e. Pelvic examination

312. A 52-year-old man with cirrhosis resulting from chronic hepatitis C presents with increasing right upper quadrant pain, anorexia, and 15-lb weight loss. The patient is mildly icteric and has moderate ascites. A friction rub is heard over the liver. Abdominal paracentesis reveals blood-tinged fluid, and CT scan shows a 4-cm solid mass in the right lobe of the liver. Which of the following is the most important initial diagnostic study?

a. Serum α-fetoprotein level
b. Colonoscopy to search for a primary neoplasm
c. Measurement of hepatitis C viral RNA
d. Upper GI endoscopy
e. Positron emission tomography scan

313. A 60-year-old male complains of hematuria and an aching pain in his right flank. Laboratory data show normal BUN, creatinine, and electrolytes. Hemoglobin is elevated at 18 g/dL and serum calcium is 11 mg/dL. A solid renal mass is found by ultrasound. Which of the following is the most likely diagnosis?

a. Polycystic kidney disease
b. Pheochromocytoma
c. Adrenal carcinoma
d. Renal adenomyolipoma
e. Renal carcinoma

314. A 64-year-old woman who is receiving chemotherapy for metastatic breast cancer has been treating midthoracic pain with acetaminophen. Over the past few days she has become weak and unsteady on her feet. On the day of admission she develops urinary incontinence. Physical examination reveals fist percussion tenderness over T8 and moderate symmetric muscle weakness in the legs. Anal sphincter tone is reduced. Which of the following diagnostic studies is most important to order?

a. Serum calcium
b. Bone scan
c. Plain radiographs of the thoracic spine
d. MRI scan of the spine
e. Electromyogram with nerve conduction studies

315. A 20-year-old male finds an asymptomatic mass in his scrotum. He denies fever, dysuria, or hematospermia. Which of the following is the most appropriate first step in evaluating this mass?

a. Palpation and transillumination
b. HCG and α-fetoprotein
c. Scrotal ultrasonography
d. Evaluation for inguinal adenopathy
e. Referral for inguinal orchiectomy

316. A 65-year-old man presents with painless hematuria. He has a 45-year history of tobacco use. He denies fever, chills, and dysuria. General physical examination is unremarkable. On rectal examination, the prostate is small, non-nodular, and nontender. A urinalysis shows 100 red blood cells per high-power field. No white cells or protein are present. Three months previously, the patient had an abdominal ultrasound for right upper quadrant pain; on review, both kidneys were normal. Which of the following is the most useful diagnostic test at this time?

a. Urine culture and sensitivity
b. PSA
c. Bladder scan
d. Cystoscopy and retrograde pyelography
e. CT scan of the kidneys

317. A 43-year-old woman complains of fatigue and night sweats associated with itching for 2 months. On physical examination, there is diffuse nontender lymphadenopathy, including small supraclavicular, epitrochlear, and scalene nodes. CBC and chemistry studies (including liver enzymes) are normal. Chest x-ray shows hilar lymphadenopathy. Which of the following is the best next step in evaluation?

a. Excisional lymph node biopsy
b. Monospot test
c. Toxoplasmosis IgG serology
d. Serum angiotensin-converting enzyme level
e. Percutaneous aspiration biopsy of the largest lymph node

318. A 19-year-old woman presents for evaluation of a nontender left axillary lymph node. She is asymptomatic and denies weight loss or night sweats. Examination reveals three rubbery firm nontender nodes in the axilla, the largest 3 cm in diameter. No other lymphadenopathy is noted; the spleen is not enlarged. Lymph node biopsy, however, reveals mixed-cellularity Hodgkin lymphoma. Liver function tests are normal. Which of the following is the best next step in evaluation?

a. Bone marrow biopsy
b. Liver biopsy
c. Staging laparotomy
d. Erythrocyte sedimentation rate
e. CT scan of chest, abdomen, and pelvis

319. A 69-year-old African American man presents with weight loss and back pain. Over the past 2 months he has developed hyperglycemia with a fasting glucose of 153 mg/dL. He does not have nocturia. His appetite is decreased; he has noticed mild constipation. The back pain is constant and keeps him awake at night. On examination he appears cachectic and pale. He does not have scleral icterus. Laboratory studies reveal a mild normochromic anemia. Liver and kidney function studies are normal. What diagnostic study is most likely to reveal the cause of his symptoms?

a. CT scan of the abdomen with IV contrast
b. Glucose tolerance test
c. Colonoscopy.
d. Stool studies for malabsorption
e. Whole-body PET scan

320. A 75-year-old man with a prior history of adenocarcinoma of the prostate treated with radical prostatectomy presents with pain in the left hip. The pain awakens him at night and has become increasingly severe over the previous 3 weeks. Plain radiographs show numerous bilateral osteoblastic lesions in the hip and sacrum, and the prostate-specific antigen level is 83 mcg/mL (normal 0 to 4). Which of the following is the treatment of choice?

a. Observation
b. Radiation therapy
c. Estrogen therapy
d. Gonadotropin-releasing hormone (GnRH) analogue
e. Chemotherapy

321. A 73-year-old woman is admitted for deep venous thrombosis and concern for pulmonary embolism. She has a history of type 2 diabetes mellitus, hypertension, and coronary artery disease. She had been admitted for a 3-vessel coronary artery bypass graft 2 weeks prior to this admission. She did well and was dismissed 5 days after the procedure. Pain and swelling of the right leg began 2 days before this admission; she has noticed mild dyspnea but no chest pain. The clinical suspicion of DVT is confirmed by a venous Doppler, and the patient is started on unfractionated heparin. Her initial laboratory studies, including CBC, are normal.

The next day her pain has improved, and helical CT scan of the chest reveals no evidence of pulmonary embolism. She is instructed in the use of low-molecular-weight heparin and warfarin; she is eager to go home. Her serum creatinine is normal. Her predischarge CBC shows no anemia, but the platelet count has dropped to 74,000. An assay for antibodies to heparin-platelet factor 4 complexes is ordered. What is the best next step in her management?

a. Dismiss the patient on low-molecular heparin, warfarin, and close outpatient followup.
b. Obtain a liver-spleen scan to look for platelet sequestration.
c. Discontinue all forms heparin, continue warfarin, and add aspirin 162 mg daily until INR becomes therapeutic.
d. Keep the patient in the hospital, discontinue unfractionated heparin, add low-molecular-weight heparin, and monitor the platelet count daily.
e. Keep the patient in the hospital, discontinue all forms of heparin, and start the patient on lepirudin by intravenous infusion.

322. A 47-year-old premenopausal woman of Mediterranean descent presents with a painless breast mass. Her mother underwent a mastectomy at age 74 because of breast cancer. Her sister has had ovarian cysts but no cancer. There is no other cancer in the family. Biopsy of the mass reveals infiltrating ductal carcinoma. The patient has two daughters and asks about genetic testing. What is the most likely cause of her malignancy?

a. A germline mutation in the p53 suppressor gene
b. A germline mutation in the *BRCA1* gene
c. A somatic mutation in the *BRCA1* gene
d. Exposure to a carcinogen such as diethylstilbestrol in utero
e. Unknown

323. A patient with bacterial endocarditis develops thrombophlebitis while hospitalized. His course in the hospital is uncomplicated. On discharge he is treated with penicillin, rifampin, and warfarin. Therapeutic prothrombin levels are obtained on 15 mg/d of warfarin. After 2 weeks, the penicillin and rifampin are discontinued. Which of the following is the best next step in management of this patient?

a. Cautiously increase warfarin dosage.
b. Continue warfarin at 15 mg/d for about 6 months.
c. Reduce warfarin dosage.
d. Stop warfarin therapy.
e. Restrict dietary vitamin K.

324. A 65-year-old male with diabetes mellitus, bronzed skin, and cirrhosis of the liver is being treated for hemochromatosis previously confirmed by liver biopsy. The patient experiences increasing right upper quadrant pain, and his serum alkaline phosphatase is now elevated. There is a 15-lb weight loss. Which of the following is the best next step in management?

a. Increase frequency of phlebotomy for worsening hemochromatosis.
b. Obtain alpha-fetoprotein level and CT scan to rule out hepatoma.
c. Obtain hepatitis B serology.
d. Obtain antimitochondrial antibody to rule out primary biliary cirrhosis.
e. Check a serum ferritin level.

325. A 66-year-old postmenopausal woman presents with a painless breast mass and is found to have a 3 cm infiltrating ductal breast cancer. Sentinel node sampling reveals metastatic cancer in the sentinel node; a formal axillary node dissection shows that 4 of 13 nodes are involved by the malignant process. Both estrogen and progesterone receptor are expressed in the tumor. There is no evidence of metastatic disease outside the axilla. In addition to lumpectomy and radiation therapy to the breast and axilla, what should her treatment include next?

a. No further treatment at this time
b. Radiation therapy to the internal mammary nodes
c. Platinum-based adjuvant chemotherapy
d. Bilateral oophorectomy
e. Adjuvant hormonal therapy (tamoxifen or aromatase inhibitor)

326. A 64-year-old African American man presents for evaluation of a painless "lump" in the left thigh. He first noticed the abnormality about 1 month previously and thinks it has increased in size; there is no prior history of trauma. On examination, you find a 5-cm soft tissue mass, firm to hard in consistency, in the soft tissue above the knee. There is no tenderness or erythema; the mass is deep to the subcutaneous tissue and appears fixed to the underlying musculature. Inguinal lymph nodes are normal. Which of the following is the most appropriate management of this patient?

a. Reexamine the lesion in 3 months, as it is probably a lipoma.
b. Obtain a bone scan.
c. Treat with cephalexin 500 mg po qid for presumed abscess.
d. Refer the patient for surgical biopsy.
e. Aspirate the mass as it is probably a hematoma.

327. A 47-year-old woman complains of fatigue, weight loss, and itching after taking a hot shower. Physical examination shows plethoric facies and an enlarged spleen, which descends 6 cm below the left costal margin. Her white cell count is 17,000 with a normal differential, the platelet count is 560,000, and hemoglobin is 18.7. Liver enzymes and electrolytes are normal; the serum uric acid level is mildly elevated. What is the most likely underlying process?

a. Myelodysplastic syndrome
b. Myeloproliferative syndrome
c. Paraneoplastic syndrome
d. Cushing syndrome
e. Gaisböck syndrome

328. A 20-year-old black male presents to the emergency room complaining of diffuse bone pain and requesting narcotics for his sickle cell crisis. Which of the following physical examination features would suggest an alternative diagnosis to sickle cell anemia (hemoglobin SS)?

a. Scleral icterus
b. Systolic murmur
c. Splenomegaly
d. Ankle ulcers
e. Leukocytosis

329. A 30-year-old black man plans a trip to India and is advised to take prophylaxis for malaria. Three days after beginning treatment, he develops pallor, fatigue, and jaundice. Hematocrit is 30% (it had been 43%) and reticulocyte count is 7%. He stops taking the medication. The next step in treatment should consist of which of the following?

a. Splenectomy.
b. Administration of methylene blue.
c. Administration of vitamin E.
d. Exchange transfusions.
e. No additional treatment is required.

330. A 26-year-old man complains of heaviness in the left testicle. There has been no recent trauma. Physical examination reveals a 3-cm painless firm mass that clearly arises from the testicle. The physical examination is otherwise unremarkable. Abdominal CT scan shows matted periaortic lymphadenopathy, with the largest node approximately 3.5 cm in size. CT of the chest shows no abnormalities. In addition to urological referral, what should be the next diagnostic study?

a. Needle aspiration biopsy of the retroperitoneal mass
b. Needle aspiration of the testicular mass
c. Measurement of alpha fetoprotein, beta HCG and lactate dehydrogenase (LDH)
d. Positron emission tomography (PET) scan
e. Measurement of carcinoembryonic antigen (CEA) and α-fetoprotein

331. A 78-year-old man complains of increasing fatigue and bone pain, especially around the knees and ankles. He has been anemic for several years, with hemoglobin of 9 to 10 g/dL and MCV of 102. His leukocyte and platelet count have been normal; he has not had lymphadenopathy or splenomegaly. He had not responded to therapeutic trials of iron and vitamin B_{12}, but has been symptomatically stable until the past month. Examination reveals pallor and spleen tip at the left costal margin. CBC reveals hemoglobin of 8.2 g/dL, but for the first time his platelet count is low (15,000); the white blood cell count is 14,000. What is the likely cause of his worsening anemia?

a. Folic acid deficiency
b. Acute myeloid leukemia
c. Myelofibrosis
d. Tuberculosis
e. Viral infection

332. A 70-year-old intensive care unit patient complains of fever and shaking chills. The patient develops hypotension, and blood cultures are positive for gram-negative bacilli. The patient begins bleeding from venipuncture sites and around his Foley catheter. Laboratory studies are as follows:

Hct: 38%
WBC: 15,000/μL
Platelet count: 40,000/μL (normal 150,000-400,000)
Peripheral blood smear: fragmented RBCs
PT: elevated
PTT: elevated
Plasma fibrinogen: 70 mg/dL (normal 200-400)

Which of the following is the best course of therapy in this patient?

a. Begin heparin.
b. Treat underlying disease.
c. Begin plasmapheresis.
d. Give vitamin K.
e. Begin red blood cell transfusion.

333. A 30-year-old female with Graves disease has been started on propyl-thiouracil. She complains of low-grade fever, chills, and sore throat. Which of the following is the most important initial step in evaluating this patient's fever?

a. Serum TSH
b. Serum T3 by RIA
c. CBC
d. Chest x-ray
e. Blood cultures

334. A 62-year-old woman has noted fever to 38.3°C (101°F) every evening for the past 3 weeks, associated with night sweats and a 15-lb weight loss. Physical examination reveals matted supraclavicular lymph nodes on the right; the largest node is 3.5 cm in diameter. She also has firm rubbery right axillary and bilateral inguinal nodes. Excisional biopsy of one of the nodes shows diffuse replacement of the nodal architecture with large neoplastic cells which stain positively for B cell markers. No Reed-Sternberg cells are seen. Which statement most accurately reflects her prognosis?

a. This is an indolent process which will respond to corticosteroids.
b. This is an aggressive neoplasm which responds poorly to chemotherapy and will likely be fatal in 6 months or less.
c. This is an aggressive neoplasm, but it may be cured with chemotherapy in up to 60% of the cases.
d. The neoplasm often responds to chemotherapy but almost always relapses.
e. Radiation therapy is curative.

335. A 37-year-old woman presents for evaluation of a self-discovered breast mass. There is no family history of breast cancer; she is otherwise healthy. Examination reveals a 1.5-cm area of firmness in the right upper outer quadrant. No skin changes are noted. You attempt to aspirate the mass, but no fluid is obtained; a mammogram is ordered and is normal. Which of the following is the most appropriate next step in management?

a. Refer the patient for further evaluation to a surgeon or comprehensive breast radiologist.
b. Reevaluate the patient in 6 months.
c. Give oral contraceptives to decrease ovulation and help shrink the lesion.
d. Recommend tamoxifen to decrease her chance of developing cancer.
e. Reassure the patient

336. A 60-year-old woman develops deep venous thrombosis after a 14-hour plane flight from New Zealand. The diagnosis is confirmed by a venous Doppler. There is no evidence of pulmonary embolism, and she is started on subcutaneous low-molecular-weight heparin. She has no family history of venous thrombosis, and she is on no medications that would increase her risk of clotting. In addition to routine monitoring of coagulation parameters and a CBC, what diagnostic tests should be ordered next?

a. Functional test for factor V Leiden (Activated protein C resistance)
b. Protein C, protein S, and antithrombin III levels
c. Antiphospholipid antibody test
d. Genetic testing for prothrombin G20210A gene mutation
e. No further testing

Questions 337 to 339

Match the clinical scenario with the likely pathogenesis. Each lettered option may be used once, more than once, or not at all.

a. Congestive heart failure caused by volume overload
b. Reaction of donor antibodies with antigens of the recipient
c. Reaction of recipient antibodies to antigens of the donor
d. IgE mediated reaction against donor IgA
e. Bacterial contamination of the transfused product
f. Activation of complement leading to intravascular hemolysis
g. Infection with intraerythrocytic parasites from the donor

337. A 46-year-old woman is transfused for upper gastrointestinal bleeding caused by peptic ulcer disease. Her past history is unremarkable except for 4 previous successful pregnancies and 3 previous spontaneous abortions. Immediately after the transfusion her hemoglobin rises to 10, the bleeding is controlled and she is dismissed from the hospital on omeprazole. One week later, however, she develops fatigue and dyspnea. Her hemoglobin has dropped to 7 g/dL. Her bilirubin, previously normal, has risen to 2.4 mg/dL (1.9 mg/dL indirect reacting), and the LDH value is 468. Stool is heme negative.

338. A 37-year-old woman receives four units of packed red blood cells after a motor vehicle accident with splenic rupture. She is otherwise healthy, without cardiac or pulmonary disease. She takes no medications. The patient does well initially, but the next day she develops shortness of breath, hypoxemia, and has diffuse crackles on her lung examination. Her neck veins are not distended and her weight is unchanged from admission. An ECG is normal, but CXR shows pulmonary edema.

339. A 22-year-old man being treated for acute lymphoblastic leukemia receives 6 units of platelets because of treatment associated thrombocytopenia. Near the end of the transfusion, the patient develops chills and fever to 39.6°C (103.3°F). His blood pressure drops to 74/46. There is no hemoglobinemia, and a direct antiglobulin (direct Coombs) test is negative.

Questions 340 to 342

Match the clinical description with the most likely diagnosis. Each lettered option may be used once, more than once, or not at all.

a. Sideroblastic anemia
b. Thalassemia
c. Iron-deficiency anemia
d. Anemia of renal disease
e. Anemia of chronic disease
f. Folate deficiency
g. Microangiopathic hemolytic anemia

340. An alcoholic patient is admitted with acute pancreatitis. He has been drinking vodka heavily for the past several months. There is no adenopathy or splenomegaly; neurological examination is normal. Hemoglobin is 7.8 with mild neutropenia and thrombocytopenia. The MCV is 114. He has this peripheral blood smear:

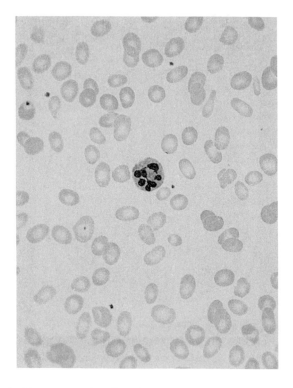

Reproduced, with permission, from Fauci A et al. *Harrison's Principles of Internal Medicine,* 17th ed. New York, NY: McGraw-Hill, 2008.

341. A 70-year-old woman of Italian origin is found to be anemic by her gynecologist. She is asymptomatic. She has a hemoglobin of 10.2, hematocrit of 30, MCV of 62, and normal serum iron studies. This is her peripheral blood smear:

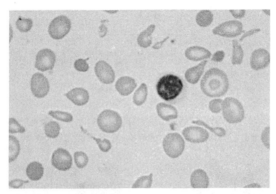

Reproduced, with permission, from Fauci A et al. *Harrison's Principles of Internal Medicine,* 17th ed. New York, NY: McGraw-Hill, 2008.

342. A 52-year-old African American diabetic requires hemodialysis for end-stage renal disease. She has hemoglobin of 9, hematocrit of 27, and normal red cell indices. The iron and iron-binding capacity are normal. Her peripheral blood smear is unremarkable.

Questions 343 and 344

Match the clinical description with the paraneoplastic syndrome most often associated with it. Each lettered option may be used once, more than once, or not at all.

a. Humoral hypercalcemia of malignancy
b. Hyponatremia caused by inappropriate ADH secretion
c. Hypoglycemia due to IGF-2
d. Migratory thrombophlebitis associated with procoagulant cytokines
e. Skin infiltration with T lymphocytes
f. Erythrocytosis due to erythropoietin overproduction

343. A 76-year-old woman presents with weight loss, depression, and anemia of chronic disease. CT of the abdomen reveals a 4-cm pancreatic mass.

344. A 58-year-old cigarette smoker develops a cough, weakness, and mental confusion. Chest CT shows a 2-cm perihilar density with hilar and mediastinal lymphadenopathy. Sputum cytology shows malignant squamous cells.

Hematology and Oncology

Answers

300. The answer is c. *(Fauci, pp 628-651.)* The patient has a microcytic anemia. A low serum iron, low ferritin, and high iron-binding capacity all suggest iron-deficiency anemia. Most iron-deficiency anemia is explained by blood loss. The patient's symptoms of constipation point to blood loss from the lower GI tract. Colonoscopy would be the highest-yield procedure. Barium enema misses 50% of polyps and a significant minority of colon cancers. Even patients without GI symptoms who have no obvious explanation (such as menstrual blood loss or multiple prior pregnancies in women) for their iron deficiency should be worked up for GI blood loss. Folate deficiency presents as a megaloblastic anemia with macrocytosis (large, oval-shaped red cells) and hypersegmentation of the polymorphonuclear leukocytes. Lead poisoning can cause a microcytic hypochromic anemia, but this would not be associated with the abnormal iron studies and low ferritin seen in this patient. Basophilic stippling or target cells seen on the peripheral blood smear would be important clues to the presence of lead poisoning. Although a bone marrow examination will prove the diagnosis by the absence of stainable iron in the marrow, the diagnosis of iron deficiency is clear from the serum studies. Thalassemia (diagnosed by hemoglobin electrophoresis) is not associated with abnormal iron studies. The most important issue is now to find the source of the iron loss.

301. The answer is c. *(Fauci, pp 633-634.)* Patients with chronic inflammatory or neoplastic disease often develop anemia of chronic disease. Cytokines produced by inflammation cause a block in the normal recirculation of iron from reticuloendothelial cells (which pick up the iron from senescent red blood cells) to the red cell precursors (normoblasts). The peptide hepcidin is felt to be the main mediator of the effect. This defect in iron reutilization causes a drop in the serum iron concentration and a normocytic or mildly microcytic anemia. The inflammatory reaction, however, also decreases the iron-binding capacity (as opposed to iron-deficiency anemia, where the iron-binding capacity is elevated), so the saturation is usually between 10% and 20%. The anemia is rarely severe (Hb rarely less than 8.5 g/dL). The hemoglobin and hematocrit will improve if the underlying process is treated. Diseases not associated with inflammation or neoplasia (ie, congestive heart failure, diabetes, hypertension, etc) do not cause anemia of chronic disease. Blood loss causes a lower serum iron level, an elevated iron-binding capacity, and a lower iron saturation. The serum ferritin (low in iron deficiency, normal or high in anemia of chronic disease) will usually clarify this situation. Vitamin B_{12} and folate deficiencies are associated with macrocytic anemia. Sideroblastic anemia can be either microcytic or macrocytic (occasionally with a dimorphic population of cells, some small and some large), but is associated with an elevated iron level. In addition, this patient's history (which suggests an inflammatory polyarthritis) would not be consistent with sideroblastic anemia. The diagnosis of sideroblastic anemia is made by demonstrating ringed sideroblasts on bone marrow aspirate. In the anemia of chronic renal insufficiency, the iron studies are normal and the red cells are normocytic.

302. The answer is b. *(Fauci, pp 355-362, 652-662.)* An elevated reticulocyte count suggests active bone marrow response either to red blood cell loss (acute bleeding) or destruction (hemolysis). Many cases of hemolytic anemia can be diagnosed from changes on the peripheral blood smear. Large polychromatophilic cells suggest reticulocytes (which can be diagnosed with a specific reticulocyte stain). Microspherocytes suggest immune-mediated hemolysis. Fragmented cells suggest microvascular damage. This patient likely has immune-mediated hemolysis due to her *Mycoplasma* infection. This is usually associated with IgM antibodies, which react better at temperatures less than 37°C (98.6°F) (and thus are called *cold-reacting antibodies*). Although the serum bilirubin is often elevated in hemolysis, it is less specific. The *Mycoplasma* antigen test would confirm recent infection with *M pneumoniae* but would not specifically explain the cause of the anemia. Evidence of G6PD deficiency and intravascular hemolysis might be sought in certain circumstances, once confirmation of hemolysis had been established by simpler tests. Liver spleen scan is not used in the diagnosis of hemolysis.

303. The answer is e. *(Fauci, pp 701-707.)* Multiple myeloma would best explain this patient's presentation. The onset of myeloma is often insidious. Pain caused by bone involvement, anemia, renal insufficiency, and bacterial pneumonia often follow. This patient presented with fatigue and bone pain, then developed bacterial pneumonia probably secondary to *Streptococcus* *pneumoniae,* an encapsulated organism for which antibody to the polysaccharide capsule is not adequately produced by the myeloma patient. There is also evidence for renal insufficiency. Hypercalcemia is frequently seen in patients with multiple myeloma and may be life threatening. Definitive diagnosis of multiple myeloma is made by demonstrating greater than 30% plasma cells in the bone marrow. None of the other findings are specific enough for definitive diagnosis. 75% of patients with myeloma will have a monoclonal M spike on serum protein electrophoresis, but 25% will produce primarily Bence-Jones proteins, which, because of their small size, do not accumulate in the serum but are excreted in the urine. Urine protein electrophoresis will identify these patients. Approximately 1% of patients with myeloma will present with a nonsecretory myeloma; the diagnosis can be made only with bone marrow biopsy. The bone scan in myeloma is usually negative. The radionuclide is taken up by osteoblasts, and myeloma is usually a purely osteolytic process. Renal biopsy might show monoclonal protein deposition in the kidney or intratubular casts but would not be the first diagnostic procedure. Rouleaux formation, although characteristic of myeloma, is neither sensitive nor specific.

304. The answer is d. *(Fauci, p 1730.)* This patient presents with the superior vena cava syndrome. Such patients have jugular venous distension but no other signs of right-sided heart failure. They have prominent facial (especially periorbital) puffiness and may complain of headache, dizziness, or lethargy. SVC syndrome is caused by a malignant tumor 90% of the time. Lung cancer and lymphoma, both of which are often associated with bulky mediastinal lymphadenopathy, predominate. Gastric cancer often metastasizes to the supraclavicular nodes (most often on the left, the so-called Virchow node) but does not usually affect the mediastinal nodes to this degree. Prompt diagnosis is necessary to prevent CNS complications or laryngeal edema. Sensitive tumors (lymphoma, small cell lung cancer) may be treated with chemotherapy, while most other cell types are treated with radiation therapy. Hypertension, emphysema, and nephrotic syndrome do not cause SVC syndrome.

305. The answer is c. *(Fauci, pp 1813-1815.)* This patient has thrombotic thrombocytopenic purpura (TTP). TTP is an acute life-threatening disorder that is characterized by the pentad of microangiopathic hemolytic anemia, nonimmune thrombocytopenia, fever, renal insufficiency, and CNS involvement (confusion or multifocal encephalopathy). Not all patients have the full pentad; the essential features are the red blood cell fragmentation (schistocytes and helmet cells) and the thrombocytopenia. TTP may be triggered by endothelial damage and is associated with deficiency of a plasma protein (ADAMTS 13) that breaks down multimers of von Willebrand factor. Plasma exchange (with the infusion of fresh frozen plasma to provide the missing ADAMTS 13 protein) can be lifesaving. The hemolytic uremic syndrome (often associated with verotoxin producing strains of E coli O157:H7) is similar but is usually not accompanied by CNS changes. The renal failure is usually more severe in HUS. Disseminated intravascular coagulation associated with sepsis can resemble TTP, but the coagulation pathway is usually activated in DIC. In TTP the prothrombin time, PTT, and fibrinogen level are normal. Antiplatelet antibodies are associated with idiopathic thrombocytopenic purpura (ITP), but this patient has multiple abnormalities, not just thrombocytopenia. Hypersplenism can cause thrombocytopenia but rarely with a platelet count of below 50,000; it is not associated with red cell fragmentation.

306. The answer is d. *(Fauci, pp 643-651.)* These neurologic deficits occur with vitamin B_{12} deficiency. This patient has a deficit of intrinsic factor after gastric surgery. Intrinsic factor is produced by gastric parietal cells and is a major factor in enhancing ileal absorption of B_{12}. Milder degrees of B_{12} malabsorption can occur after partial gastrectomy, probably due to decreased release of B_{12} from food. Folic acid deficiency causes identical megaloblastic changes in the blood but is not associated with the neurologic deficit (loss of proprioception) that occurs with B_{12} deficiency. Thiamine deficiency causes beriberi; Vitamin K deficiency causes a coagulopathy associated with ecchymoses and prolongation of prothrombin time. Riboflavin deficiency is rare and causes corneal and oral inflammation. These vitamins do not depend on gastric factors for their absorption.

307. The answer is c. *(Fauci, pp 687-700.)* Chronic lymphocytic leukemia is the most common of all leukemias, with incidence increasing with age. Patients are usually asymptomatic, but may complain of weakness, fatigue, or enlarged lymph nodes. The diagnosis is made by peripheral blood smear, as mature small lymphocytes constitute almost all the white blood cells seen. Smudge cells are often present. No other process produces a lymphocytosis of this morphology and magnitude. The leukemic cells in acute leukemia are immature blast cells that are easily distinguished from the normal-appearing mature lymphocytes of CLL. Both chronic myelogenous leukemia and the leukemoid reaction associated with illness such as TB are associated with increased numbers of a variety of cells of the myeloid series (mature polymorphonuclear leukocytes, metamyelocytes, myelocytes, etc). The peripheral blood is said to resemble a dilute preparation of bone marrow. The presence of basophilia would suggest CML. Infectious mononucleosis would be rare at this age and causes large "atypical" lymphocytes that are easily distinguished from mature lymphocytes on peripheral smear.

308. The answer is c. *(Fauci, pp 363-369, 723-728.)* This woman's lifelong history of excessive bleeding suggests an inherited bleeding problem, as does the positive family history. The prolonged PTT indicates a deficiency of factors VIII, IX, XI, or XII, but the commonest of these deficiencies (classic hemophilia A and Christmas disease, or hemophilia B) are vanishingly rare in women. Furthermore, the continued oozing from dental sites and the absence of ecchymoses or hemarthroses suggest a platelet function disorder, as does the prolonged bleeding time. Von Willebrand disease is an autosomal dominant condition that leads to both platelet and factor VIII dysfunction and is the likeliest diagnosis in this patient. Although factor VIII concentrates can be used for life-threatening bleeding, most will respond to desmopressin, which raises the von Willebrand factor level in the most common form (the so-called type 1 form) of this disease. Mild von Willebrand disease is fairly common (1 in 250 individuals). Fresh frozen plasma and whole blood are much less effective ways to deliver factor VIII. Platelet transfusion would not be as effective as correction of the von Willebrand factor level.

309. The answer is b. *(Fauci, pp 551-562.)* Cigarette smokers have a 15- to 25-fold increased incidence of both squamous cell carcinoma and small cell undifferentiated (oat cell) carcinoma of the lung. Both of these neoplasms tend to be central (ie, perihilar); the presence of obstructive lung disease increases the risk of lung cancer over and above the smoking history. Of the choices given, squamous cell carcinoma is the likeliest explanation for this patient's hemoptysis. Bronchoscopy would likely show the lesion and allow a tissue diagnosis to be made. Adenocarcinoma of the lung is the commonest lung cancer seen in nonsmokers, women, and younger patients. Its incidence is increased in smokers (probably twofold), but not to the degree seen with squamous cell carcinoma and small cell undifferentiated carcinoma. Adenocarcinoma is typically peripheral with pleural involvement (rather than the central involvement seen in this case). Bronchoalveolar cell carcinoma arises from alveolar epithelium, is typically peripheral, and may resemble a nonhealing pneumonia (it may even have air bronchograms like a pneumonia). Bronchial adenomas (carcinoid being the most common type) are often central but are usually smaller and are less common than squamous cell carcinomas. Their incidence is not increased by cigarette smoking. The hilar lymphadenopathy in sarcoidosis is bilateral and, unless the bronchial mucosa is involved (5% of cases), is not associated with hemoptysis.

310. The answer is c. (*Fauci, pp 663-671.*) This patient has an unexplained pancytopenia. If all three elements (red blood cells, white blood cells, and platelets) are affected, the cause is usually in the bone marrow (although peripheral destruction from hypersplenism can cause pancytopenia as well). In this patient without a history of liver disease or palpable splenomegaly on physical examination, a bone marrow production problem is the most likely culprit. Although B_{12} deficiency can cause pancytopenia, usually a macrocytic anemia is the most prominent feature; a serum B_{12} level would be reasonable, but the most productive approach would be to examine the bone marrow. Leukemia can present without leukocytosis (so-called aleukemic leukemia), but the most likely diagnosis would be aplastic anemia. In the elderly patient, myelodysplastic syndrome (MDS) may present with pancytopenia. Decreased levels of erythropoietin can cause decreased RBC production, but will not cause pancytopenia. A corticosteroid trial is not warranted.

311. The answer is e. (*Fauci, pp 604-607.*) The first step in this patient's evaluation is a pelvic examination to check for ovarian cancer. Pelvic fullness, vague discomfort, constipation, and early satiety are often the first symptoms of this disease. Ascites may be present on initial evaluation. Abdominal ultrasound would follow. Unexplained ascites should be approached diagnostically; an empiric trial of diuretics would be inappropriate and would not help ascites due to infection or neoplasm. The CA 125 cancer antigen supports the diagnosis of ovarian cancer, but it is not sensitive or specific. If the pelvic examination and ultrasound were negative, colonoscopy (rather than sigmoidoscopy) might be indicated to evaluate the patient's constipation.

312. The answer is a. (*Fauci, pp 580-585.*) This patient has probably developed hepatocellular carcinoma as a complication of his macronodular cirrhosis. HCC is a feared complication of patients with cirrhosis resulting from hepatitis B, hepatitis C, and hemochromatosis (although it occurs with modestly increased frequency in patients with alcoholic cirrhosis as well). The incidence in high-risk patients is 3% per year. An α-fetoprotein (AFP) level greater than 500 mcg/L is suggestive, and greater than 1000 mcg/L virtually diagnostic, of this tumor. Most patients will die within 6 months if untreated;

resection of the tumor is often difficult due to the underlying liver disease. Liver transplantation can be curative in selected patients. If the α-fetoprotein is unexpectedly normal, CT-guided biopsy of the lesion would be more productive than a blind search (EGD, colonoscopy) for a primary tumor. PET scans are very expensive and would be unlikely to provide information that would change his management.

313. The answer is e. (*Fauci, pp 589-593.*) Renal carcinoma is twice as common in men as women and tends to occur in the 50- to 70-year age group. Many patients present with hematuria or flank pain, but the classic triad of hematuria, flank pain, and a palpable flank mass occurs in only 10% to 20% of patients. Paraneoplastic syndromes such as erythrocytosis, hypercalcemia, hepatic dysfunction, and fever of unknown origin are common. Surgery is the only potentially curable therapy; the results of treatment with chemotherapy or radiation therapy for nonresectable disease have been disappointing. Interferon-α and interleukin-2 produce responses (but no cures) in 10% to 20% of patients. Newer tyrosine kinase inhibitors (eg, sunitinib) are active against renal cell cancers and hold promise for more effective treatment. The prognosis for metastatic renal cell carcinoma is dismal. Pheochromocytoma can cause erythrocytosis and occasionally hypercalcemia but would not cause hematuria nor an intrarenal mass. Polycystic kidney disease can cause erythrocytosis because of erythropoietin production by the cysts but would cause numerous bilateral cysts, not a solid mass. Renal adenomyolipoma is a benign tumor that can present as a solitary renal mass on ultrasound. It has a characteristic CT appearance due to fat in the tumor. Neither renal adenomyolipoma nor adrenal carcinoma would cause erythrocytosis or hypercalcemia.

314. The answer is d. (*Fauci, pp 1732-1733.*) Spinal cord compression is an oncologic emergency. Major neurological deficit is often irreversible and severely compromises the patient's remaining quality of life. Vertebral and then epidural involvement precede the neurological findings; the thoracic cord is involved 70% of the time. The patient is often given high-dose dexamethasone before being sent for MRI. In the presence of neurological compromise, the definitive test, MRI scan, should be performed as quickly as possible. Multiple epidural metastases are noted in 25% of patients; their presence can affect treatment (eg, the extent of radiation therapy fields). If no neurological abnormalities are present, most experts recommend plain radiographs of the painful vertebra as the initial diagnostic test. A radionuclide bone scan would reveal the vertebral involvement but would not show the degree of spinal cord compromise. Electromyogram and nerve conduction studies would be normal in spinal cord disease. Bone scan and thoracic spine films are less specific than MRI. Hypercalcemia might cause confusion but not spinal cord signs.

315. The answer is a. (*Fauci, pp 601-604.*) The first step in evaluating a scrotal mass is to determine whether the mass is in the testis or outside it. Most solid masses arising from within the testis are malignant. Palpation of the scrotal mass and transillumination (holding a flashlight directly against the posterior wall of the scrotum) will distinguish testicular lesions from other masses within the scrotum, such as hydrocele. Ultrasonography will confirm a solid testicular mass. The tumor markers β-HCG and α-fetoprotein are not used in the initial evaluation of a scrotal mass, but will be important for staging if a solid mass suggestive of testicular carcinoma is found. β-HCG or AFP will be elevated in about 70% of patients with disseminated nonseminomatous testicular cancer. Seminomas are associated with normal tumor cell markers. The lymphatic drainage of the testis is into the periaortic nodes, not to the inguinal nodes. The periaortic nodes must be assessed radiographically, usually by CT scanning, if a testicular neoplasm is found. Orchiectomy is often used diagnostically, but it is not the best initial diagnostic step.

316. The answer is d. (*Fauci, pp 589-592.*) Unexplained gross hematuria requires evaluation. Patients who have gross hematuria in association with clear-cut urinary tract infection are usually treated and followed with a repeat urinalysis to confirm clearing of the RBCs, but this patient has no symptoms of urinary tract infection. Although benign causes (prostatitis, renal stones) are most common, as many as 15% of patients with gross hematuria will have bladder or ureteral cancer. Cigarette smoking increases the risk of bladder cancer two- to fourfold. Exposure to aniline dyes, chronic cyclophosphamide treatment, external beam radiation, and *Schistosoma* infection of the bladder are other risk factors. This patient should be referred to a urologist for cystoscopy to rule out transitional cell carcinoma of the bladder; the urologist will usually do a contrast retrograde pyelogram to assess for a ureteral cancer as well. If no lesion is found, CT scanning of the kidneys would be indicated despite the previous negative sonogram. The bladder scan is an ultrasonographic technique that assesses the volume of urine in the bladder. It does not visualize the bladder mucosa. Hematuria is uncommon in prostate cancer, which can be associated with an elevated PSA.

317. The answer is a. (*Fauci, pp 370-372.*) The long-term nature of these symptoms, the fact that the nodes are nontender, and their location (including scalene and supraclavicular) all suggest the likelihood of malignancy. Although infectious mononucleosis and toxoplasmosis can cause diffuse lymphadenopathy, these infections are usually associated with other evidence of infection such as pharyngitis, fever, and atypical lymphocytosis in the peripheral blood. It would be unusual for the lymphadenopathy associated with these infections to persist for 2 months. Serum angiotensin-converting enzyme level is a nonspecific test for sarcoidosis but is also elevated in other granulomatous diseases and is not sensitive or specific enough to be used as an initial diagnostic test. Lymphadenopathy associated with sarcoidosis requires a biopsy for diagnosis. In this patient, an excisional biopsy is necessary primarily to rule out the malignancy, particularly lymphoma. Needle aspiration biopsy, useful for the diagnosis of metastatic carcinoma, is insufficient to diagnose suspected lymphoma, where assessment of the lymph node architecture is important.

318. The answer is e. (*Fauci, pp 691, 698-699.*) The staging of Hodgkin disease is important so that proper treatment can be planned. Stage I (single lymph node bearing area) or stage II (more than one lymph node site on the same side of the diaphragm) patients with good prognostic features may be treated with radiation therapy. Those with stage III (affected lymph nodes on both sides of the diaphragm) or stage IV (extranodal disease) are treated with combination chemotherapy. CT or MRI of the abdomen and pelvis will show evidence of lymph node involvement below the diaphragm. Staging laparotomy with splenectomy, formerly done to provide pathology of the periaortic nodes and spleen, is rarely done today. Gallium scans can be useful in difficult cases. Bone marrow biopsy can later be performed to exclude bone marrow disease, which would imply stage IV, if less invasive studies have not clarified the proper stage. Liver biopsy is rarely indicated and the ESR is a nonspecific test.

319. The answer is a. (*Fauci, pp 586-589.*) Anorexia, weight loss, and back pain are common presenting symptoms of adenocarcinoma of the pancreas. Some patients present with new-onset diabetes. Although diabetes itself can cause weight loss, this would usually be associated with nocturia. Polyphagia rather than anorexia would characterize the weight loss of diabetes and malabsorption. In this patient, a CT scan would likely show a mass in the pancreas.

Although cancer in the head of the pancreas can present with obstructive jaundice, cancer of the body or tail of the pancreas is often associated with normal liver enzymes. This patient's symptoms are not suggestive of colon cancer, and the anemia associated with colon cancer is usually microcytic. Although PET scan may be used to stage certain cancers, it is rarely indicated as an initial test when cancer is suspected. Malabsorption is associated with diarrhea, not constipation. A glucose tolerance test will not add to the evaluation of this patient with known diabetes.

320. The answer is d. (*Fauci, pp 593-600.*) Patients with metastatic prostatic carcinoma are treated with endocrine therapy to shrink primary and secondary lesions by depriving prostatic tissue of circulating androgens. Estrogens are no longer recommended because of the high incidence of cardiovascular events. Most patients now receive a GnRH analogue or surgical castration; whether an antiandrogen (such as flutamide) provides additional benefit is currently a matter of debate. The bisphosphonate zoledronic acid can decrease pain and skeletal-related complications in patients with bony metastases and may be added to hormonal therapy. Radiotherapy is used for localized disease, but is less effective than hormonal therapy. The survival benefit of chemotherapy, if any, is small.

321. The answer is e. (*Fauci, p 721.*) Heparin is the commonest cause of drug-induced thrombocytopenia. Between 10% and 15% of patients receiving unfractionated heparin develop thrombocytopenia. The drop in platelet count is attributed to the production of an antibody against a complex of heparin and platelet factor 4. Low-molecular-weight heparin can also cause thrombocytopenia, although less frequently than unfractionated heparin. Usually the platelet count drops 5 to 10 days after heparin is started. In this case, however, the patient likely had been exposed to heparin at the time of her CABG. With previous exposure, the thrombocytopenia can begin within hours of the reinstitution of any form of heparin.

Although low-molecular-weight heparin causes HIT less frequently than unfractionated heparin, all heparin products must be discontinued in the patient with HIT. In all patients with an active clot and those with HITT (heparin-induced thrombocytopenia with thrombosis), a direct thrombin inhibitor must be started and used as a bridge to full potency warfarin therapy. The chief consequence of HIT is not bleeding but accelerated clotting resulting from the aggregation of platelet-heparin complexes in the circulation. HITT is a feared complication of HIT. Even with proper treatment, the amputation rate (owing to intra-arterial clotting) is as high as 40%, and the death rate as high as 25%.

322. The **answer is e.** *(Fauci, pp 492-498.)* Although much is being learned about the genetic mechanisms that underlie the susceptibility to cancer, most cancers are still considered "sporadic." Many are attributed to a combination of genetic factors (often acquired) and environmental carcinogens, such as ambient radiation. Only 20% of women who develop breast cancer have a positive family history of this disease. Of these, only 5% to 10% have an autosomal dominant mutation in *BRCA1* or *BRCA2*. Genetic testing, which is quite expensive, should be reserved for women who have had multiple family members (usually in different generations) with premenopausal breast cancer or ovarian cancer. Women of Ashkenazi Jewish origin have a particularly high carriage rate for *BRCA*.

The p53 tumor suppressor gene is disordered in the Li-Fraumeni syndrome, which is associated with tumors in numerous organs, generally in very young patients. Other specific genetic defects have been discovered in colon cancer (the familial adenomatous polyposis and hereditary nonpolyposis colorectal cancer syndromes), in retinoblastoma, and a few other rare familial cancer syndromes. Intrauterine exposure to DES is associated with cancer of the vagina, not breast.

323. **The answer is c.** *(Fauci, pp 743-745.)* Rifampin induces the cytochrome P450 that metabolizes warfarin; higher doses of warfarin are required to overcome this effect. When rifampin is stopped, the dose of warfarin necessary to produce a therapeutic prothrombin time will decrease. Barbiturates also accelerate the metabolism of warfarin. Many drugs interfere with the metabolism and clearance of warfarin. Drugs such as nonsteroidal anti-inflammatories can compete with warfarin for albumin-binding sites and will lead to an increased prothrombin time. The list of medications that can either increase or decrease the effect of warfarin is long; all patients given this drug should be advised to contact their physician before taking any new drug. They should also be counseled about over-the-counter drugs (aspirin and NSAIDs) and even health food supplements (such as ginkgo biloba) which can affect the prothrombin time in these patients. A stable intake of vitamin K containing foods (ie, green leafy vegetables) is recommended.

324. **The answer is b.** *(Fauci, pp 580-586.)* Patients with hemochromatosis and cirrhosis have a very high incidence of hepatocellular carcinoma. The incidence of this complication is 30% and increases with age. Weight loss and abdominal pain suggest hepatoma in this patient. A CT scan or ultrasound and measurement of alpha-fetoprotein are indicated. The picture of right upper quadrant pain and elevated alkaline phosphatase would not suggest acute hepatitis (which causes an elevation of transaminases) or worsening of the cirrhosis caused by hemochromatosis. Primary biliary cirrhosis (associated with antimitochondrial antibodies) can cause an obstructive biliary disease, but would be much less likely in this patient.

325. The answer is e. *(Fauci, pp 566-570.)* This woman is at high risk of recurrent breast cancer, an ultimately fatal event. Adjuvant therapy has been shown to decrease the chance of recurrence by 40%. This translates into a proven survival advantage for the woman; the advantages of treatment far outweigh the risk of side effects. Therefore, no therapy or only local therapy (eg, radiation therapy) would represent inadequate treatment.

Postmenopausal women who are ER or PR positive are generally treated with adjuvant hormonal therapy. Premenopausal women, or women whose tumor does not contain ER or PR, will usually need adjuvant chemotherapy. Both tamoxifen (an estrogen receptor antagonist) and aromatase inhibitors (eg, letrozole, anastrozole) are effective in decreasing the rate of recurrence. Although aromatase inhibitors may be slightly more effective than tamoxifen, they are much more expensive, can produce troublesome side effects, and unlike tamoxifen do not improve bone density. This choice is often based on the preference of the patient and her oncologist. In a woman 5 or more years after menopause, the ovaries produce inconsequential amount of estrogens. Therefore oophorectomy, sometimes used in the premenopausal woman, is an inappropriate choice for this patient.

326. The answer is d. *(Fauci, pp 330-331, 610-611.)* Although lipomas are the commonest soft tissue mass, they are soft, move with the subcutaneous tissue, and grow very slowly. Any atypical or enlarging soft tissue mass should be further evaluated, either by CT or MRI scan or by biopsy, because this is how soft tissue sarcomas present. Bone scan is usually normal. The size, firmness, and fixity to deep tissues are all worrisome features in this patient. An abscess would be soft and fluctuant, and hematomas are painful and associated with trauma. Therefore a biopsy should be requested even if the CT scan is reassuring. An open biopsy would be the preferred approach. Sixty percent of soft tissue sarcomas arise in the extremities, with the lower extremities three times as common as the upper extremities. Several histological types are possible and are not predictable from clinical features; malignant fibrous histiocytomas are most common. The only curative approach is complete surgical resection. Radiation and chemotherapy have a role in adjuvant or palliative therapy. Occasional patients with favorable metastatic disease enter long-term remission with aggressive therapy. Soft tissue sarcomas metastasize hematogenously, most often to the lungs; lymph node metastases would not be expected.

327. The answer is b. *(Fauci, pp 671-677.)* This patient has polycythemia vera, a clonal proliferative disorder of the bone marrow in which all three cell lines (red blood cells, platelets, and myelocytes) are overproduced. The other classic myeloproliferative disorders are chronic myelogenous leukemia, essential thrombocytosis, and myelofibrosis. It is important to distinguish myeloproliferative syndromes (where one or more cell lines proliferate) from myelodysplastic syndromes (where one or more cell lines—usually red cells—are deficient). In myelodysplastic disorders, white blood cells and platelets are normal, at least initially. These patients present with anemia, often in association with mild macrocytosis and other features of altered marrow maturation (ringed sideroblasts, hypolobulated polys, etc). Splenomegaly and cellular overproduction are not features of the myelodysplastic syndromes. Cushing syndrome can cause facial plethora but would not account for the splenomegaly or hematological changes. Gaisböck syndrome causes erythrocytosis with a normal red cell mass (resulting from diminished plasma volume) but does not cause splenomegaly, leukocytosis, or thrombocytosis. Polycythemia vera does not occur as part of a paraneoplastic process.

328. The answer is c. *(Fauci, pp 372-375, 637-639.)* Splenomegaly is not typical of sickle cell anemia. Recurrent splenic infarcts usually occur during childhood and lead to a small, infarcted spleen with functional asplenia. These patients often have Howell-Jolly bodies on peripheral blood smear (indicative of asplenia) and have an increased incidence of infection with encapsulated organisms. The presence of an enlarged spleen in a patient with sickled cells on peripheral blood smear is most often seen in hemoglobin SC disease. Any hemolytic anemia can result in an unconjugated hyperbilirubinemia and low-grade icterus. Anemia results in a hyperdynamic circulation and a systolic ejection murmur. Ankle ulcers and other chronic skin ulcers may be persistent problems in patients with SS disease, particularly in those with severe anemia. Patients with sickle cell crisis often present with leukocytosis, related both to stress and to the asplenia.

329. The answer is e. *(Fauci, pp 652-662.)* This patient has developed a hemolytic anemia secondary to an antimalarial drug. Toxins or drugs such as primaquine, sulfamethoxazole, and nitrofurantoin cause hemolysis in patients with G6PD deficiency, which occurs most commonly in African Americans. Since the *G6PD* gene is carried on the X chromosome, most affected patients are males. The drugs that cause hemolysis in G6PD deficiency are oxidizing agents. Oxidant stress on red blood cells is normally counteracted by reduced glutathione. NADPH (which is required to regenerate reduced glutathione after it has been oxidized) is produced by the hexose monophosphate shunt. G6PD is the first enzyme in this metabolic pathway. If this enzyme is less active, the cell cannot replace reduced glutathione and succumbs to oxidizing stress. Clinically this can range from mild to life-threatening hemolysis. In mild cases, no treatment is necessary; once the offending drug is eliminated, the hemolysis resolves.

330. The answer is c. *(Fauci, pp 601-604.)* This patient has testicular carcinoma. A solid mass arising from the testis (ie, not an extratesticular scrotal mass) is almost always malignant. Bulky retroperitoneal lymphadenopathy is characteristic of the metastatic pattern of testicular cancer. The evaluation first involves staging the tumor with CT rather than PET scanning. Stage 1 is confined to the testicle, Stage II involves retroperitoneal or periaortic lymphadenopathy, and Stage III implies distant spread to mediastinal or supraclavicular nodes, lung, or brain. The intensity of treatment is decided by placing the patient into good, intermediate, or poor prognostic groups. This is based on histological type (determined from the radical inguinal orchiectomy), stage, and tumor markers (AFP, beta HCG, and LDH). Diagnosis is often confirmed by orchiectomy as needle biopsy or aspiration is usually not diagnostic. In general, favorable prognosis features include seminomatous histology, absent or (in the case of nonseminomatous tumors) low levels of serum tumor markers, absence of metastases beyond the retroperitoneal nodes, and testicular site of origin (extragonadal tumors carry a less favorable outlook). Favorable prognosis seminomas are often cured with orchiectomy and retroperitoneal radiation therapy. Chemotherapy is usually necessary to cure nonseminomatous tumors, but even intermediate prognosis nonseminomatous tumors can be cured 80% of the time. Other cancers may also be associated with tumor markers (CEA in colon and alpha-fetoprotein in hepatoma).

331. The answer is b. *(Fauci, pp 668-671.)* The patient has probably had myelodysplastic syndrome (MDS) for years. This commonly causes anemia with mild macrocytosis in the elderly. Some of these patients will transform into acute myeloid leukemia. The leukemic cells can expand the marrow and cause diffuse bone pain (especially over the sternum and around the knees). Although 20% of patients with MDS may have mild splenomegaly, the newly detected spleen tip and the rapidly worsening pancytopenia suggest that leukemic cells are squeezing out the normal hematopoietic cells. Patients with secondary AML (ie, AML that arises from a preexisting hematopoietic disease) have a grave prognosis and respond poorly to combination chemotherapy. Folic acid deficiency would not cause leukocytosis. Viral infection and tuberculosis may present subacutely but not this chronically.

332. The answer is b. *(Fauci, pp 728-731, 937-938.)* This patient with gram-negative bacteremia has developed disseminated intravascular coagulation, as evidenced by multiple-site bleeding, thrombocytopenia, fragmented red blood cells on peripheral smear, prolonged PT and PTT, and reduced fibrinogen levels from depletion of coagulation proteins. Initial treatment is directed at correcting the underlying disorder—in this case, infection. Although heparin was formerly recommended for the treatment of DIC, it is now used rarely and only in unusual circumstances (such as acute promyelocytic leukemia). For the patient who continues to bleed, supplementation of platelets and clotting factors (with fresh frozen plasma or cryoprecipitate) may help control life-threatening bleeding. Red cell fragmentation and low platelet count can be seen in microangiopathic disorders such as TTP, but in these disorders the coagulation pathway is not activated. Therefore, in TTP the prothrombin time, partial thromboplastin time and plasma fibrinogen levels will be normal. Plasmapheresis, vitamin K therapy, and RBC transfusion will not correct the underlying cause.

333. The answer is c. *(Fauci, p 664.)* Propylthiouracil often causes a mild leukopenia that does not require discontinuation of the drug. Drug-induced agranulocytosis, however, is a life-threatening complication occurring in 0.1% to 0.2% of patients on antithyroid medications and requires immediate discontinuation of the drug. Agranulocytosis is an immune-mediated disorder; the absolute neutrophil count is often extremely depressed (usually less than 100). Generally the neutrophil count will recover 5 to 7 days after the offending drug has been discontinued. During this time the patient is at grave risk of septicemia. Although blood cultures and CXR may be indicated in this patient prior to the administration of antibiotics, the most important initial step is evaluating the white blood cell count. Evaluation of thyroid function (with TSH or T3) will not diagnose the agranulocytosis.

334. The answer is c. *(Fauci, pp 687-700.)* This is a classic presentation of diffuse large cell lymphoma. These neoplasms usually present with a rapidly enlarging nodes and B symptoms (fever, night sweats, >10% weight loss). Extranodal disease (eg, gastric involvement) is occasionally seen, whereas extralymphatic disease is unusual in the more indolent small cell lymphomas. Although Hodgkin disease can also present in this fashion, the histological features and B-cell markers are those of a non-Hodgkin lymphoma.

Untreated large cell lymphomas are progressive and rapidly fatal. Usually, however, they respond to combination therapy (multidrug chemotherapy, often combined with the anti-CD 20 antibody rituximab). As opposed to indolent lymphomas, which respond but almost always relapse, most large cell lymphomas are cured with therapy. Exceptions are mantle cell lymphomas and primary central nervous system lymphomas, which are more refractory to therapy.

335. The answer is a. *(Fauci, pp 564-565.)* A breast mass, even in a young woman, requires definitive evaluation. Although most such masses are benign, breast cancer is still the most common cause of cancer death in this age group. Risk factor assessment cannot provide sufficient reassurance. A negative mammogram never rules out breast cancer. Either excisional biopsy or, in selected hands, fine needle aspiration with follow-up, will be needed to detect cases of breast cancer before metastases outside the breast have occurred. Reassurance and reevaluation in 6 months may lead to delay in diagnosis of breast cancer. Neither oral contraceptives nor tamoxifen are indicated prior to a definitive diagnosis.

336. The answer is e. *(Fauci, p 363-369, 733.)* Testing for thrombophilia is generally reserved for patients who develop unprovoked venous thromboses, especially when those events occur before age 50 in a patient with a positive family history of abnormal clotting. This patient should simply be treated with low-molecular-weight heparin followed by 3 to 6 months of warfarin in the standard fashion. If she develops recurrent DVT, thrombophilia testing would be considered.

The prothrombin gene mutation (G20210A) and factor V Leiden are the commonest genetic factors associated with DVT, but they cause only a modestly increased risk of DVT and their presence may not change the management of the patient. Patients with factor V Leiden who are taking oral contraceptives have a 35-fold increased risk of DVT, but OCPs should be avoided if possible in women with any prior history of DVT. Protein C, S, and AT III deficiencies confer a much greater risk, but are significantly less common. Their presence will usually be identified by the history including family history. Remember that these genetic conditions have been associated with an increased risk of venous, not arterial, thrombosis. Only the antiphospholipid antibody syndrome and elevated homocysteine levels have been associated with arterial thromboses.

337 to 339. The answers are 337-c, 338-b, 339-e. *(Fauci, pp 707-713.)* Although the risk of the transmission of viral agents with transfusions is very low (probably less than one in a million for hepatitis C and HIV), other types of transfusion reactions still occur. Febrile and allergic reactions occur between 1% and 4% of the time. Life-threatening reactions associated with ABO and Rh incompatibility occur rarely and are usually due to mislabeling of the blood product. These reactions fix complement, cause intravascular hemolysis, and occur acutely during the transfusion. Delayed hemolytic reactions to minor antigens on the donor red blood cells occur more commonly. This type of reaction often occurs in multiparous women or in multiply transfused patients who have previously been exposed to foreign antigens. Within several days to a week, antigenic memory cells in the patient produce antibodies against the transfused cells, which express this antigen. Delayed hemolytic reactions are rarely life threatening.

Transfusion-related acute lung injury (TRALI) is a form of noncardiogenic pulmonary edema that, while self-limited, can lead to respiratory failure and the need for mechanical ventilation. It is caused by antibodies in the *donor* plasma that bind to HLA antigens on the recipient's white blood cells. The recipient's leukocytes agglutinate and are trapped in the capillaries of the lungs. Aspiration pneumonia can mimic TRALI but usually has other features (eg, purulent sputum, fever) to suggest it. The lung examination and CXR do not distinguish TRALI from volume overload resulting from multiple transfusions, but this young woman, with volume depletion from blood loss and no history of heart disease, is much more likely to have TRALI.

Bacteria can contaminate blood products, especially platelets, which must be stored at room temperature and can be held for 5 days. In the past, many of these septic reactions were associated with contamination of the skin plug that enters the collection apparatus when the blood is being obtained. Now many reactions are attributed to gram-negative rods, including *Yersinia,* which can cause asymptomatic bacteremia in the donor. The septic response occurs acutely during or immediately after the transfusion, in association with the direct infusion endotoxins and other bacterial products. The clinical features are similar to acute ABO incompatibility (which can cause fever and hypotension as well) but without evidence of acute intravascular hemolysis. The transfusion should be immediately stopped and antibiotics administered.

340 to 342. The answers are 340-f, 341-b, 342-d. (Fauci, pp 355-363, 628-643, 643-651.) The most useful way to categorize an anemia is according to the mean corpuscular volume. Although overlap can occur (ie, the anemia of chronic disease can be either normocytic or microcytic, sideroblastic anemia can be microcytic, macrocytic, or normocytic), the MCV is still the best place to start.

Causes of macrocytic anemia include megaloblastic anemias (cobalamin and folate deficiency), vigorous reticulocytosis, hypothyroidism, chronic liver disease, and myelodysplastic syndrome. Only megaloblastic anemias have hypersegmentation of the neutrophils, oval-shaped red blood cells and slow maturation of cellular nuclei (eg, megaloblastic cellular changes in the bone marrow). These changes result from impaired DNA synthesis; both cobalamin and folate are involved in the methyl transfer reactions that synthesize thymidine for DNA synthesis. B_{12} and folate deficiency cannot be distinguished on the blood smear, but this patient's alcoholism and the normal neurological examination (only cobalamin deficiency causes clinically important neurological changes) suggest folate deficiency.

Common causes of microcytic anemia include iron deficiency, thalassemia, and (sometimes) the anemia of chronic disease and sideroblastic anemia. Both iron-deficiency anemia and anemia of chronic disease are associated with a low serum iron level. In iron-deficiency anemia, the TIBC is high and the iron saturation is usually less than 10%. In anemia of chronic disease, the iron-binding capacity is low and the saturation is usually between 10% and 20%. In borderline cases, a serum ferritin level will usually make the distinction (it is low in iron-deficiency anemia and normal or high in anemia of chronic disease). This patient has a Mediterranean heritage, severe microcytosis (out of proportion to her relatively mild anemia) and target cells on her peripheral smear, all features of thalassemia. If she has beta-thalassemia, a hemoglobin electrophoresis with quantitative hemoglobin A2 and F levels will confirm the diagnosis. Alpha thalassemia, seen most often in African Americans, is harder to diagnose definitively.

The anemia of renal disease is normocytic and normochromic, as are most anemias associated with bone marrow production problems (aplastic anemia, leukemia) and most hemoglobinopathies. In renal failure, the red cells themselves are normal but are not stimulated to proliferate because of inadequate amounts of erythropoietin. White cell and platelet counts are usually normal, although there are disorders of function in both these cell lines. This anemia responds to erythropoietin supplementation.

343 and 344. The answers are 343-d, 344-a. *(Fauci, pp 554, 587, 622.)* The classic Trousseau syndrome consists of migratory superficial thrombophlebitis. A single episode of tenderness and inflammation in a superficial vein is common and usually benign, but recurrent unprovoked episodes should prompt a search for an underlying neoplasm. Cancer of the pancreas is the classic and most common cause, but any mucin-producing carcinoma can produce this syndrome.

Humoral hypercalcemia of malignancy resembles hyperparathyroidism, but the substance produced by the cancer is parathormone-related peptide (PTHrP), which does not cross-react with PTH on modern assays. PTHrP is an oncofetal protein involved in squamous differentiation in the fetus. For this reason squamous cancers (lung, head and neck, cervix) are the usual causes. Adenocarcinomas are relatively uncommon causes of this syndrome. This patient's mental status changes are probably caused by hypercalcemia.

Neurology

Questions

345. A 30-year-old male complains of unilateral headaches. He was diagnosed with migraine headaches at age 24. The headaches did not respond to triptan therapy at that time, but after 6 weeks the headaches resolved. He has had 3 or 4 spells of severe headaches since then. Currently his headaches have been present for the past 2 weeks. The headaches start with a stabbing pain just below the right eye. Usually the affected eye feels "irritated" (reddened with increased lacrimation). He saw an optometrist during one of the episodes and a miotic pupil was noted. Each pain lasts from 60 to 90 minutes, but he may have several discrete episodes each day. The neurological examination, including cranial nerve examination, is now normal. What is your best approach to treatment at this time?

a. Prescribe oral sumatriptan for use at the onset of headache.
b. Prednisone 60 mg daily for 2 to 4 weeks.
c. Obtain MRI scan of the head with gadolinium contrast.
d. Begin propranolol 20 mg bid.
e. Refer for neuropsychiatric testing.

346. A 47-year-old dentist consults you because of tremor, which is interfering with his work. The tremor has come on gradually over the past several years and seems more prominent after the ingestion of caffeine; he notices that, in the evening after work, an alcoholic beverage will decrease the tremor. No one in his family has a similar tremor. He is otherwise healthy and takes no medications. On examination his vital signs are normal. Except for the tremor, his neurological examination is normal; in particular there is no focal weakness, rigidity, or bradykinesia. When he holds out his arms and extends his fingers, you detect a rapid fine tremor of both hands; the tremor goes away when he rests his arms at his side. What is the next best step in the management of this patient?

a. MRI scan to visualize the basal ganglia
b. Electromyogram and nerve conduction studies to more fully characterize the tremor
c. Therapeutic trial of propranolol
d. Therapeutic trial of primidone
e. Neurology referral to rule out motor neuron disease

347. A 35-year-old previously healthy woman complains of a severe, excruciating headache and then has transient loss of consciousness. There are no focal neurologic findings. Which of the following is the best next step in evaluation?

a. CT scan without contrast
b. CT scan with contrast
c. Cerebral angiogram
d. Holter monitor
e. Therapeutic trial of nortriptyline

348. A 58-year-old male complains of the sudden onset of syncope. It occurs without warning and with no sweating, dizziness, or light headedness. He believes episodes tend to occur when he turns his head too quickly or sometimes when he is shaving. Physical examination is unremarkable. He has no carotid bruits, and cardiac examination is normal. Which of the following is the best way to make a definitive diagnosis in this patient?

a. ECG
b. Carotid massage with ECG monitoring
c. Holter monitor
d. Electrophysiologic study to evaluate the AV node
e. Carotid duplex ultrasonogram

349. An 82-year-old woman is evaluated for progressive dementia. She is on no medications; the family has not noticed urinary incontinence or seizure activity. Her MMSE score is 21 out of 30; she has no focal weakness or reflex asymmetry on physical examination. MR scan shows a 2.4 cm partly calcified, densely enhancing mass near the falx (see below). There is no surrounding edema or mass effect. What is the best approach to this patient's management?

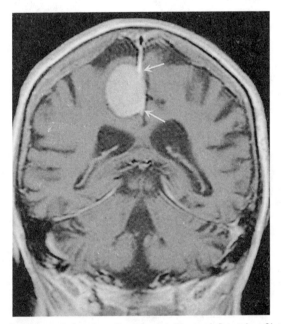

Reproduced, with permission, from Fauci A et al. *Harrison's Principles of Internal Medicine*, 17th ed. New York, NY: McGraw-Hill, 2008.

a. Neurosurgical resection of the mass
b. Radiation therapy to the mass
c. Serial CT scans and cholinergic treatment for the dementia if indicated
d. Ventriculoperitoneal shunting
e. Phenytoin and watchful waiting

350. A 30-year-old male complains of bilateral leg weakness and clumsiness of fine movements of the right hand. Five years previously he had an episode of transient visual loss. On physical examination, there is hyperreflexia with Babinski sign, and cerebellar dysmetria with poor finger-to-nose movement. When the patient is asked to look to the right, the left eye does not move normally past the midline. Nystagmus is noted in the abducting eye. A more detailed history suggests the patient has had several episodes of gait difficulty that have resolved spontaneously. He appears to be stable between these episodes. He has no systemic symptoms of fever or weight loss. Which of the following is the most appropriate next test to order?

a. Lumbar puncture
b. MR scan with gadolinium infusion
c. Quantitative CSF IgG levels
d. Testing for oligoclonal bands in cerebrospinal fluid
e. CT scan of the head with intravenous contrast

351. A 76-year-old woman consults you because of leg discomfort. Her legs are comfortable during the day, but in the evening she develops an uncomfortable creepy-crawly sensation that keeps her awake for hours. The feeling is temporarily relieved by movement; she will awaken, pace around, and sometimes run water on her legs to achieve relief. Which of the following is the best initial treatment for her condition?

a. Zolpidem 5 mg po at bedtime
b. Trazodone 50 mg po at bedtime
c. Stretching exercises of the legs
d. Pramipexole 0.125 mg po in the evening
e. Cyclobenzaprine 10 mg po at bedtime

352. A 50-year-old male complains of slowly progressive weakness over several months. Walking has become more difficult, as has using his hands. There are no sensory, bowel, or bladder complaints; he denies problems with thinking, speech, or vision. Examination shows distal muscle weakness with muscle wasting and fasciculations. There are also upper motor neuron signs, including extensor plantar reflexes and hyperreflexia in wasted muscle groups. Which of the following tests is most likely to be abnormal in this patient?

a. Cerebrospinal fluid white blood cell count
b. Sensory conduction studies
c. CT scan of the brain
d. Electromyography
e. Thyroid studies and vitamin B_{12} level

353. A 22-year-old woman seeks advice for the treatment of headaches. The first of these headaches began at age 16, but their frequency has increased to 2 to 3 per month over the past year. The headaches are not preceded by an aura. The headaches are usually bilateral, are throbbing, and are so intense that she has to go home from work. Loud noise and physical activity make the pain more severe. Each headache lasts until the evening; she will awaken the next morning without pain or nausea, and will be able to return to work. She takes acetaminophen at the onset of the headache but without benefit. She is on no other medications including oral contraceptives. Neurological examination is benign. What is the best step in the management of these headaches?

a. Topiramate starting at a dose of 25 mg twice daily
b. An oral triptan such as sumatriptan at the onset of pain
c. Combination acetaminophen/hydrocodone at the onset of pain
d. Long acting propranolol 40 mg daily, increasing until the headaches are completely prevented
e. Gabapentin 300 mg daily at bedtime, increasing until the headaches are controlled

354. A 20-year-old woman complains of weakness that is worse in the afternoon, worse during prolonged activity, and improved by rest. When fatigued, the patient is unable to hold her head up or chew her food. On physical examination, she has no loss of reflexes, sensation, or coordination. Which of the following is the likely pathogenesis of this disease?

a. Antiacetylcholine receptor antibodies causing neuromuscular transmission failure
b. Destruction of anterior horn cells by virus
c. Progressive muscular atrophy caused by spinal degeneration
d. Demyelinating disease
e. Defect in muscle glycogen breakdown

355. A 65-year-old man develops a severe headache and right-sided weakness. He has a history of osteoarthritis, gout, and hypertension. He regularly keeps his follow-up visits and is compliant with his medications, which include lisinopril 10 mg po q AM for hypertension, allopurinol 300 mg po q AM to prevent gout, and acetaminophen for his joint pains. Review of his recent office record shows that his mean blood pressure has been 124/78. On physical examination the patient is drowsy but arousable. His blood pressure is 164/90 and his pulse rate is 56. He has a right homonymous hemianopsia and a mild right hemiparesis. Sensory examination is difficult due to poor cooperation. Cardiac examination shows no S_3 or S_4 gallop and a regular rhythm. He has no ecchymoses or evidence of abnormal bruising. His ECG is normal without left ventricular hypertrophy. CT of the head without IV contrast shows an acute hemorrhage in the left parietal lobe; the basal ganglia and thalamus are uninvolved. What is the likely pathogenesis of the neurological problem?

a. Small vessel vasculitis
b. Intimal damage to penetrating cerebral vessels
c. Trauma from domestic abuse
d. Coagulopathy
e. Amyloid deposition in the cerebral vasculature

356. Three weeks after an upper respiratory illness, a 25-year-old male develops weakness of his legs over several days. On physical examination he has 4/5 strength in his arms but only 2/5 in the legs bilaterally. There is no sensory deficit, but motor reflexes in the legs cannot be elicited. During a 2-day observation period the weakness ascends, and he begins to notice increasing weakness of the hands. He notices mild tingling, but the sensory examination continues to be normal. The workup of this patient is most likely to show which of the following?

a. Acellular spinal fluid with high protein
b. Abnormal EMG/NCV showing axonal degeneration
c. Positive edrophonium (Tensilon) test
d. Elevated CK
e. Respiratory alkalosis on arterial blood gas

357. A 32-year-old woman presents to you for evaluation of headache. The headaches began at age 18, were initially unilateral and worse around the time of her menses. Initially the use of triptans 2 or 3 times a month would provide complete relief. Over the past several years, however, the headaches have become more frequent and severe. Triptans provide only partial relief; the patient requires a combination of acetaminophen, caffeine, and butalbital to achieve some improvement. Prophylactic medications including beta-blockers, tricyclics, and topiramate have been unsuccessful in preventing the headaches, and she has been to the emergency room three times over the past 2 weeks for a "pain shot." The general physical examination is unremarkable. Her funduscopic examination shows no evidence of papilledema, and a careful neurological examination is likewise normal. What is the most likely explanation for her headache syndrome?

a. Status migranosus
b. Medication overuse headache
c. Space occupying intracerebral lesion
d. CNS vasculitis
e. Pseudotumor cerebri

358. A 76-year-old woman presents with numbness and mild weakness in the legs. She has noticed mild numbness in the fingertips bilaterally. The symptoms have been slowly progressive over the past year. She rarely goes to the doctor and takes no medications. Neurological examination shows sensory loss to light touch distal to the knees and wrists in a symmetric pattern. Joint position and vibratory sensation are normal. Ankle reflexes are absent, and she has mild distal weakness. Which of the following is the most likely abnormality on laboratory testing?

a. Hyperglycemia
b. Macrocytic anemia with a low vitamin B_{12} level
c. Oligoclonal bands on CSF analysis
d. Low T_4, elevated TSH
e. Positive antiacetylcholine receptor antibody titers

359. A 68-year-old man with a history of hypertension and coronary artery disease presents with right-sided weakness, sensory loss, and an expressive aphasia. Neuroimaging studies are shown. In the emergency department the patient's blood pressure is persistently 160/95. Which of the following is the best next step in management of this patient's blood pressure?

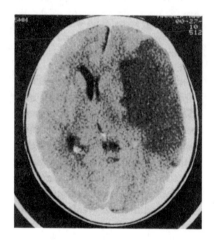

a. Administer IV nitroprusside.
b. Administer oral clonidine 0.1 mg po until the blood pressure drops below 140/90.
c. Observe the blood pressure.
d. Administer IV mannitol.
e. Administer IV labetolol.

360. A 45-year-old woman presents to her physician with an 8-month history of gradually increasing limb weakness. She first noticed difficulty climbing stairs, then problems rising from a chair, and, finally, lifting her arms above shoulder level. Aside from some difficulty swallowing, she has no ocular, bulbar, or sphincter problems and no sensory complaints. Family history is negative for neurological disease. Examination reveals significant proximal limb and neck muscle weakness with minimal atrophy, normal sensory findings, and normal deep tendon reflexes. Which of the following is the most likely diagnosis in this patient?

a. Polymyositis
b. Cervical myelopathy
c. Myasthenia gravis
d. Mononeuritis multiplex
e. Limb-girdle muscular dystrophy

361. A 55-year-old diabetic woman suddenly develops weakness of the left side of her face as well as of her right arm and leg. She also has diplopia on left lateral gaze. Where is the responsible lesion?

a. Right cerebral hemisphere
b. Left cerebral hemisphere
c. Right side of the brainstem
d. Left side of the brainstem
e. Right median longitudinal fasciculus

362. A 26-year-old woman presents for follow-up of her multiple sclerosis. She has had two separate episodes of optic neuritis and has noticed stutteringly progressive weakness in her lower extremities. She has a mild neurogenic bladder. Her symptoms have been stable over the past 4 months. MRI scanning reveals several plaques in the periventricular white matter (see MR scan below) and several other plaques in the brainstem. What is the best next step in her management?

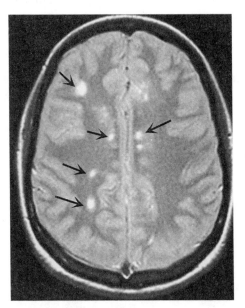

Reproduced, with permission, from Fauci A et al. *Harrison's Principles of Internal Medicine,* 17th ed. New York, NY: McGraw-Hill, 2008.

a. Intravenous methylprednisolone 1 g daily for 3 days
b. Oral cyclophosphamide
c. Oral anticholinergics for the urinary incontinence and observation of the demyelinating process
d. Interferon-beta
e. Intravenous mitoxantrone every 3 months

363. A 72-year-old woman presents with poor coordination and frequent falls. She smokes 1 pack of cigarettes per day and uses alcohol modestly. She takes raloxifene for osteoporosis and a daily multiple vitamin. She has lost 10 pounds of weight over the past 6 weeks and notices some diminution of appetite. Her general physical examination shows evidence of mild temporal muscle wasting and diminished breath sounds over both lung fields. On neurological examination her strength, sensation (including vibratory sensation), and reflexes are normal. She walks with an uncoordinated unsteady gait. On testing of coordination in the upper extremities, she displays past pointing and poor rapid alternating movements. The findings are symmetrical. In the lower extremities, her heel-shin testing also reveals poor coordination symmetrically. What is the most likely cause of her condition?

a. Tumor in the right lobe of the cerebellum
b. Multiple small infarcts in the basal ganglia
c. Paraneoplastic cerebellar degeneration
d. Alcohol abuse
e. Posterior column degeneration as a result of vitamin deficiency

364. A 40-year-old woman complains of headache associated with visual disturbance. Which of the following histories suggests migraine headache as the likely diagnosis?

a. Numbness or tingling of the left face, lips, and hand lasting for 5 to 15 minutes, followed by throbbing headache
b. An increasingly throbbing headache associated with unilateral visual loss and generalized muscle aches
c. A continuous headache associated with sleepiness, nausea, ataxia, and incoordination of the right upper limb
d. An intense left retro-orbital headache associated with transient left-sided ptosis and rhinorrhea
e. A visual field defect that persists following cessation of a unilateral headache

365. A 74-year-woman consults you because of tremor and difficulty completing her daily tasks on time. She has hypertension and takes hydrochlorothiazide 25 mg every morning. She does not smoke and uses alcohol infrequently. On examination, her BP is 126/84; her vital signs are otherwise unremarkable. Eye movements are normal as are her reflexes and motor strength. She moves slowly; her timed get-up-and-go test takes 24 seconds (normal 10 seconds). She has a slow resting tremor with a frequency of about 3/second; the tremor is more prominent on the right than the left. The tremor decreases with intentional movement. Her handwriting has deteriorated and is small and crabbed. Which therapy is most likely to improve her functional disabilities?

a. Switching her antihypertensive to propranolol 20 mg po bid
b. Benztropine mesylate 0.5 mg po tid
c. Lorazepam 0.5 mg po tid
d. Ropinirole beginning at a dose of 0.25 mg tid
e. Carbidopa/levodopa beginning at a dose of one-half of a 25 mg/100 mg tablet tid

366. A 72-year-old woman is found unconscious at home by her daughter. In the emergency room the patient does not respond to verbal or noxious stimuli. Which of the following is the most likely cause of her condition?

a. Hypoglycemia
b. Left posterior cerebral artery occlusion
c. Lacunar infarct in the right internal capsule
d. Middle cerebral artery occlusion
e. Anterior cerebral artery occlusion

367. A 37-year-old factory worker develops increasing weakness in the legs; coworkers have noted episodes of transient confusion. The patient has bilateral foot drop and atrophy; mild wrist weakness is also present. His CBC shows an anemia with hemoglobin of 9.6 g/dL; examination of the peripheral blood smear shows basophilic stippling. Which of the following is the most likely cause of this patient's symptoms?

a. Amyotrophic lateral sclerosis
b. Lead poisoning
c. Overuse syndrome
d. Myasthenia gravis
e. Alcoholism

368. A 53-year-old woman presents with increasing weakness, most noticeable in the legs. She has noticed some cramping and weakness in the upper extremities as well. She has more difficulty removing the lids from jars than before. She has noticed some stiffness in the neck but denies back pain or injury. There is no bowel or bladder incontinence. She takes naproxen for osteoarthritis and is on alendronate for osteoporosis. She smokes one pack of cigarettes daily. The general physical examination reveals decreased range of motion in the cervical spine. On neurological examination, the patient has 4/5 strength in the hands with mild atrophy of the interosseous muscles. She also has 4/5 strength in the feet; the weakness is more prominent in the distal musculature. She has difficulty with both heel walking and toe walking. Reflexes are hyperactive in the lower extremities. Sustained clonus is demonstrated at the ankles. What is the best next step in her management?

a. Obtain MRI scan of the head.
b. Begin riluzole.
c. Obtain MRI scan of the cervical spine.
d. Check muscle enzymes including creatine kinase and aldolase.
e. Refer for physical therapy and gait training exercises.

369. A 73-year-old man has had 3 episodes of visual loss in the right eye. The episodes last 20 to 30 minutes and resolve completely. He describes the sensation as like a window shade being pulled down in front of the eye. He has a history of hypertension and tobacco use. He denies dyspnea, chest pain, palpitations, or unilateral weakness or numbness. On examination the patient appears healthy; his vital signs are normal and the neurological examination is unremarkable. An ECG shows normal sinus rhythm without evidence of ischemia or hypertrophy. Initial laboratory studies are normal. Both noncontrast CT scan of the head and MR scan of the brain are normal. What is the best next step in this patient's management?

a. Begin anticoagulation with low-molecular-weight heparin and warfarin.
b. Obtain an echocardiogram.
c. Check for antiphospholipid antibodies and homocysteine levels.
d. Order a carotid duplex ultrasonogram and begin antiplatelet therapy.
e. Begin lamotrigine for probable nonconvulsive seizure.

Questions 370 and 371

Match the clinical description with the most likely disease process. Each lettered option may be used once, more than once, or not at all.

a. Parkinson disease
b. Wilson disease
c. Huntington disease
d. Dystonia
e. Essential tremor
f. Tic
g. Sydenham chorea

370. An 18-year-old male admitted to the hospital because of psychotic behavior is found to have a proximal "wing-beating" tremor, dystonia, and incoordination. Serum transaminases are moderately elevated; brownish corneal deposits are noted on slit-lamp examination.

371. A 37-year-old man is brought to the doctor by his family because of intellectual decline over the past 2 months. Examination reveals slow writhing movements with dystonic posturing. His father died of a similar illness.

Questions 372 to 374

For each of the clinical descriptions, select the most likely diagnosis. Each lettered option may be used once, more than once, or not at all.

a. Senile dementia of the Alzheimer type
b. Vascular (multi-infarct) dementia
c. Vitamin B_{12} deficiency
d. Dementia with Lewy bodies
e. Creutzfeldt-Jakob disease
f. Normal pressure hydrocephalus

372. An 80-year-old develops steady, progressive memory and cognitive deficit over 2 years. He has normal blood pressure and no focal neurologic findings, and workup for "treatable" causes of dementia is negative.

373. A 70-year-old male with history of hypertension and diabetes presents with a stepwise loss of intellectual function. Prior episodes have been associated with unilateral weakness and difficulty swallowing. A unilateral Babinski sign is found on neurological examination.

374. A 50-year-old presents with rapidly progressive change in mental status over 3 months. Numerous myoclonic jerks accompany the dementia; the EEG shows repetitive high-voltage polyphasic discharges

Questions 375 and 376

Match each clinical description with the correct diagnosis. Each lettered option may be used once, more than once, or not at all.

a. Pneumococcal meningitis
b. Cryptococcal meningitis
c. Coxsackievirus (aseptic) meningitis
d. Pyogenic brain abscess
e. *Listeria monocytogenes* meningitis
f. Herpes simplex encephalitis
g. Cerebral cysticercosis

375. A 50-year-old woman is on high-dose corticosteroids and immuno-suppressives because of renal transplant rejection. She presents with a 10-day history of fever, headache, and confusion. Lumbar puncture reveals 25 lymphocytes per microliter and a very high CSF protein. India ink stain is positive.

376. A 28-year-old alcoholic has recently been treated for lung abscess. Three days before this admission, the patient develops headache, fever, and mild right-sided weakness. His MRI scan is shown below.

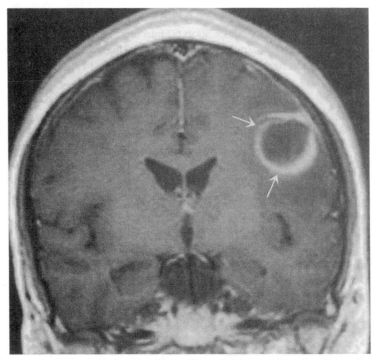

Reproduced with permission, from Kasper DL et al. *Harrison's Principles of Internal Medicine,* 16th ed. New York: McGraw-Hill, 2005.

Questions 377 and 378

Match each symptom or sign with the appropriate diagnosis. Each lettered option may be used once, more than once, or not at all.

a. Tension headache
b. Cluster headache
c. Migraine headache
d. Temporal arteritis
e. Brain tumor
f. Sinusitis
g. Temporomandibular joint dysfunction
h. Tic douloureux

377. A 42-year-old executive complains of a bandlike tightness across the temples and neck, worse in the afternoon, usually relieved by aspirin or acetaminophen. Neurological examination is normal.

378. An 82-year-old woman complains of worsening headaches and episodes of transient visual loss and diplopia. When she chews, her jaw muscles ache until she stops chewing. Examination reveals a tender nodular right temporal artery. She has a mild normocytic anemia; sedimentation rate is 95.

Questions 379 and 380

Match each symptom with the appropriate diagnosis. Each lettered option may be used once, more than once, or not at all.

a. Absence (petit mal) seizure
b. Complex partial seizure
c. Simple partial seizure
d. Atonic seizure
e. Myoclonic seizure
f. Nonconvulsive seizure (pseudoseizure)

379. The patient recalls having episodes when he smells a pungent odor, becomes sweaty, and loses consciousness. His wife describes a period of motor arrest followed by repetitive picking movements that last about a minute. The patient does not fall or lose muscle control.

380. The teacher of a 14-year-old child recounts episodes where the child stares into space and does not respond to verbal commands for a few seconds. These episodes occur several times per day. An EEG shows 3-per-second spike and slow wave discharges.

Questions 381 and 382

For each symptom of cerebrovascular disease, select the site of the lesion. Each lettered option may be used once, more than once, or not at all.

a. Vertebral artery
b. Middle cerebral artery
c. Midbasilar artery
d. Anterior cerebral artery
e. Penetrating branch, middle cerebral artery
f. Superior cerebellar artery

381. A 37-year-old smoker who takes birth control pills presents with sudden weakness and numbness of the right side of her body. She has a severe expressive aphasia and tends to neglect the deficit on her right side.

382. A 79-year-old diabetic presents with right-sided weakness. The weakness is equal in the right face, arm, and leg. Sensation, speech, and comprehension are intact.

Neurology

Answers

345. The answer is b. (*Fauci, pp 95-107.*) The history is classic for cluster headache, an often debilitating periodic pain syndrome. The typical cluster lasts for weeks and then remits. Like classic migraines, cluster headaches are unilateral and can be associated with autonomic symptoms (including Horner syndrome) on the symptomatic side. The following chart helps you to distinguish cluster headache from migraine:

	Cluster headache	Migraine headache
Aura	no	sometimes
Duration of pain	30 min-3 hours	4-72 hours
Gender	male	female
Activity	pt paces in agitation	pt prefers to lie quietly in the dark
Eyes	unilateral lacrimation and rhinorrhea	photophobia, otherwise normal

Treatment of cluster headache involves two principles: (1) aborting the cluster and (2) relieving the headache when it occurs. Prednisone is usually given to abort the cluster; 40 to 60 mg per day is given for weeks and then tapered over a month or two. Propranolol and tricyclic antidepressants (which are given for migraine prevention) are much less helpful in the patient with cluster headache. Verapamil and carbamazepine are sometimes used if prednisone is ineffective. It is harder to relieve the individual headache in cluster disorder because each episode of pain is of shorter duration than in migraine. Triptans or high-flow oxygen (7-10 L per minute via face mask) may be effective. The pain in cluster headache is very severe, and suicides have occurred when the patient enters another stereotypical cluster. Proper diagnosis and treatment are therefore crucial. Neuroimaging studies are not indicated unless atypical features or focal neurological findings are present. Neuropsychiatric testing is expensive and would not be indicated in this patient with classic cluster headache.

346. The answer is c. *(Fauci, pp 2560-61.)* This patient's action tremor (ie, brought out by sustained motor activity) and otherwise normal neurological examination are diagnostic of essential tremor. Fifty percent of patients will have a positive family history (benign familial tremor). The tremor is termed "benign" to separate it from Parkinson disease and other progressive neurological diseases and because it does not affect other areas of function; however, about 15% of patients (especially those in professions that require fine motor control) will be functionally impaired. An identical rapid fine action tremor can be seen in normal persons after strenuous motor activity or with anxiety. Hyperthyroidism, caffeine overuse, alcohol withdrawal, and use of sympathomimetic drugs (such as cocaine and amphetamines) can cause an identical tremor and can exacerbate the tremor in familial cases.

Neurological imaging is normal in patients with essential tremor. The EMG is nonspecific. This patient has no features (eg, weakness, fasciculations) to suggest motor neuron disease. Patients are managed with medications, especially beta-blockers, to decrease the severity of the tremor. Most neurologists feel that nonselective beta-blockers (blocking both beta-1 and beta-2 receptors) are most effective. They can be used on an "as needed" basis (ie, before performance of fine tasks) if the patient is not troubled by the tremor at other times. Primidone is also effective but is associated with more side effects, especially at higher doses.

347. The answer is a. *(Fauci, pp 1726-1729.)* An excruciating headache with syncope requires evaluation for subarachnoid hemorrhage. The headache that precedes or accompanies SAH is often described as a "thunderclap" headache, meaning that it reaches its maximum intensity in seconds. This description is unusual in migraine (where the headache usually reaches maximum intensity in 5-30 minutes) and mandates CT scanning or lumbar puncture. In about 90% of patients, there will be enough blood to be visualized on a noncontrast CT scan. If the scan is normal, a lumbar puncture is the next step to establish the presence of subarachnoid blood. A contrast CT scan sometimes obscures the diagnosis because, in an enhanced scan, normal arteries may be mistaken for subarachnoid blood. Cerebral angiogram will be necessary if SAH is present to assess for a berry aneurysm but would not be the best initial test. Holter monitor might be helpful in unexplained syncope but would not address the severe headache. Nortriptyline can be used to prevent migraine recurrence, but this patient's headache does not suggest migraine; overlooking the possibility of SAH would be a serious mistake.

348. The answer is b. *(Fauci, pp 139-143.)* When syncope occurs in an older patient as a result of head turning, wearing a tight shirt collar, or shaving over the neck area, carotid sinus hypersensitivity should be considered. It usually occurs in men above the age of 50. Baroreceptors of the carotid sinus are activated and pass impulses through the glossopharyngeal nerve to the medulla oblongata. Some consider the process to be quite rare. Gentle massage of one carotid sinus at a time may show a period of asystole or hypotension. This should be performed in a controlled setting with monitoring and atropine available. Most cases of carotid sinus hypersensitivity are not associated with significant carotid stenosis; if a carotid bruit is heard on physical examination, however, a duplex study should precede carotid massage. More expensive studies, such as Holter monitoring or electrophysiologic study, would be unnecessary if carotid sinus massage demonstrates the diagnosis.

349. The answer is c. *(Fauci, pp 2605-2606.)* This patient has an asymptomatic meningioma, the commonest CNS tumor. The radiographic picture of a densely enhancing tumor near the surface of the brain is essentially diagnostic, and biopsy is not necessary. An occasional patient will have bony overgrowth of the skull as a result of the hypervascular tumor; the patient may notice a change in the contour of the skull. Almost all meningiomas are benign and grow slowly. Many are discovered incidentally during CNS imaging for other problems. While large or symptomatic meningiomas are usually treated with surgical resection, this patient's tumor should be followed at 3 to 6 month intervals with serial CT scans. Radiation therapy is ineffective. Ventriculoperitoneal shunting would be indicated only if neuroimaging studies showed hydrocephalus. Phenytoin is used if seizures occur; seizures are less common in meningioma than in glial tumors that arise within the brain parenchyma. This patient's tumor would not account for her intellectual decline (bilateral cortical disease is necessary to affect higher intellectual function), and craniotomy with resection in the very elderly often causes more problems that it treats.

350. The answer is b. *(Fauci, pp 2613, 2611-2621.)* This patient's episode of transient blindness was likely a result of optic neuritis. This transient loss of vision in one eye occurs in 25% to 40% of multiple sclerosis patients (A similar presentation can occur in SLE, sarcoidosis, or syphilis). In addition, the patient gives a history of a relapsing-remitting process. There are abnormal signs of cerebellar and upper motor neuron disease. Signs and symptoms therefore suggest multiple lesions in space and time, making multiple sclerosis the most likely diagnosis. All patients with suspected multiple sclerosis should have an MR of the brain. MR is sensitive in defining demyelinating lesions in the brain and spinal cord. Disease-related changes are found in more than 95% of patients who have definite evidence for MS. Most patients do not need lumbar puncture or spinal fluid analysis for diagnosis, although 70% have elevated IgG levels, and myelin basic protein does appear in the CSF during exacerbations. When the diagnosis is in doubt, lumbar puncture is indicated. Pleocytosis of greater than 75 cells per microliter or finding polymorphonuclear leukocytes in the CSF makes the diagnosis of MS unlikely. In some cases, chronic infection such as with syphilis or HIV may be in the differential of MS. Quantitative IgG levels would not be specific enough for diagnosis. Oligoclonal banding of CSF IgG is determined by agarose gel electrophoresis, but this is not the first test chosen. Two or more bands are found in 70% to 90% of patients with MS. CT scans are much less sensitive than MRIs in picking up demyelinating lesions, especially in the posterior fossa and cervical cord.

351. The answer is d. *(Fauci, p 176.)* This woman has restless leg syndrome, a common sensory complaint in the elderly. It is characterized by ill-defined leg discomfort that occurs in the evening when the patient is reclining or at night when the patient is trying to sleep. The uncomfortable sensation is relieved by movement. Examination is normal or shows at most mild distal sensory loss. There are no motor or reflex changes. Although most often idiopathic, RLS can be associated with iron-deficiency or renal insufficiency. Although several agents (benzodiazepines, opioids) can provide symptomatic relief, dopamine-enhancing drugs are most effective. Levodopa-carbidopa is effective but may lead to rebound effects, so direct dopamine agonists (pramipexole, ropinirole) are now preferred. Soporifics such as zolpidem or trazodone are usually ineffective. RLS is a sensory, not a motor, syndrome; so muscle stretching exercises or muscle relaxants rarely provide symptom relief.

352. The answer is d. *(Fauci, pp 2572-2574.)* The disease described involves motor neurons exclusively. Amyotrophic lateral sclerosis affects both upper and lower motor neurons. In this patient, there is upper and lower motor neuron involvement without sensory deficit. Lower motor neuron signs include focal weakness, focal wasting, and fasciculations. Upper motor neuron signs include an extensor plantar response and an increased tendon reflex in a weakened muscle. Peripheral neuropathy and dementia do not occur in ALS. Muscular dystrophy, polymyositis, and the neuromuscular junction disorder myasthenia gravis cause (usually proximal) muscle weakness but not the atrophy and upper motor neuron signs seen in this patient. EMG in the patient with ALS shows widespread denervation and fibrillation potentials with preserved nerve conduction velocities. Sensory testing is normal. There is no inflammatory reaction in the CSF. CT or MRI of the brain may be necessary to rule out a mass in the region of the foramen magnum. In most patients, a CT of the cervical spine is necessary to rule out a structural lesion of the spine, which could mimic ALS. Thyroid studies and vitamin B_{12} levels may be useful in peripheral neuropathy but not in motor neuron disease.

353. The answer is b. (*Fauci, pp 96-100.*) Although the classic migraine is unilateral and is preceded by an aura, many patients experience migraines without aura (formerly termed "common" migraines). This patient's female gender, the onset of the headaches in adolescence, the severity of the pain, and the worsening with light, noise, or activity are all suggestive of migraine. Muscle contraction headaches are often bilateral but occur more frequently (often every afternoon), are less intense (rarely debilitating) and are usually relieved by simple analgesics. Medication overuse headaches are often bilateral but occur more frequently (usually daily); this patient's occasional use of acetaminophen is insufficient to cause medication overuse headache. Space occupying lesions can cause bilateral headaches, but the headaches occur more frequently, at increasing severity (as the lesion expands), often worsen at night or with Valsalva maneuver, and are usually associated with (sometimes subtle) focal abnormalities on neurological examination.

Triptans are very effective medications to abort migraines and are usually the first agents tried in patients either with or without aura. Parenteral or nasal triptans are favored if the patient needs rapid relief or if vomiting precludes the use of oral medications. It is often necessary to try two of three different agents to find which one works best for the individual patient. If the headaches occur frequently or are debilitating despite triptan treatment, prophylactic medications are called for. These medications are administered daily in order to prevent the migraines from occurring; they are ineffective if used at the onset of the headache. Beta-blockers, tricyclic antidepressants and certain anticonvulsants (topiramate, valproate) are the usual prophylactic agents that are tried. Gabapentin is less effective. Narcotics such as hydrocodone are often less effective than triptans and carry the risk of habituation if used frequently.

354. The answer is a. (*Fauci, pp 2672-2677.*) The disease process described is myasthenia gravis, a neuromuscular disease marked by muscle weakness and fatigability. Myasthenia gravis results from a reduction in the number of junctional acetylcholine receptors as a result of autoantibodies. Antibodies cross-link these receptors, causing increased endocytosis and degradation in lysosomes. A decreased number of available acetylcholine receptors results in decreased efficiency of neuromuscular transmission. Successive nerve impulses result in the activation of fewer muscle fibers and produce fatigue. Myasthenia presents with weakness and fatigability, particularly of cranial muscles, causing diplopia, ptosis, nasal speech, and dysarthria. Asymmetric limb weakness also occurs. Diseases of the central nervous system (poliomyelitis, Friedreich ataxia, or multiple sclerosis, as in choices b, c, and d) cause changes in reflexes, sensation, or coordination. ALS, a pure motor disorder, causes fasciculations and muscle atrophy as a result of lower motor neuron involvement. McArdle disease, a glycogen storage disease, causes muscle cramping and occasionally rhabdomyolysis with heavy exertion but only very rarely with usual daily activities.

Ten percent of myasthenia patients have thymic tumors. Surgical removal of a thymoma is necessary because of local tumor spread. Even in the absence of tumor, 85% of patients clinically improve after thymectomy. It is now consensus that thymectomy be performed in all patients with generalized MG who are between puberty and age 55.

355. The answer is e. (*Fauci, pp 2531-2534.*) This patient has the classic presentation of an intraparenchymal (intracerebral) hemorrhage, that is, sudden onset of headache with progressive hemiparesis and the development of obtundation caused by brainstem compression. Although approximately 25% of ischemic strokes are associated with headache, a severe and progressive headache usually indicates intracerebral bleeding. The usual cause is poorly controlled hypertension, but this patient's compliance with his antihypertensive regimen, the lack of an S$_4$ gallop and the absence of left ventricular hypertrophy militate against this diagnosis. In addition, hypertensive bleeds are usually in the central structures of the brain (eg, thalamus, basal ganglia, cerebellum) whereas this patient has a lobar hemorrhage (ie, blood in the parietal lobe). This is the classic presentation of cerebral amyloid angiopathy, a disease of the elderly associated with congophilic deposits in the cerebral vessels. The vessels are weakened and typically cause recurrent lobar hemorrhages. Rarely is there evidence of systemic amyloidosis. The prognosis is poor and treatment usually unsuccessful. True CNS vasculitis is usually associated with a chronic or subacute course and evidence of systemic involvement. Trauma and coagulopathy are usually associated with fracture or ecchymosis.

356. The answer is a. *(Fauci, pp 2667-2670.)* This patient presents with an acute symmetrical polyneuropathy characteristic of Guillain-Barré syndrome. This demyelinating process is often preceded by a viral illness. Characteristically, there is little sensory involvement; about 30% of patients require ventilatory assistance. Loss of deep tendon reflexes, especially in the lower extremities, is an important clue to the lower motor neuron involvement that characterizes GBS. Guillain-Barré syndrome is characterized by an elevated CSF protein with few if any white blood cells. EMG would show a demyelinating (not an axonal) process with nonuniform slowing and conduction block. A positive edrophonium test is characteristic of myasthenia gravis, but this patient's loss of tendon reflexes would not occur in MG. Arterial blood gases in Guillain-Barré syndrome might show a respiratory acidosis (not respiratory alkalosis) secondary to hypoventilation. CK levels are normal, as there is no involvement of muscle in this disease process. Research laboratories show antiganglioside antibodies in 50% of patients with Guillain-Barré syndrome.

357. The answer is b. *(Fauci, pp 103-105.)* Patients who use medications for headache more than twice weekly are at risk of medication overuse headache. Any analgesic, including triptans themselves, can be the culprit. In this setting, the migraine may "transform" into a chronic daily headache. Medication overuse headaches usually start in the morning and improve but do not completely resolve with analgesic therapy. The patient must completely discontinue the offending drug for 2 to 12 weeks for the headaches to resolve. Treating headaches during the period of abstinence can be very difficult. The physician should be vigilant about the development of another cause of headache (mass lesion, inflammatory disorder) in a patient with transformed migraines. CNS imaging and laboratory workup, not generally recommended in the patient with typical migraine, is sometimes indicated. In this patient, however, the most likely diagnosis is still medication overuse headache.

Status migranosus (continuous migraine) and CNS vasculitis are much less common than medication overuse headache. Pseudotumor cerebri ("benign" intracranial hypertension) usually causes papilledema.

358. The answer is a. *(Fauci, pp 2651-2654, 2656-2657.)* The insidious onset of a distal and progressive sensory loss is characteristic of diabetic neuropathy. In many metabolic neuropathies, the longest nerve fibers are affected first, leading to the stocking-glove pattern of sensory loss. Autonomic changes can accompany the sensory loss. Some diabetics will have vascular changes in the vasa nervorum which can lead to asymmetric peripheral or cranial neuropathies; these are often reversible, while the distal neuropathy is usually progressive. It is not rare for neuropathy to be a presenting symptom of type 2 diabetes, particularly if the patient has not had prior glucose testing. Other conditions associated with peripheral neuropathy include medication side effect, toxins, uremia, neoplasm, vitamin deficiency, and amyloidosis. EMG with nerve conduction velocity testing will categorize neuropathy into axonal and demyelinating varieties and will often provide important diagnostic information. In vitamin B_{12} deficiency, posterior column function (eg, vibratory sensation) would be affected out of proportion to small pain and temperature fibers. Although the relaxation phase of muscle stretch reflexes is delayed in hypothyroidism, thyroid deficiency does not cause a sensory neuropathy. Multiple sclerosis (which can cause oligoclonal bands) is an upper motor neuron disease that would not cause distal weakness or hyporeflexia. Myasthenia gravis does not affect sensation or reflexes.

359. The answer is c. *(Fauci, pp 2513-2516.)* Although hypertension is an important cause of stroke, it should not be aggressively treated in the setting of acute cerebral ischemia. Since cerebral autoregulation is disrupted in acute stroke, a drop in blood pressure can decrease perfusion and worsen the so-called ischemic penumbra. Generally, blood pressure elevation up to 185/110 is not treated. Some stroke specialists recommend more aggressive blood pressure control in acute intracranial hemorrhage, but this patient has an ischemic (not hemorrhagic) stroke. Mannitol is of minimal benefit in cerebral edema associated with acute stroke.

360. The answer is a. *(Fauci, pp 2696-2703.)* Polymyositis is an acquired myopathy characterized by subacute symmetrical weakness of proximal limb and trunk muscles that progresses over several weeks or months. When a characteristic skin rash occurs, the disease is known as dermatomyositis. In addition to progressive proximal limb weakness, the patient often experiences dysphagia and neck muscle weakness. Up to half of cases with polymyositis-dermatomyositis have additional features of connective tissue diseases (rheumatoid arthritis, lupus erythematosus, scleroderma, Sjögren syndrome). Laboratory findings include an elevated serum CK level, an EMG showing myopathic potentials with fibrillations, and a muscle biopsy showing necrotic muscle fibers and inflammatory infiltrates. Polymyositis is clinically distinguished from the muscular dystrophies by its less prolonged course and lack of family history. It is distinguished from myasthenia gravis by its lack of ocular muscle involvement, absence of variability in strength over hours or days, lack of response to cholinesterase inhibitor drugs, and the characteristic EMG findings. Cervical myelopathy usually causes hyperreflexia. Mononeuritis multiplex causes asymmetric signs, usually with sensory loss, and does not affect swallowing.

361. The answer is d. *(Fauci, pp 193-194.)* This patient has weakness of the left face and the contralateral (right) arm and leg, commonly called a *crossed hemiplegia*. Such crossed syndromes are characteristic of brainstem lesions. In this case, the lesion is an infarct localized to the left inferior pons caused by occlusion of a branch of the basilar artery. The infarct has damaged the left sixth and seventh cranial nerves or nuclei in the left pons with resultant diplopia on left lateral gaze and left facial weakness. Also damaged is the left descending corticospinal tract, proximal to its decussation in the medulla; this damage causes weakness in the right arm and leg. This classic presentation is called the Millard-Gubler syndrome. Hemispheric lesions cause motor and sensory loss all on the same side (contralateral to the lesion). A lesion in the median longitudinal fasciculus causes third and sixth cranial nerve dysfunction but not motor deficit of the face or body.

362. The answer is d. *(Fauci, pp 2611-2621.)* Interferon-beta is standard therapy used to prevent progressive disease in relapsing-remitting multiple sclerosis. Both interferon-beta 1b and several forms of interferon-beta 1a are available and are similarly effective. Glatiramer acetate (Copaxone) is also approved for MS. While patients who receive any one of these treatments have 30% fewer exacerbations and fewer new MRI lesions, the treatments do not cure the disease. Interferon-beta can cause side effects, particularly a flulike syndrome that usually resolves within several months. Acute exacerbations of MS are treated with high dose methylprednisolone followed by tapering oral prednisone. This treatment improves symptoms during a relapse but does not appear to affect the long-term course of the disease. This patient, however, is not having an acute exacerbation of her disease. Steadily progressive MS, especially primary progressive disease, when the disease never remits but worsens inexorably, is a difficult management problem. Immunosuppressives such as cyclophosphamide and mitoxantrone are often tried. Such patients often progress to debility and mortality from urinary infection, aspiration pneumonia, or infected pressure ulcers. Simply providing this patient who has worsening disease with symptomatic treatment would be inappropriate.

363. The answer is c. (*Fauci, pp 2525-2528, 2565-2571, 2672.*) This patient has evidence of bilateral cerebellar dysfunction. A focal lesion in one lobe of the cerebellum (eg, cerebellar tumor or infarct) would be expected to cause dyscoordination on the same side of the body (ipsilateral) as the lesion. Midline cerebellar lesions (most commonly alcoholic cerebellar degeneration) cause midline signs (especially gait ataxia) out of proportion to the findings in the extremities. Infarcts in the basal ganglia would cause extrapyramidal signs with rigidity and uncontrolled movements in addition to dyscoordination. Posterior column disease would cause sensory abnormalities (especially to proprioception and vibratory sensation) rather than problems with coordination.

Paraneoplastic cerebellar degeneration is one of the commonest CNS manifestations of remote cancer. It may be associated with small cell carcinoma of the lung, breast or female genital cancers, and lymphomas. Patients usually have antibodies to neuronal antigens (Hu, Ri, Yo, Tr antigens); these autoantibodies can be detected by obtaining a panel of neuronal autoantibodies. With her weight loss, evidence of obstructive lung disease, and smoking history, this patient most likely harbors a small cell lung cancer. The prognosis of patients with paraneoplastic cerebellar degeneration is poor; most become debilitated before their death. Other neurological syndromes that raise suspicion for remote cancer include encephalopathy with sensory neuropathy, opsoclonus-myoclonus syndrome (erratic conjugate jerking eye movements in association with myoclonic jerks) and Lambert-Eaton myasthenic syndrome.

364. The answer is a. (*Fauci, pp 95-107.*) The differential diagnosis of headaches associated with neurological or visual dysfunction is important because it encompasses a variety of disorders, some quite serious and others relatively benign. Classic (or neurological) migraine usually begins in childhood or early adult life. Typically, the onset of an episode is marked by the progression of a neurological disturbance over 5 to 15 minutes, followed by a unilateral (or occasionally bilateral) throbbing headache for several hours up to a day. The most common neurological disturbance involves formed or unformed flashes of light that impair vision in one of the visual fields (scintillating scotoma). Other neurological symptoms seen with migraine include unilateral numbness and tingling of the face, lips, and hand; weakness of an arm or leg; mild aphasia; and mental confusion. The transience of the neurological symptoms distinguishes migraine from other, more serious conditions that cause headaches. Persistence of a visual field defect, speech disturbance, or hemiparesis suggests a focal lesion (eg, arteriovenous malformation with hemorrhage or infarct). In the case of persistent ataxia, limb incoordination, and nausea, one should consider a posterior fossa (possibly cerebellar) mass lesion. Monocular visual loss in an elderly patient with throbbing headaches should initiate a search for cranial (temporal) arteritis. This should include a sedimentation rate (usually elevated) and a temporal artery biopsy (which would show a giant cell arteritis). Fifty percent of these patients have the generalized muscle aches and morning stiffness of polymyalgia rheumatica. Unilateral orbital or retro-orbital headaches that occur daily for a period of 2 to 8 weeks are characteristic of cluster headaches. These headaches are often associated with ipsilateral injection of the conjunctiva, nasal stuffiness, rhinorrhea, and, less commonly, miosis, ptosis, and cheek edema. Although both migraine and cluster headaches may respond to treatment with triptans or ergotamine, they are considered to be distinct entities.

365. The answer is e. (*Fauci, pp 2549-2559.*) Parkinson disease (PD) is marked by depletion of dopamine-rich cells in the substantia nigra. The resulting decrease in striatal dopamine is the basis for the classic symptoms of rigidity, bradykinesia, tremor, and postural instability. Many experts consider bradykinesia to be the fundamental feature of PD. Although tremor is often the first manifestation, about 20% of patients do not have a tremor. When present, the tremor occurs at rest, is slower than most other tremors, and decreases with intentional activity (so that a watch repairman with PD is often able to function normally).

The most effective treatment for PD is levodopa. Levodopa is converted to dopamine in the substantia nigra and then transported to the striatum, where it stimulates dopamine receptors. This is the basis for the drug's clinical effect on PD. Levodopa is usually administered with carbidopa (a dopa decarboxylase inhibitor) in one pill. This prevents levodopa's destruction in the blood and allows it to be given at a lower dose that is less likely to cause nausea and vomiting. The major problems with levodopa have been (1) limb and facial dyskinesias in most patients on chronic therapy and (2) the fact that levodopa treats PD only symptomatically and the disease process of neuronal loss in the substantia nigra continues despite drug treatment. Direct dopamine agonists (such as ropinirole or pramipexole), although less potent than dopamine itself, are often used as the first drug in younger patients. Side effects (in particular, motor fluctuations) are often less troublesome. Anticholinergic agents, such as benztropine mesylate, work by restoring the balance between striatal dopamine and acetylcholine; they are particularly effective in decreasing the degree of tremor. In the elderly, however, they often cause CNS side effects (especially confusion) and would not be a good choice in this elderly woman. Propranolol will help essential tremor but has no benefit in Parkinson disease. Chronic benzodiazepine use should be avoided because of the risk of habituation as well as confusion and falls in the elderly.

366. The answer is a. *(Fauci, pp 1714-1719.)* Focal disorders of the cerebral hemisphere do not cause coma unless the brainstem is compressed by edema or mass effect. Coma implies either severe metabolic derangement of the brain (ie, hypoglycemia, hyponatremia, intoxication), brainstem dysfunction (affecting the reticular activating system of the pons), or else bilateral hemispheric insults. Posterior cerebral artery occlusion will cause an occipital lobe infarction with homonymous hemianopsia but should not affect the level of consciousness. Similarly, a lacunar infarct will cause a pure motor or pure sensory stroke but not global brain dysfunction. Although the patient with a middle cerebral artery stroke may be unable to speak, she should be awake and alert. Anterior cerebral artery occlusion causes motor and sensory deficits of the contralateral leg and foot but does not impair global brain function.

367. The answer is b. *(Fauci, p 1808.)* Lead poisoning often causes a peripheral neuropathy with primary motor involvement. It can superficially resemble ALS, but upper motor neuron signs (such as hyperreflexia) are not seen in lead poisoning. In addition the cognitive changes of lead encephalopathy are not seen in ALS, in peripheral nerve injuries (eg, carpal or tarsal tunnel syndromes), or in myasthenia. Alcoholism can cause peripheral neuropathy but would not cause this patient's prominent motor weakness or the basophilic stippling. The presence of any anemia in a patient with peripheral neuropathy should prompt the search for an underlying cause. Lead lines may be seen at the gingiva-tooth border. Laboratory testing focuses on protoporphyrin levels (free erythrocyte or zinc) and blood lead levels. Industries often associated with lead exposure include battery and ceramic manufacturing, the demolition of lead-painted houses and bridges, plumbing, soldering, and, occasionally, exposure to the combustion of leaded fuels.

368. The answer is c. *(Fauci, pp 115-117, 2572-2576.)* Cervical spondylosis (arthritis) or midline disc protrusion can cause cervical myelopathy, which can mimic amyotrophic lateral sclerosis. The neck pain and stiffness can be mild, and the patient can have both lower motor neuron signs such as atrophy, reflex loss, and even fasciculations in the arms and upper motor neuron signs such as hyperreflexia and clonus (from cord compression) in the legs. Therefore, the diagnosis of ALS is never made without imaging studies of the cervical cord, as compressive cervical myelopathy is a remediable condition. Disease in the cortex would never cause this combination of bilateral upper and lower neuron disease, so an MRI scan of the brain would be superfluous. Myopathies such as polymyositis or metabolic myopathy cause more proximal than distal weakness and would not be associated with hyperreflexia. You should think of disease of the neuromuscular junction (eg, myasthenia gravis) or muscle when the neurological examination is normal except for weakness. Simply referring the patient for physical or occupational therapy would leave her potentially treatable cervical spine disease undiagnosed. Decompressive surgery can improve symptoms and halt progressive loss of function in cervical myelopathy.

369. The answer is d. *(Fauci, pp 186-187, 2521.)* This patient has suffered several transient ischemia attacks with the classic description of amaurosis fugax. Although the traditional symptom duration of less than 24 hours is often cited, most TIAs last less than 1 hour, usually 15 or 20 minutes. Many patients whose symptoms last for several hours are found to have ischemic strokes on MRI imaging. TIAs carry a high risk of neurological morbidity and should be promptly evaluated and treated. Five percent of patients will have a full-blown stroke within the next 2 weeks.

Assessing the extracranial carotid arteries for evidence of atherosclerosis is crucial in patients with anterior circulation TIAs. If a common or internal carotid stenosis of 70% or greater is found, carotid endarterectomy has been proven to decrease the risk of subsequent stroke. Lesions of the external carotid artery do not cause CNS symptoms. Cardiogenic sources of clots (ie, atrial fibrillation, mitral valve disease, intracardiac tumors) usually cause large vessel ischemic strokes rather than TIAs; so echocardiography would be less important in this patient. The use of anticoagulants in acute stroke has diminished greatly and is primarily used in cases of demonstrated cardiogenic emboli. For the typical atherosclerotic process, antiplatelet therapy is preferred. Testing for thrombophilia is rarely helpful in patients with TIA. These tests may be helpful in patients with large vessel strokes and no identifiable source of the stroke. Amaurosis fugax would not be a manifestation of seizure disorder.

370 and 371. The answers are 370-b, 371-c. (*Fauci, pp 2449-2451, 2561-2562.*) Any movement disorder in a young person suggests Wilson disease. This is an autosomal recessive disorder of cellular copper transport that results in copper deposition in tissue. Copper deposition in the basal ganglia causes tremor and rigidity. Copper deposition in the eye produces the Kayser-Fleischer ring. Deposition in the liver causes cirrhosis and hepatitis.

Huntington disease is characterized by the combination of dementia and rapid, nonrhythmic movements. The disease is autosomal dominant in inheritance and is caused by an expansion of CAG trinucleotide repeats. Huntington disease often presents in the third or fourth decade of life and progresses inexorably to debility and death. Slow, writhing movements (athetosis) are seen oftener than the quick jerking movements of chorea. Psychiatric manifestations are prominent in one-third of patients.

372 to 374. The answers are 372-a, 373-b, 374-e. (*Fauci, pp 2536-2549.*) The 80-year-old patient with progressive, steady memory loss and cognitive dysfunction over 2 years has not been found to have a reversible cause of dementia by standard workup. The great majority of such patients have senile dementia of the Alzheimer type. At present, there is no definitive method of premortem diagnosis, but characteristic histologic findings of neurofibrillary tangles and neuritic plaques would be noted at autopsy.

The 70-year-old with hypertension and previous focal deficits is most likely to have vascular dementia. This is associated with progressive stepwise deterioration, usually the result of recurrent bilateral cerebral infarcts. Focal findings, including hemiparesis, extensor plantar responses, and pseudobulbar palsy, are common.

The patient with rapidly progressive dementia and myoclonus must be evaluated for Creutzfeldt-Jakob disease. This transmissible disease is associated with an abnormal conformation of prion-related protein in the CNS. A related condition (variant CJD) was associated with the ingestion of tainted beef in Europe and the United Kingdom and affected more than 190 patients.

375 and 376. The answers are 375-b, 376-d. (*Fauci, pp 1251-1253.*) The patient on high-dose corticosteroids with a positive CSF India ink stain has cryptococcal meningitis. Cryptococcal meningitis patients usually have a lymphocytic meningitis, with a very high CSF protein and low CSF sugar. Cryptococcal meningitis usually begins insidiously with headache and mental status changes. Bacterial or viral meningitis and herpetic encephalitis typically have a more acute onset.

The patient with focal findings and a history of pyogenic lung infection has a brain abscess. Organisms can gain access to the pulmonary veins and then be spread hematogenously to various organs of the body, bypassing the normal sieving effect of the pulmonary capillaries. Lumbar puncture is contraindicated in the presence of mass effect, but would usually show only a small number of white blood cells, a high protein, and elevated CSF pressure.

377 and 378. The answers are 377-a, 378-d. (*Fauci, pp 100-101, 2126-2127.*) Tension headaches are the leading cause of chronic headaches, and 90% are bilateral. These headaches are described as dull, constricting, and bandlike. Associated muscular tenderness may be present.

Temporal arteritis may cause scalp tenderness localized to the involved vessel. It is primarily a disease of the elderly. Blindness caused by occlusion of the ophthalmic artery is the feared complication. Temporal artery biopsy is often needed to confirm the diagnosis, since treatment with oral steroids is fraught with complications in this age group.

379 and 380. The answers are 379-b, 380-a. (*Fauci, pp 2498-2512.*) Complex partial seizures, also known as psychomotor seizures, are characterized by complex auras with psychic experiences followed by periods of impaired consciousness with abnormal motor behavior. Common psychic experiences include illusions, visual or auditory hallucinations, feelings of familiarity (*déjà vu*) or strangeness (*jamais vu*), and fear or anxiety. Motor components include automatisms (eg, lip smacking) and so-called automatic behavior (walking around in a daze, undressing in public). The brain lesion is usually in the temporal lobe, less commonly in the frontal lobe, and is often manifest as a focal epileptiform abnormality on EEG. Postictal confusion or drowsiness is the rule.

Absence, or petit mal, seizure is the most characteristic epilepsy of childhood, with onset usually between age 4 and the early teens. Attacks, which may occur as frequently as several hundred times a day, consist of sudden interruptions of consciousness. The child stares, stops talking or responding, often displays eye fluttering, and may show automatisms such as lip smacking and fumbling movements of the fingers. Attacks end in 2 to 10 seconds with the patient fully alert and able to resume activities. The characteristic EEG abnormality associated with absence attacks is 3-per-second spike-and-wave activity.

381 and 382. The answers are 381-b, 382-e. (*Fauci, pp 2523-2524.*) Occlusion of the entire middle cerebral artery results in contralateral hemiplegia, hemianesthesia, and homonymous hemianopsia. When the dominant hemisphere is involved, aphasia is present. When the nondominant hemisphere is involved, apraxia and neglect often occur. When only a penetrating branch of the middle cerebral artery is affected, the syndrome of pure motor hemiplegia is produced; the infarct involves only the posterior limb of the internal capsule, impairing motor fibers to the face, arm, and leg. Occlusion of a penetrating artery causes a lacunar infarct.

Dermatology

Questions

383. A 20-year-old woman complains of skin problems and is noted to have erythematous papules on her face with blackheads (open comedones) and whiteheads (closed comedones). She has also had cystic lesions. She is prescribed topical tretinoin, but without a totally acceptable result. You are considering oral antibiotics, but the patient requests oral isotretinoin, which several of her college classmates have used with benefit. Which of the following statements is correct?

a. Intralesional triamcinolone should be avoided due to its systemic effects.
b. Systemically administered isotretinoin therapy cannot be considered unless concomitant contraceptive therapy is provided.
c. Antimicrobial therapy is of no value since bacteria are not part of the pathogenesis of the process.
d. The teratogenic effects of isotretinoin are its only clinically important side effects.
e. The patient will not benefit from topical antibiotics since she did not respond to topical retinoids.

384. A 22-year-old male presents with a 6-month history of a red, non-pruritic rash over the trunk, scalp, elbows, and knees. These eruptions are more likely to occur during stressful periods and have occurred at sites of skin injury. The patient has tried topical hydrocortisone without benefit. On examination, sharply demarcated plaques are seen with a thick scale. Pitting of the fingernails is present. There is no evidence of synovitis. What is the best first step in the therapy of this patient's skin disease?

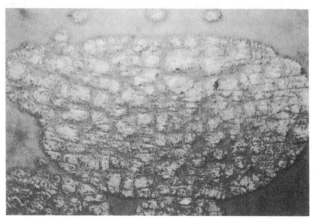

Reproduced, with permission, from Fauci A et al. *Harrison's Principles of Internal Medicine,* 17th ed. New York, NY: McGraw-Hill, 2008.

a. Photochemotherapy (PUVA)
b. Oral methotrexate
c. Topical calcipotriene
d. Oral cyclosporine
e. Topical fluticasone

385. A 25-year-old complains of fever and myalgias for 5 days and now has developed a macular rash over his palms and soles with some petechial lesions. The patient recently returned from a summer camping trip in Tennessee. Which of the following is the most likely cause of the rash?

a. Contact dermatitis
b. Sexual exposure
c. Tick exposure
d. Contaminated water
e. Undercooked pork

386. A 17-year-old female presents with a pruritic rash localized to the wrist. Papules and vesicles are noted in a bandlike pattern, with slight oozing from some lesions. Which of the following is the most likely cause of the rash?

a. Herpes simplex
b. Shingles
c. Atopic dermatitis
d. Seborrheic dermatitis
e. Contact dermatitis

387. A 35-year-old woman develops an itchy rash over her back, legs, and trunk several hours after swimming in a lake. Erythematous, edematous papules and plaques are noted. The wheals vary in size. There are no mucosal lesions and no swelling of the lips. What is the best first step in management of her symptomatic rash?

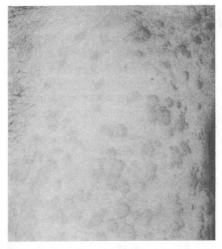

Reproduced, with permission, from Fauci A et al. *Harrison's Principles of Internal Medicine,* 17th ed. New York, NY: McGraw-Hill, 2008.

a. Subcutaneous epinephrine
b. Intravenous glucocorticoids
c. Oral antihistamines (H1 blockers)
d. Aspirin
e. Oral doxycycline

388. A 64-year-old woman presents with diffuse hair loss. She says that her hair is "coming out by the handfuls" after shampooing. She was treated for severe community-acquired pneumonia 2 months ago but has regained her strength and is exercising regularly. She is taking no medications. Examination reveals diffuse hair loss. Several hairs can be removed by gentle tugging. The scalp is normal without scale or erythema. Her general examination is unremarkable; in particular, her vital signs are normal, she has no pallor or inflammatory synovitis, and her reflexes are normal with a normal relaxation phase. What is the best next step in her management?

a. Reassurance
b. Measurement of serum testosterone and DHEA-S levels
c. Topical minoxidil
d. Topical corticosteroids
e. CBC and antinuclear antibodies

389. A 30-year-old black female has a 2-month history of nonproductive cough and a painful skin eruption in the lower extremities. She denies fever or weight loss. Physical examination shows several nontender raised plaques around the nares and scattered similar plaques around the base of the neck. In the lower extremities she has several erythematous tender nonulcerated nodules, measuring up to 4 cm in diameter. Chest x-ray reveals bilateral hilar adenopathy and a streaky interstitial density in the right upper lobe. What is the best way to establish a histological diagnosis?

a. Punch biopsy of one of the plaques on the neck
b. Incisional biopsy of one of the lower extremity nodules
c. Sputum studies for AFB and fungi
d. Mediastinoscopy and biopsy of one of the hilar or mediastinal nodes
e. Serum angiotensin-converting enzyme assay

390. A 72-year-old woman presents with pruritus for the past 6 weeks. She is careful to moisturize her skin after her daily shower and uses soap sparingly. She has never had this symptom before. The itching is diffuse and keeps her awake at night. Over this time she has lost 15 lb of weight and has noticed diminished appetite. She has previously been healthy and takes no medications. Physical examination shows no evidence of rash; a few excoriations are present. She appears fatigued and shows mild temporal muscle wasting. The general examination is otherwise unremarkable. What is the best next step in her management?

a. Topical corticosteroids
b. Oral antihistamines
c. Psychiatric referral for management of depression
d. Skin biopsy at the edge of one of the excoriations
e. Laboratory testing including CBC, comprehensive metabolic panel, and thyroid studies

391. A 53-year-old female presents to the clinic with an erythematous lesion on the dorsum of her right hand. The lesion has been present for the past 7 months and has not responded to corticosteroid treatment. She is concerned because the lesion occasionally bleeds and has grown in size during the past few months. On physical examination you notice an 11-mm erythematous plaque with a small central ulceration. The skin is also indurated with mild crusting on the surface. Which of the following is true about this process?

a. It is a malignant neoplasm of the keratinocytes with the potential to metastasize.
b. It is an allergic reaction resulting from elevation of serum IgE.
c. It is a chronic inflammatory condition, which can be complicated by arthritis of small and medium-sized joints.
d. It is a malignant neoplasm of the melanocytes with the potential to metastasize.
e. It is the most common skin cancer.

392. A 50-year-old woman develops pink macules and papules on her hands and forearms in association with a sore throat. The lesions are target-like, with the centers a dusky violet. What causes of this disorder are most likely in this patient?

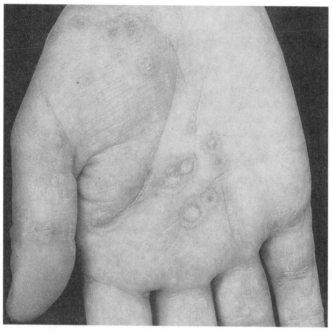

Reproduced with permission from Wolff K et al. *Fitzpatrick's Color Atlas & Synopsis of Clinical Dermatology*, 5th ed. New York, NY: McGraw-Hill, 2005.

a. Tampons and superficial skin infections
b. Drugs and herpesvirus infections
c. Rickettsial and fungal infections
d. Anxiety and emotional stress
e. Harsh soaps and drying agents

393. A 25-year-old female with blonde hair and fair complexion complains of a mole on her upper back. The lesion is 8 mm in diameter, darkly pigmented, and asymmetric, with an irregular border (see illustration below). Which of the following is the best next step in management?

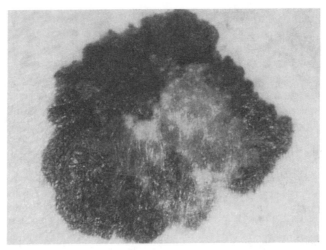

Reproduced, with permission, from Fauci A et al. *Harrison's Principles of Internal Medicine*, 17th ed. New York, NY: McGraw-Hill, 2008.

a. Tell the patient to avoid sunlight.
b. Follow the lesion for any evidence of growth.
c. Obtain metastatic workup.
d. Obtain full-thickness excisional biopsy.
e. Obtain shave biopsy.

394. A 39-year-old male with a prior history of myocardial infarction complains of yellow bumps on his elbows and buttocks. Yellow-colored cutaneous plaques are noted in those areas. The lesions occur in crops and have a surrounding reddish halo. Which of the following is the best next step in evaluation of this patient?

a. Biopsy of skin lesions
b. Lipid profile
c. Uric acid level
d. Chest x-ray
e. Liver enzymes

395. A 15-year-old girl complains of low-grade fever, malaise, conjunctivitis, runny nose, and cough. After this prodromal phase, a rash of discrete pink macules begins on her face and extends to her hands and feet. She is noted to have small red spots on her palate. What is the most likely cause of her rash?

a. Toxic shock syndrome
b. Gonococcal bacteremia
c. Reiter syndrome
d. Rubeola (measles)
e. Rubella (German measles)

396. A 17-year-old girl noted a 2-cm annular pink, scaly lesion on her back. Over the next 2 weeks she develops several smaller oval pink lesions with a fine collarette of scale. They seem to run in the body folds and mainly involve the trunk, although a few occur on the upper arms and thighs. There is no adenopathy and no oral lesions. Which of the following is the most likely diagnosis?

a. Tinea versicolor
b. Psoriasis
c. Lichen planus
d. Pityriasis rosea
e. Secondary syphilis

397. A 45-year-old man with Parkinson disease has macular areas of erythema and scaling behind the ears and on the scalp, eyebrows, glabella, nasolabial folds, and central chest. Which of the following is the most likely diagnosis?

a. Tinea versicolor
b. Psoriasis
c. Seborrheic dermatitis
d. Atopic dermatitis
e. Dermatophyte infection

398. A 20-year-old white man notes an uneven tan on his upper back and chest. On examination, he has many circular, lighter macules with a barely visible scale that coalesce into larger areas. Which test is most likely to establish the diagnosis?

a. Punch biopsy
b. Potassium hydroxide (KOH) microscopic examination
c. Dermatophyte test medium (DTM) culture for fungus
d. Serological test for syphilis
e. Tzanck smear

399. A 33-year-old fair-skinned woman has telangiectasias of the cheeks and nose along with red papules and occasional pustules. She also appears to have conjunctivitis with dilated scleral vessels. She reports frequent flushing and blushing. Drinking red wine produces a severe flushing of the face. There is a family history of this condition. Which of the following is the most likely diagnosis?

a. Carcinoid syndrome
b. Porphyria cutanea tarda
c. Lupus vulgaris
d. Rosacea
e. Seborrheic dermatitis

400. A 46-year-old construction worker is brought to the clinic by his wife because she has noticed an unusual growth on his left ear for the past 8 months (see photo below). The patient explains that, except for occasional itching, the lesion does not bother him. On physical examination, you notice an 8-mm pearly papule with central ulceration and a few small dilated blood vessels on the border. What is the natural course of this lesion if left untreated?

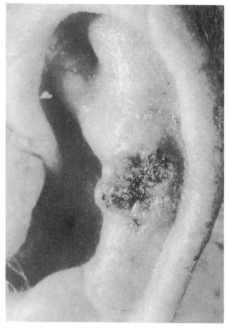

Reproduced with permission from Braunwald et al. *Harrison's Principles of Internal Medicine*, 16th ed. New York, NY: McGraw-Hill, 2004.

a. This is a benign lesion and will not change.
b. Local invasion of surrounding tissue.
c. Regression over time.
d. Local invasion of surrounding tissue and metastasis via lymphatic spread.
e. Disseminated infection resulting in septicemia.

401. A 25-year-old postal worker presents with a pruritic, nonpainful skin lesion on the dorsum of his hand. It began like an insect bite but expanded over several days. On examination, the lesion has a black, necrotic center associated with severe local swelling. The patient does not appear to be systemically ill, and vital signs are normal. Which of the following is correct?

a. The lesion is ecthyma gangrenosum, and blood cultures will be positive for *Pseudomonas aeruginosa*.
b. A skin biopsy should be performed and Gram stain examined for gram-positive rods.
c. The patient has been bitten by *Loxosceles reclusa*, the brown recluse spider.
d. The patient has the bubo of plague.
e. The patient has necrotizing fasciitis and needs immediate surgical debridement.

402. A 25-year-old who has been living in Washington, DC, presents with a diffuse vesicular rash over his face and trunk. He also has fever. He has no history of chickenpox and has not received the varicella vaccine. Which of the following information obtained from history and physical examination suggests that the patient has chickenpox and not smallpox?

a. There are vesicular lesions on the palms and soles.
b. Vesicular lesions are concentrated on the trunk.
c. The rash is most prominent over the face.
d. All lesions are at the same stage of development.
e. The patient experienced high fever several days prior to the rash.

403. A 68-year-old man complains of several blisters arising over the back and trunk for the preceding 2 weeks. He takes no medications and has not noted systemic symptoms such as fever, sore throat, weight loss, or fatigue. The general physical examination is normal. The oral mucosa and the lips are normal. Several 2 to 3 cm bullae are present over the trunk and back. A few excoriations where the blisters have ruptured are present. The remainder of the skin is normal, without erythema or scale. What is the best diagnostic approach at this time?

a. Culture of vesicular fluid for herpes viruses
b. Trial of corticosteroids
c. Biopsy of the edge of a bulla with some surrounding intact skin
d. CT scan of the chest and abdomen looking for occult malignancy
e. Combination of oral H_1 and H_2 antihistamines

404. A 63-year-old retired farmer presents to the clinic complaining of red scaly spots on his head for the past 9 months. Physical examination is remarkable for numerous erythematous hyperkeratotic papules and plaques. The lesions are confined to the head and forehead and have poorly defined borders. Which of the following is the most appropriate next step in management of this patient?

a. Punch biopsy of one of the lesions
b. Application of hydrocortisone cream to affected areas and follow-up in 4 weeks
c. Reassurance that this is a benign finding and follow-up in 6 months
d. Application of fluocinide cream to affected areas and follow-up in 4 weeks
e. Application of 5-fluorouracil cream to affected areas and follow-up in 4 weeks

405. A 21-year-old female presents with an annular pruritic rash on her neck. She explains that the rash has been present for the past 3 weeks and that her roommate had a similar rash not long ago. Physical examination is remarkable for a 20-mm scaling, erythematous plaque with a serpiginous border. Which of the following is the most appropriate initial treatment for this condition?

a. Griseofulvin
b. Oral cephalexin
c. Topical mupirocin ointment
d. Topical ketoconazole
e. Hydrocortisone cream

406. A 34-year-old homosexual male with a history of HIV presents to the clinic complaining of a wheezing and multiple violaceous plaques and nodules on his trunk and extremities. Physical examination of the oral mucosa reveals similar findings on his palate, gingiva, and tongue. Chest x-ray is also significant for pulmonary infiltrates. What is the most likely pathogenesis of this process?

a. Proliferation of neoplastic T cells
b. Infection with human herpesvirus 6
c. Infection with *Mycobacterium avium* due to decreasing CD4 count
d. Angioproliferative disease caused by infection with human herpesvirus 8
e. Disseminated HSV infection

Dermatology

Answers

383. The answer is b. (*Fauci, pp 319-320.*) In general, the treatment of acne is based on the stage of the disease. Comedonal acne is first managed with topical retinoids. Mild to moderate disease usually requires the use of topical antibiotics, and moderate to severe acne is often managed with oral antibiotics, usually tetracycline derivatives. The more severe papulonodular forms may require the addition of isotretinoin supplemented with intralesional steroids for cystic lesions.

Isotretinoin has a high potential for teratogenicity and should not be used in women in their childbearing years unless contraception (preferably dual contraception) is being practiced. The drug also causes hypertriglyceridemia, musculoskeletal pains, and drying of mucous membranes. It should be reserved for severe or refractory acne. Intralesional triamcinolone is effective for occasional cystic lesions and does not cause systemic side effects. Antimicrobial therapy is of value, in part due to its suppressive effect on *Propionibacterium acnes*. The combination of topical retinoids and topical antibiotics has been shown to be better than topical retinoids alone.

384. The answer is e. (*Fauci, pp 315-316.*) The rash described is classic for psoriasis, a common chronic inflammatory skin disorder. Its characteristic features include sharply-bordered papules or plaques with silver scale, usually located on the knees, elbows, and scalp. Stress, certain medications such as lithium, and skin injury commonly exacerbate the disease. The distribution of the described rash would make contact dermatitis unlikely. In the differential of psoriasis are lichen planus (polygonal pruritic purple papules with lacy mucous membrane lesions), pityriasis rosea (herald patch occurs first on trunk in Christmas tree pattern), and dermatophytes (usually less well demarcated; affecting skin, hair, and nails). Topical corticosteroids of moderate or high potency are the first agents to try in psoriasis without joint involvement. Topical vitamin D analogues such as calcipotriene or calcitriol may be combined with topical steroids in refractory cases, but they are less effective and much more expensive than topical steroids. Psoralen and UVA phototherapy (PUVA) are reserved for difficult cases because of an increased risk of squamous cell carcinoma of the skin. Methotrexate, cyclosporine, and immune response modifiers such as etanercept are useful in difficult cases but carry a higher risk of side effects.

385. The answer is c. *(Fauci, pp 122-128, 1061.)* The rash described is most consistent with Rocky Mountain spotted fever, for which a tick is the intermediate vector. Secondary syphilis could present with a macular rash in the same distribution, but the associated symptoms would be atypical. Always think of these two diagnoses when a rash begins on the palms and soles. Contact dermatitis would not cause petechial lesions. The skin lesions in disseminated gonococcal infection can be distal, but are usually few in number and are pustular. Giardiasis does not cause a rash. Trichinosis, typically associated with periorbital edema and severe myalgias, can cause splinter hemorrhages and a maculopapular rash, but would rarely show the distal involvement seen in this patient.

386. The answer is e. *(Fauci, pp 311-314.)* Contact dermatitis causes pruritic plaques or vesicles localized to an area of contact. In this case, nickel in a bracelet or wristband would be the inciting agent. Contact dermatitis may produce vesicles with weeping lesions. The process is related to direct irritation of the skin from a chemical or physical irritant. It may also be immune mediated. Zoster would be painful and occur in a dermatomal distribution. Herpes simplex produces grouped vesicles, but they are painful and also unlikely to occur around the wrist. Atopic dermatitis usually affects skin creases (especially the antecubital fossae) and the hands. It may be vesicular but is more often associated with skin thickening (lichenification) as a result of constant scratching. Seborrheic dermatitis presents as red, scaly nonpruritic lesions localized to the eyebrows, nasolabial folds, scalp, and retroauricular areas.

387. The answer is c. *(Fauci, pp 324, 330, 2065-2067.)* Urticaria, or hives, is a common dermatologic problem characterized by pruritic, edematous papules, and plaques that vary in size and come and go, often within hours. Mast cells may be stimulated by heat, cold, pressure, water, or exercise. Immunologic mechanisms can also cause mast cell degranulation. Folliculitis caused by *Pseudomonas aeruginosa* can cause a rash, often after exposure to hot tubs. The lesions are not as diffuse, with a line of demarcation depending on the water level, and are usually pustular. "Hot tub" dermatitis begins 8 to 48 hours after exposure to contaminated water (ie, long enough for superficial infection to develop). Systemic antibiotics are seldom necessary, and tetracyclines would be the wrong choice against pseudomonads.

Avoidance of the offending agent, when it is identifiable, is most important in management of urticaria. Oral antihistamines provide symptomatic relief. Agents such as aspirin or alcohol, which aggravate cutaneous vasodilation, are contraindicated. Glucocorticoids play a minimal role in management of urticaria unless the process is severe and unremitting. Epinephrine plays no role unless there is concomitant anaphylaxis.

388. The answer is a. *(Fauci, pp 301, 322, 345.)* This patient's diffuse hair loss after a severe illness is caused by telogen effluvium. Normal hair follicles go through a life cycle. Approximately 5% are in the death (telogen) phase where the hair shaft is released. In telogen effluvium, the hair follicles are "shocked" by the systemic stress, and many enter the telogen phase at the same time. The diagnosis is made by careful history and physical examination. CBC, ANA, and hormonal levels will be normal. The patient will recover fully in a month or two, although a wig may be necessary to hide cosmetically troubling alopecia in the meantime. Diffuse hair loss may be seen with many drugs or with systemic illnesses such as hypothyroidism, systemic lupus, syphilis, or iron deficiency, but there is no evidence of any of these illnesses in this patient. Male pattern baldness (androgen-dependent alopecia) is seen in normal men, in some older women, and in women with androgen excess, but the hair loss affects the crown and frontal region rather than the scalp diffusely. The dramatic and acute hair loss of telogen effluvium does not occur in male pattern baldness.

389. The answer is a. *(Fauci, pp 2135-2142.)* This patient probably has sarcoidosis; rarely tuberculosis or granulomatous fungal infections can cause the same syndrome. The painful nodules on the legs represent erythema nodosum, a hypersensitivity reaction associated with this patient's illness. Erythema nodosum can be associated with sarcoidosis, TB, inflammatory bowel disease, several infectious processes or can be idiopathic. Biopsy of one of these lesions would reveal a nonspecific panniculitis (inflammation of the subcutaneous fat) and would not be helpful diagnostically. Biopsy of one of the plaques, however, would reveal noncaseating granulomas characteristic of sarcoidosis and would be helpful in ruling out the less likely infectious pathogens. Skin biopsy is safer and less expensive than an invasive procedure. In the absence of sputum production, fever, or weight loss, AFB and fungal studies would be unlikely to be productive. The serum ACE assay is nonspecifically elevated in many systemic granulomatous diseases and plays a minor role in the assessment and management of a patient with sarcoidosis.

390. The answer is e. *(Fauci, 319, 330, 1769, 1919.)* In 20% of cases, diffuse itching is a manifestation of systemic illness. Renal insufficiency, obstructive liver disease (especially primary biliary cirrhosis), hematological conditions such as polycythemia vera or lymphoma, and thyroid disorders can all present in this fashion. Although most patients with pruritus will have dry skin (xerosis) or dermatitis (usually the primary dermatitis is apparent from the examination), this patient's weight loss and anorexia should prompt a search for an underlying disorder. Topical agents, oral antihistamines, or doxepin (a tricyclic antidepressant with potent H_1 and H_2 blocking effects) can be used for symptomatic purposes but should not replace a search for an underlying cause in this elderly patient with new onset of symptoms. Excoriations are nonspecific manifestations of scratching; unless a specific primary lesion (eg, papule, vesicle) is found, skin biopsy will rarely be helpful in the evaluation of pruritus.

391. The answer is a. *(Fauci, pp 308-312, 541-548.)* Cutaneous squamous cell carcinoma (SCC) is a malignant neoplasm of the keratinocytes; it can grow rapidly and may metastasize (1%-3% of cases). Clinically, SCC commonly presents as an ulcerated erythematous nodule or superficial erosion on the skin. SCC can occur anywhere on the body but is most common on areas of sun-damaged skin, including the lower lip. Elevation of serum IgE is associated with urticaria, which presents as pruritic, red wheals. Psoriasis is a chronic inflammatory disease characterized by well-marginated erythematous papules and plaques covered by a silvery scale. A complication of this disease is asymmetric arthritis of the distal and proximal interphalangeal joints. Ulceration is not seen in psoriatic plaques. Melanomas are malignant neoplasms of the melanocytes that have the potential to metastasize. Metastasis and prognosis are related to depth of invasion. Melanomas, however, usually have areas of definite hyperpigmentation. Basal cell carcinoma (BCC) is the most common skin cancer, accounting for 70% to 80% of nonmelanoma skin cancers. They usually have a characteristic rolled or undermined border with telangiectasias around the lesion. Local invasion can be a serious problem with BCCs, but they almost never metastasize.

392. The answer is b. *(Fauci, pp 129, 311, 1097.)* Target lesions, especially with nonblanching violet or petechial centers, are classic manifestations of erythema multiforme. Blanchable lesions and blisters may be found as well. Common causes of erythema multiforme include drugs and herpesvirus infections (especially herpes simplex or Epstein-Barr virus). It is most important to identify the offending agent, as continuation of a causative drug can lead to oral involvement, systemic illness and the full-blown Stevens-Johnson syndrome. The rash may take 4 to 6 weeks to resolve. Readministration of the causative agent should be scrupulously avoided. Phenytoin, sulfa drugs, barbiturates, and penicillin are common causes. The rash, with its target lesions, should not be confused with toxic shock syndrome, which causes a blanchable erythema. Rocky mountain spotted fever causes a distal petechial rash as a result of endothelial damage. Neurodermatitis and xerotic eczema would not cause target lesions.

393. The answer is d. (*Fauci, pp 541-545.*) The lesion has characteristics of melanoma (Remember the ABCDs: *a*symmetry, irregular or ill-defined *b*order, dark black or variegated *c*olor, and *d*iameter greater than 6 mm). A full-thickness excisional biopsy is required for diagnosis and should not be delayed. Shave biopsy of a suspected melanoma is always contraindicated. Diagnosis is urgent; the lesion cannot be observed over time. Once the diagnosis of melanoma is made, the tumor must then be staged to determine prognosis and treatment.

394. The answer is b. (*Fauci, pp 331-332, 2419.*) The description and location of these lesions are suggestive of eruptive xanthomas. Eruptive xanthomas occur primarily on buttocks or extensor surfaces and are associated with elevated triglycerides. Tophaceous gout can result in deposits of monosodium urate, usually in the skin around joints of the hands and feet, that may also be yellow (usually yellowish-white) in color. The cutaneous lesions of sarcoidosis are reddish-brown waxy papules, usually on the face. Obstructive liver disease can occasionally cause palmar xanthomas, which are seen as yellow plaques along the palmar creases.

Xanthomatous skin lesions can be important cutaneous clues for underlying lipid disorders. Xanthelasma, yellowish plaques on the inner aspect of the upper eyelids, are nonspecific but may be associated with hyperlipidemia 50% of the time. Tendon xanthomas are important clues for the presence of familial hypercholesterolemia. Tuberous xanthomas, which often present as plaques or even polypoid nodules over pressure points, usually mean significant hypercholesterolemia. Eruptive xanthomas, again, are associated with triglyceride levels above 1000 mg/dL. Treatment of the hypertriglyceridemia usually results in resolution of lesions. Biopsy of a xanthoma would show lipid-containing macrophages, but is usually not necessary for diagnosis.

395. The answer is d. *(Fauci, pp 1214-1220.)* The patient presents with the classic picture of measles (rubeola). Coryza, conjunctivitis, cough, and fever characterize the measles prodrome. The pathognomonic Koplik spots (pinpoint elevations connected by a network of minute vessels on the soft palate) usually precede onset of the rash by 24 to 48 hours and may remain for 2 or 3 days. After the prodrome of 1 to 7 days, discrete red macules and papules begin behind the ears and spread to the face and trunk, and then distally over the extremities. Toxic shock syndrome produces a diffuse, sunburn-like rash with mucosal hyperemia (sometimes causing a "strawberry" tongue). Gonococcal bacteremia is more likely to cause pustular skin lesions in association with tenosynovitis. Reiter syndrome (characterized by arthritis, urethritis, and conjunctivitis) may be associated with ulcers of the mouth, tongue, or penis. In rubella, a maculopapular rash is associated with petechial lesions of the soft palate. Cervical lymphadenopathy is a prominent feature.

396. The answer is d. *(Fauci, pp 315-316, 318, 321, 1040-1041.)* The description of this papulosquamous disease is classic for pityriasis rosea. This disease occurs in about 10% of the population, usually in young adults. Pityriasis rosea primarily affects the trunk and proximal extremities. Pityriasis rosea is usually asymptomatic, although some patients have an early, mild viral prodrome (malaise and low-grade fever), and itching may be significant. Drug eruptions, fungal infections, and secondary syphilis may mimic this disease. Fungal infections (tinea) are rarely as widespread and sudden in onset; potassium hydroxide (KOH) preparation will be positive. Syphilis usually is characterized by lymphadenopathy, oral patches, and lesions on the palms and soles (a VDRL test will be strongly positive at this stage). Psoriasis, with its thick, scaly plaques on extensor surfaces, should not cause confusion. A rare condition called guttate parapsoriasis should be suspected if the rash lasts more than 2 months, since pityriasis rosea usually clears spontaneously in 6 weeks. Lichen planus is a papulosquamous disorder, but it causes intensely pruritic polygonal plaques, often with intraoral involvement. It would not cause a "Christmas tree" pattern on the back as seen in this patient.

397. The answer is c. *(Fauci, pp 315, 1263-1265.)* The patient has the typical areas of involvement of seborrheic dermatitis. This common dermatitis appears to be worse in many neurological diseases. It is also very common and severe in patients with AIDS. In general, symptoms are worse in the winter. *Pityrosporum ovale* appears to play a role in seborrheic dermatitis and dandruff, and the symptoms improve with the use of certain antifungal preparations (eg, ketoconazole) that decrease this yeast. Mild topical steroids also produce an excellent clinical response.

The pattern of involvement provides an important diagnostic clue in dermatology. Tinea versicolor usually affects the neck and shoulders. Psoriasis often involves the scalp, elbows, knees, and buttocks but rarely affects the eyebrows and nasolabial creases. Atopic dermatitis is most prominent in the antecubital and popliteal fossae. Dermatophytes are more varied in their localization (scalp, inguinal areas, interdigital folds of the feet) but would rarely localize to the areas affected in this patient.

398. The answer is b. *(Fauci, pp 311-312, 1263.)* The diagnosis is tinea versicolor, which can be easily confirmed by a KOH microscopic examination. Routine fungal cultures will not grow this yeast. A Wood light examination will often show green fluorescence, but it may be negative if the patient has recently showered. Tzanck smear is used on vesicles to detect herpes infection. A punch biopsy would show the fungus, but is unnecessary, and the fungus might be missed unless special stains are performed. The described rash would not be seen in secondary syphilis.

399. The answer is d. *(Fauci, p 320.)* Rosacea is a common problem in middle-aged, fair-skinned people. Sun damage appears to play an important role. Stress, alcohol, and heat contribute to the flushing. Men may develop rhinophyma (connective tissue overgrowth, particularly of the nose). Low-dose oral tetracycline, erythromycin, and metronidazole control the symptoms. Topical erythromycin and metronidazole also work well. The carcinoid syndrome causes flushing but not papules and pustules and is usually associated with gastrointestinal symptoms; it is quite rare. PCT can cause telangiectasias and can be associated with alcohol consumption, but patients with this disease usually have increased facial hair growth and fragile skin in sun-exposed areas as well. The butterfly-shaped macular rash of lupus does not cause pustules; usually the patient has other evidence of active disease, especially synovitis. Seborrheic dermatitis affects the eyebrows and nasolabial folds more prominently than the cheeks and nose.

400. The answer is b. *(Fauci, pp 310, 545-548.)* This is a classic description of basal cell carcinoma. Basal cell carcinoma is a malignant neoplasm of the epidermal basal cells that clinically presents as a pearly papule or nodule with a central ulceration, raised borders, and telangiectasias. Basal cell carcinomas are locally invasive and rarely metastasize; distant spread is reported in fewer than 0.1% of these cancers. Invasion of surrounding tissue and metastasis are more frequently seen in squamous cell carcinoma. Squamous cell carcinoma is malignant neoplasm of the keratinocytes; it is much more aggressive than basal cell carcinoma, grows rapidly, and may metastasize via lymphatic spread. Bacterial infections such as meningococcemia and necrotizing fasciitis could result in septicemia without appropriate treatment but are acute, not chronic, conditions.

401. The answer is b. *(Fauci, pp 800-803, 1343-1347.)* The possibility of cutaneous anthrax in this postal worker is the most important consideration in the era of bioterrorism concern. The lesion described would be characteristic of cutaneous anthrax—beginning as a small papule that is painless and progressing to a black, necrotic lesion over several days. A skin biopsy would show the very characteristic gram-positive rods of anthrax. Cutaneous anthrax has been shown to occur in postal workers who have handled letters containing anthrax spores, and can also occur in those who handle infected animals or their wool or hides. Unlike inhalational anthrax, these patients do not appear severely ill at the outset of the infection. Ecthyma gangrenosum also produces a black, necrotic skin lesion. These lesions occur in patients who are bacteremic and systemically ill from *P aeruginosa*. The brown recluse spider's bite can also produce a black necrotic ulcer. The bite is painful and usually spreads rapidly. The bubo of plague produces a tender lymphadenitis. The patient with plague or necrotizing fasciitis is acutely ill with fever and other signs of systemic inflammatory response syndrome.

402. The answer is b. *(Fauci, pp 1113-1114, 1348.)* Although there have been no cases of smallpox in the world since 1977, the threat of bioterrorism has forced physicians to be vigilant about the disease's reemergence. It will be important for students and physicians to recognize the distinguishing characteristics of smallpox versus chickenpox. Lesions are more likely to occur on palms and soles in smallpox. In chickenpox, lesions are more concentrated on the trunk, whereas in smallpox they are likely to be more concentrated on the face. In smallpox, lesions are characteristically in the same stage of development. In chickenpox, lesions are more superficial, come out in crops, and are in many different stages of development. In smallpox, patients are much more systemically ill, and give a history of fever and prostration for several days prior to the development of the rash. In chickenpox, fever usually occurs at the time of the appearance of the rash.

403. The answer is c. *(Fauci, 328-329, 336-340.)* Blistering diseases are potentially serious conditions. Blisters that are smaller than 0.5 cm are termed vesicles; larger lesions are called bullae. The proper diagnosis and treatment of bullous disorders are paramount in order to prevent disability and even death from burn-like denudation of the skin and associated infection. Although many skin diseases such as allergic contact dermatitis, erythema multiforme, and bullous impetigo can cause blisters, this patient is more likely to have bullous pemphigoid or pemphigus. These are immunologically mediated disorders; skin biopsy with immunofluorescence staining will reveal antibodies at the basal layer of the epidermis (bullous pemphigoid) or within the epidermis (pemphigus). Mucosal, especially oral, involvement is characteristic of pemphigus. Immunosuppressive agents including systemic corticosteroids are often necessary to treat these conditions. Antihistamines, sometimes helpful if itching is prominent, will not treat the underlying condition. It is no longer felt that bullous dermatoses are indicative of underlying malignancy, so a "shotgun" search for occult malignancy is not recommended. Dermatitis herpetiformis and porphyria cutanea tarda are other skin diseases that can be associated with blisters.

404. The answer is e. *(Fauci, pp 487, 541-548; Wolff, pp 262-264.)* Actinic keratoses are premalignant lesions of the skin with the potential to degenerate into squamous cell carcinoma. If left untreated, up to 20% of these lesions can become malignant. Diagnosis is usually made clinically through history and physical examination of the skin; biopsy is rarely necessary unless clinical features (ulceration, induration) suggest that malignant degeneration has already occurred. Actinic keratoses often present as erythematous hyperkeratotic papules or plaques on sun-exposed areas. They have poorly defined borders and are easier to feel because of their scaly texture. Treatment can be done with either cryotherapy (liquid nitrogen) or application of topical 5-fluorouracil. Cryotherapy is the preferred method when there are a few lesions. However, when there are many lesions with poorly defined borders, 5-fluorouracil may be used. Topical corticosteroids such as hydrocortisone or fluocinolone would not be used for treatment of actinic keratoses.

405. The answer is d. *(Fauci, pp 318, 1263-1265.)* Tinea corporis (ringworm) is a dermatophyte that causes a superficial infection of the skin. Tinea corporis clinically presents as an erythematous scaly plaque with a central clearing and serpiginous border. It is usually acquired through contact with an infected individual or animal. Initial treatment involves application of topical antifungals such as ketoconazole, clotrimazole, miconazole, toconazole, econazole, naftifine, terbinafine, or ciclopirox olamine cream. More severe infection that is unresponsive to topical therapy, or one involving the scalp, nails, or beard area, should be treated systematically with oral griseofulvin, itraconazole, or terbinafine. Cephalexin and mupirocin are antibacterial agents used for superficial infections of the skin caused by *Staphylococcus aureus* such as folliculitis or impetigo. Hydrocortisone is a weak corticosteroid that can actually exacerbate a fungal infection. Potassium hydroxide (KOH) skin prep would confirm the diagnosis.

406. The answer is d. *(Fauci, p 1186-1188; Wolff, pp 536-540.)* This patient has Kaposi sarcoma (KS). In HIV-infected individuals, KS is associated with human herpesvirus 8 (HHV-8). KS lesions are derived from the proliferation of endothelial cells in blood/lymphatic microvasculature. They present as violaceous patches, plaques, and/or nodules on the skin, mucosa, and/or viscera. The pulmonary infiltrates observed on the chest x-ray of this patient are the result of visceral KS affecting the lungs. Proliferation of neoplastic T cells is seen in cutaneous T cell lymphomas such as mycosis fungoides. Human herpesvirus 6 (HHV-6) is the cause of exanthema subitum (roseola) in children. It consists of 2- to 3-mm pink macules and papules on the trunk following a fever. *Mycobacterium avium* causes pulmonary infection in HIV patients with a CD4 count <50/µL. Immunodeficient patients or patients with HIV who are infected with HSV can present with the disseminated form of the disease. However, these lesions consist of a vesicular rash that is different from the violaceous plaques observed in KS.

General Medicine and Prevention

Questions

407. A 53-year-old woman presents to the emergency room with a minor injury and is found to have a blood pressure of 150/102, possibly elevated as a result of pain. On follow-up at your office, her BP on two occasions is 142/94 despite good dietary habits and reasonable exercise. Her history and physical are normal except that she has had a hysterectomy. Basic laboratory evaluation reveals no significant abnormalities. Based on recent recommendations of the JNC 7 (The Seventh Report of the Joint National Committee on Prevention, Detection, Evaluation, and Treatment of High Blood Pressure) which of the following is accurate information to give her?

a. At age >50, high diastolic BP becomes a more important cardiovascular risk factor than high systolic BP.
b. The new classification of prehypertension fits her latest BP readings; continue close follow-up.
c. Thiazide diuretics would be a good initial choice for her.
d. Initiating therapy with two antihypertensives would be preferred based on her current BP.
e. Estrogen-replacement therapy would be helpful in delaying her need for antihypertensives.

408. A 69-year-old woman complains of gradually worsening vision over the last 2 years. She can no longer read the newspaper on her porch in the early evening, and sometimes has difficulty seeing faces and distinguishing colors. She has hypertension and smokes cigarettes, but does not have diabetes. Her only regular medication is lisinopril. Funduscopic examination is shown in the figure. What is the next best step in the evaluation of this patient?

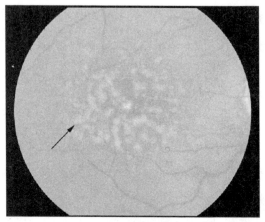

Reproduced, with permission, from Ho A et al. *Retina: Color Atlas & Synopsis of Clinical Ophthalmology.* New York, NY: McGraw-Hill; 2003.

a. Determination of fasting blood sugar and hemoglobin A1C.
b. Referral to an optometrist for tonometry
c. Recommendation that she stop smoking cigarettes, take antioxidants, and see an ophthalmologist
d. Referral to an ophthalmologist for cataract extraction
e. MRI scan of the brain with particular attention to the pituitary

409. A 60-year-old white man has just moved to town and needs to establish care. He had a "heart attack" last year. Preferring a "natural" approach, he has been very conscientious about low-fat, low-cholesterol eating habits, and a significant exercise program. He has gradually eliminated a number of prescription medications (he does not recall their names) that he was on at the time of hospital discharge. Past history is negative for hypertension, diabetes, or smoking. The lipid profile you obtain shows the following:

Total cholesterol: 194 mg/dL
Triglycerides: 140 mg/dL
HDL: 42
LDL (calculated): 124
ECG shows Q waves in leads II, II, and avF

Which of the following recommendations would most optimally treat his lipid status?

a. Continue current dietary efforts and exercise.
b. Add an HMG-CoA reductase inhibitor (statin drug) to reduce LDL cholesterol to less than 100.
c. Add a fibric acid derivative such as gemfibrozil.
d. Review previous medications and resume an angiotensin-converting enzyme inhibitor.
e. Begin aspirin 81 mg daily.

410. A 60-year-old man had an anterior myocardial infarction 3 months ago. He currently is asymptomatic and has normal vital signs and a normal physical examination. He is on an antiplatelet agent and an ACE inhibitor. What other category of medication would typically be prescribed for secondary prevention of myocardial infarction?

a. Alpha-blocker
b. Beta-blocker
c. Calcium-channel blocker
d. Nitrates
e. Naproxen sodium

411. A patient with type 2 diabetes mellitus is found to have a blood pressure of 152/98. She has never had any ophthalmologic, cardiovascular, or renal complications of diabetes or hypertension. Which of the following is the currently recommended goal for blood pressure control in this case?

a. Less than 160/90
b. Less than 145/95
c. Less than 140/90
d. Less than 130/80
e. Less than 120/70

412. A 58-year-old man has a history of hypertension and asks about reducing his risk for myocardial infarction. A lipid profile shows low HDL cholesterol at 32 mg/dL. Which of the following is an important recommendation in attempting to raise the HDL?

a. Aspirin, one tablet each day
b. Low cholesterol diet
c. Vitamin E, 400 U each day
d. DHEA (dehydroepiandrosterone) supplementation
e. Exercise

413. A 32-year-old diabetic woman who takes an estrogen-containing oral contraceptive and drinks three beers per day is found to have a triglyceride level greater than 1000 mg/dL. She is at greatest risk for which of the following complications?

a. Acute pancreatitis
b. Sudden cardiac death
c. Acute peripheral arterial occlusion
d. Acute renal insufficiency
e. Myositis

414. A 42-year-old banker sees you as a new patient. He states that he is healthy and takes no regular medications. His examination is normal except for a blood pressure of 150/94. When questioning him about alcohol use, he admits that he goes out drinking with friends about 2 Saturdays each month to relieve stress. At these times he will often have 8 to 10 mixed alcohol drinks. He and his wife have recently had several arguments about this habit, and she has threatened to divorce him if he doesn't change his ways. Despite this he has been unable to change. On one occasion he was arrested for driving while intoxicated. Nonetheless he has continued to be successfully employed, has never been hospitalized for an alcohol-related problem, and has never had symptoms of alcohol withdrawal. Which of the following statements is true regarding treatment of this patient?

a. Advice from a physician to reduce his alcohol consumption is likely to be successful.
b. The patient should be advised that complete abstinence from alcohol and referral to a mutual aid group is the best strategy in treating his alcohol-related problem.
c. Abstinence from alcohol may necessitate treatment of his blood pressure because he is currently using alcohol to treat stress.
d. Medications for alcohol dependence are not usually helpful.
e. The fact that this patient has had no symptoms of alcohol dependence proves that he does not abuse alcohol.

415. A 32-year-old stockbroker sees you because she has felt anxious almost every day for the past 9 months. She feels "keyed up" at work. At times she has difficulty concentrating and has made several minor errors in clients' accounts. For the past year she has frequently had trouble falling asleep at night despite the fact that she always feels tired. She does not fall asleep during the day at inopportune times. She takes supplemental calcium but no other medications. She denies substance or alcohol abuse. Her vital signs and physical examination are normal. CBC and chemistry panel are normal. What is the most likely diagnosis?

a. Hyperthyroidism
b. Hyperparathyroidism
c. Generalized anxiety disorder
d. Obstructive sleep apnea
e. Frontal lobe dementia

416. A 25-year-old PhD candidate recently traveled to Central America for 1 month to gain information regarding the socioeconomics of that region. While there, he took ciprofloxacin twice a day for 5 days for diarrhea. However, over the 2 to 3 weeks since coming home, he has continued to have occasional loose stools plus vague abdominal discomfort and bloating. There has been no rectal bleeding. Which of the following therapies is most likely to relieve this traveler's diarrhea?

a. Another course of ciprofloxacin
b. Doxycycline
c. Metronidazole
d. Trimethoprim-sulfamethoxazole
e. Oral glucose-electrolyte solution

417. A 42-year-old pediatric nurse practitioner seeks your advice regarding his immunization needs. He is healthy and takes no regular medications. He had well-documented chickenpox as a child. He received a tetanus-diphtheria booster 5 years ago and influenza vaccine 4 months ago. Influenza A activity has been reported in your community in the last 2 weeks. Which of the following immunizations would you recommend for this patient at this time?

a. An influenza booster
b. Tetanus-diphtheria-acellular pertussis (Tdap)
c. Pneumococcal vaccine
d. Herpes zoster vaccine
e. Meningococcal vaccine

418. You see a debilitated 80-year-old woman who requires nursing home placement in the early summer. She had had no immunizations for many years except for a pneumococcal vaccine 3 years ago when discharged from the hospital after a stay for pneumonia. Appropriate admission orders to the nursing home include which of the following?

a. Influenza vaccine
b. *Haemophilus influenzae* B immunization
c. Hepatitis B immunization series
d. Pneumococcal revaccination
e. Tetanus-diphtheria toxoid booster

419. Evidence-based guidelines support which of the following cancer screening evaluations?

a. Chest x-ray in a 50-year-old male cigarette smoker
b. Mammography in a 35-year-old woman with a history of fibrocystic breast disease
c. Prostate specific antigen in a 80-year-old man with a brother who has prostate cancer
d. Colonoscopy in an asymptomatic 50-year-old man with no family history of colon cancer
e. CA-125 in a 45-year-old woman with a sister who was just diagnosed with ovarian cancer

420. A 26-year-old medical student plans a 3-week mission trip to Mexico. She will be staying with local villagers and working indoors in a rural area 30 minutes from Mexico City. She has previously been vaccinated for hepatitis B. Of the following choices, which vaccination is most important?

a. Inactivated poliovirus vaccine (IPV) booster
b. Hepatitis A vaccine
c. Rabies vaccine
d. Meningococcal vaccine
e. Dengue vaccine

421. A 28-year-old laborer sees you because of low back pain. Ten days ago he strained his back while moving a refrigerator. Despite taking acetaminophen, his pain has worsened. He has difficulty sleeping because of the pain and for the past 3 days he has spent most of the day in bed. He has not had fever, leg numbness or weakness, or bladder or bowel problems. He takes no regular prescription medications. On examination he has difficulty getting on and off the examination table because of back pain. He has normal vital signs including a normal temperature. There is evidence of bilateral paraspinous muscle spasm. The patient is able to walk on his heels and toes and has negative straight leg raising test bilaterally. What is the next best step in the treatment of this patient?

a. Two view lumbar spine
b. MRI scan of the lumbar spine
c. Continued bed rest
d. Massage and nonsteroidal anti-inflammatories
e. Epidural corticosteroids

422. You have been asked to perform preoperative consultation on a 66-year-old man who will be undergoing transurethral resection of the prostate for urinary retention. Of the following findings, which is of most concern in predicting a cardiac complication in this patient undergoing noncardiac surgery?

a. Age over 65
b. Current cigarette use at one pack per day
c. Serum creatinine 2.2 mg/dL
d. History of three alcoholic drinks/day with ALT (SGOT) 60 mg/dL
e. LDL cholesterol of 135 mg/dL

423. A 42-year-old male is persuaded by his wife to come to you for general checkup. She hints of concern about alcohol use. Therefore, you ask the CAGE questions as an initial screen. These include which of the following?

a. Concern expressed by family
b. Previous Alcoholics Anonymous contact
c. Alcohol intake greater than two drinks per 24 hours
d. Use of an eye-opener (early-morning alcoholic beverage)
e. Presence of excess extremity shakiness

424. A 78-year-old woman comes to your office with symptoms of insomnia nearly every day, fatigue, weight loss of over 5% of body weight over the past month, loss of interest in most activities, and diminished ability to concentrate. Physical examination is normal. Which treatment is most likely to improve her symptomatology?

a. Antidepressant
b. Donepezil
c. Iron supplement
d. Prednisone
e. Thyroid supplement

425. A 65-year-old woman was hospitalized for pulmonary embolus and eventually discharged on warfarin (Coumadin) with a therapeutic INR. During the next 2 weeks as an outpatient, she was started back on her previous ACE inhibitor antihypertensive, given temazepam for insomnia, treated with ciprofloxacin for a urinary tract infection, started on over-the-counter famotidine (Pepcid) for GI symptoms, and told to stop the OTC naproxen she was taking. Follow-up INR was 5.0. Which of the following drugs most likely potentiated the effects of warfarin and led to the high INR?

a. ACE inhibitor
b. Temazepam
c. Ciprofloxacin
d. Famotidine (Pepcid)
e. Naproxen discontinuation

426. A 20-year-old college basketball player is brought to the university urgent care clinic after developing chest pain and palpitations during practice. There is no dyspnea or tachypnea. He denies family history of cardiac disease, and social history is negative for alcohol or drug use. Cardiac auscultation is unremarkable, and ECG shows only occasional PVCs. Which of the following is the most appropriate next step in evaluation and/or management?

a. Obtain urine drug screen.
b. Arrange treadmill stress test.
c. Obtain Doppler ultrasound of deep veins of lower legs.
d. Institute cardioselective beta-blocker therapy.
e. Institute respiratory therapy for exercise-induced bronchospasm.

427. A 92-year-old woman with type 2 diabetes mellitus has developed cellulitis and gangrene of her left foot. She requires a lifesaving amputation, but refuses to give consent for the surgery. She has been ambulatory in her nursing home but states that she would be so dependent after surgery that life would not be worth living for her. She has no living relatives; she enjoys walks and gardening. She is competent and of clear mind. Which of the following is the most appropriate course of action?

a. Perform emergency surgery.
b. Consult a psychiatrist.
c. Request permission for surgery from a friend of the patient.
d. Follow the patient's wishes.
e. Obtain a court order to override the patient's wishes.

428. A 42-year-old man sees you because of obesity. He played football in high school and at age 18 weighed 250 pounds. He has gradually gained weight since. Many previous attempts at dieting have resulted in transient weight loss of 10 to 15 pounds, which he then rapidly regains. He has been attending Weight Watchers for the last 3 months and has successfully lost 4 pounds. Recent attempts at exercise have been limited because of bilateral knee pain and swelling. On examination height is 6 ft 0 in, weight 340 pounds, BMI 46. Blood pressure with a large cuff is 150/95. Baseline laboratory studies including CBC, biochemical profile, thyroid stimulating hormone and lipids are normal with the exception of fasting serum glucose which is 145 mg/dL. What is the next best step?

a. Discuss bariatric surgery with the patient.
b. Refer to a commercial weight-loss program.
c. Recommend a 1000 calorie per day diet.
d. Prescribe sibutramine.
e. Recommend a low-fat diet.

429. A 54-year-old man sees you for follow-up of hypertension and a seizure disorder that is well-controlled. He established as a new patient 2 months ago and is back for his second office visit with you. At the time of his initial visit he admitted to a 35-year history of smoking 2 packages of cigarettes per day. At that time he indicated that he was not interested in stopping smoking, and seemed irritated when you suggested that he quit. Today his blood pressure is well controlled and there are no new medical issues. With regard to discussing cessation of cigarette smoking during today's visit, what is the next best step?

a. Do not discuss cessation of cigarette smoking because it will likely upset him again.
b. Do not discuss cessation of cigarette smoking, because there is no real benefit to cessation of cigarette smoking after smoking this long.
c. Ask him if he is still smoking, and if so advise him to quit and assess his willingness to do so.
d. Recommend bupropion.
e. Recommend that he switch to smokeless tobacco.

430. A 70-year-old man with unresectable carcinoma of the lung metastatic to liver and bone has developed progressive weight loss, anorexia, and shortness of breath. The patient has executed a valid living will that prohibits the use of feeding tube in the setting of terminal illness. The patient becomes lethargic and stops eating altogether. The patient's wife of 30 years now insists on enteral feeding for her husband. Which of the following is the most appropriate course of action?

a. Respect the wife's wishes as a reliable surrogate decision maker.
b. Resist the placement of a feeding tube in accordance with the living will.
c. Ask the daughter to make the decision.
d. Place a feeding tube until such time as the matter can be discussed with the patient.
e. Request a court order to place a feeding tube.

431. After being stung by a yellow jacket, a 14-year-old develops the sudden onset of hoarseness and shortness of breath. An urticarial rash is noted. Which of the following is the most important first step in treatment?

a. An antihistamine
b. Epinephrine
c. Venom immunotherapy
d. Corticosteroids
e. Removal of the stinger

432. A 40-year-old male is found to have a uric acid level of 9 mg/dL on a comprehensive blood chemistry profile. The patient has never had gouty arthritis, renal disease, or kidney stones. The patient has no evidence on history or physical examination of underlying chronic or malignant disease. What is the best approach to this patient?

a. The risk of urolithiasis requires the institution of prophylactic therapy such as allopurinol.
b. Asymptomatic hyperuricemia is associated with an increased risk of gouty arthritis, but benefits of prophylaxis do not outweigh risks in this patient.
c. Further investigation beyond history and physical is needed to assess for lymphoproliferative disease.
d. Hyperuricemia is associated with cardiovascular disease; its treatment will lower this risk.
e. A 24-hour excretion in urine of uric acid will identify those persons with asymptomatic hyperuricemia who need treatment.

433. A 38-year-old obese female with history of chronic venous insufficiency and peripheral edema was admitted to the hospital the previous night for cellulitis involving both lower legs. She has had recurrent such episodes, treated successfully in the past with various antibiotics, including cefazolin, nafcillin, ampicillin/sulbactam, and levofloxacin. Intravenous levofloxacin was again chosen due to the perceived ease in transitioning to a once-daily oral outpatient dose. Normal saline at 50 mL/h is administered. Past history is otherwise significant only for hypertension, which is being treated at home with HCTZ 25 mg, lisinopril 40 mg, and atenolol 100 mg, all once each morning. Admission BP was 144/92 and the orders were written to continue each of these antihypertensives at one tablet po qd. The only other inhospital medication is daily prophylactic enoxaparin. As you round at 6 PM on the day following admission, the nurse contacts you emergently stating that she has just finished giving evening medicines and the patient's BP is unexpectedly 90/50. Pulse rate is 92. There is no chest pain, dyspnea, or tachypnea. What is most likely cause of her hypertension?

a. An allergic reaction either to the antibiotic or to one of the antihypertensives
b. A vasovagal reaction secondary to pain
c. Hypovolemia due to the cellulitis
d. Acute pulmonary embolism
e. Medication error

434. A 44-year-old Hispanic woman comes to clinic for a general checkup due to concern about a family history of diabetes and high blood pressure. Her height is 62 in, weight 50 kg (110 lb), waist circumference 33 inches (85 cm), blood pressure 138/88. Laboratory evaluation reveals fasting glucose of 120 mg/dL. Lipid profile shows total cholesterol 240 mg/dL, HDL 38 mg/dL, and triglycerides 420 mg/dL; LDL cannot be calculated. She does not smoke, use alcohol, or take any medications. Which of the following is correct regarding the identification of the metabolic syndrome in this patient?

a. Metabolic syndrome is not present in this case due to the absence of abdominal obesity.
b. Metabolic syndrome is not present because the blood pressure is not sufficiently elevated to be a risk factor.
c. Metabolic syndrome is not present because the glucose is not sufficiently elevated to be a risk factor.
d. Metabolic syndrome is present based on the risk factors given.
e. Metabolic syndrome cannot be identified until the LDL is determined.

Questions 435 to 437

The initial choice of an antihypertensive or the addition of further agent(s) to the regimen may depend on concomitant factors. For each of the cases below, indicate the medication choice that would give the best additional benefit in addition to blood pressure control. Each lettered option may be used once, more than once, or not at all.

a. Alpha-blocker
b. Beta-blocker
c. Calcium-channel blocker
d. Angiotensin-converting enzyme inhibitor
e. Centrally acting alpha agonist
f. Diuretic

435. A 67-year-old African American man complains of tendency toward urinary retention. Digital rectal examination reveals enlarged prostate.

436. An obese 54-year-old white woman has a hemoglobin A1C of 9.5 and elevated urine microalbumin.

437. A 62-year-old man has a history of a myocardial infarction and has chronic stable angina.

Questions 438 to 440

The choice of an antihypertensive agent may involve trying to avoid an adverse effect on a comorbid condition. For each of the patients with known hypertension below, indicate the medication choice that needs to be avoided above all others. Each lettered option may be used once, more than once, or not at all.

a. Angiotensin-converting enzyme inhibitor
b. Beta-blocker, noncardioselective
c. Calcium-channel blocker
d. Diuretic
e. Hydralazine

438. A 40-year-old white man has three episodes over the past 2 years of debilitating acute arthritis involving ankle or foot joints.

439. A 70-year-old man with COPD quit smoking 5 years ago, but is now beginning to experience cramps in his calf muscles upon walking one block. Diminished popliteal and pedal pulses are noted on examination.

440. A 24-year-old single woman has delayed seeing a doctor over the past 3 months due to lack of insurance; she has experienced amenorrhea and nausea.

Questions 441 to 444

For each patient below, what are appropriate screening tests? Each lettered option may be used once, more than once, or not at all.

a. DNA or RNA amplification tests for chlamydia obtained from the cervix
b. Intermediate strength tuberculin skin test
c. Abdominal ultrasonography
d. Chest x-ray
e. Rapid plasma reagin (RPR)

441. A 23-year-old asymptomatic unmarried woman who is in a monogamous relationship

442. A 67-year-old male smoker

443. A 22-year-old male nurse's aide who is beginning employment at a hospital

444. A 70-year-old woman admitted to a nursing home

General Medicine and Prevention

Answers

407. The answer is c. *(JNC 7 Express, p xiii.)* A key point in the JNC 7 is that a thiazide diuretic should be used in most patients with uncomplicated hypertension when diet and lifestyle modifications are not sufficient. Other major points include (1) systolic BP >140 is a more important cardiovascular risk factor than diastolic BP in persons over age 50; (2) individuals normotensive at age 55 still have a 90% lifetime risk of developing hypertension; (3) CVD risk doubles, beginning at 115/75, for each rise in BP of 20/10; (4) a new category of prehypertension has been designated with systolic BP 120 to 139 or diastolic BP 80 to 89, with emphasis on healthy diet and lifestyle modifications; (5) if BP >20/10 above goal is present at the outset, consider initiating therapy with two agents. Estrogen-replacement therapy does not lower blood pressure.

408. The answer is c. *(Fauci, pp 188-191.)* The ophthalmologic examination shows drusen. These pale yellowish retinal lesions can often be seen with a handheld ophthalmoscope. Drusen are caused by deposition of acellular debris between the retinal epithelium and Bruch membrane. These lesions are the hallmark of age-related macular degeneration, which is the leading cause of blindness in older adults in the United States. Evidence suggests that antioxidants (such as beta-carotene, vitamin C, or vitamin E) and zinc can prevent the progression of age-related macular degeneration. About 15% of patients with macular degeneration have a "wet form" which leads to more severe visual loss and which is treated by photocoagulation. Ophthalmologic evidence of open angle glaucoma consists of an increased cup-to-disc ratio. Glaucoma is diagnosed by the characteristic optic nerve appearance and visual field loss. Many (but not all) patients with open angle glaucoma have an elevated intraocular pressure which can be detected by tonometry. Diabetic retinopathy is characterized by microaneurysms and neovascularization and is treated by photocoagulation and optimizing blood sugar control. Cataracts are a common cause of vision loss in the elderly, but do not cause retinal abnormalities. Pituitary tumors can cause visual field defects and/or papilledema, but do not cause drusen.

409. The answer is b. (*NCEP ATP III, pp 2-4, 7-9, 12-14.*) The National Cholesterol Education Program Adult Treatment Panel III recommendations include lowering the LDL cholesterol to <100 mg/dL in those with known coronary heart disease (secondary prevention). The 2004 update to these guidelines adds an optional goal of LDL <70 mg/dL in very high risk patients. In this case, with dietary efforts and exercise already well-established and unlikely to reduce LDL further, a statin drug is indicated. These typically lower LDL by 20% to 50%. Gemfibrozil is used primarily for hypertriglyceridemia; this patient's triglyceride level is normal (<150 mg/dL). ACE inhibitors have no significant effect on lipids. In men, aspirin has been shown to reduce mortality from myocardial infarction. However, it does not lower cholesterol.

410. The answer is b. (*Fauci, pp 1521-1524.*) Beta-blockers are documented to lower the risk of myocardial reinfarction, whereas calcium channel-blockers may increase the risk. Alpha-blockers have been associated with an increased risk of congestive heart failure. ACE inhibitors are beneficial in this setting and should be continued. Despite their decades-long use for the symptomatic treatment of angina, nitrates are not indicated for secondary prevention of infarction. Recently, long-term use of some nonsteroidal anti-inflammatory drugs (including naproxen sodium) has been associated with an increased risk of myocardial infarction.

411. The answer is d. (*JNC 7 Express, pp 7, 15.*) Goals for blood pressure control and lipid levels are typically more stringent in the diabetic compared to the nondiabetic. The goal blood pressure for diabetics and patients with renal disease is <130/80. Blood pressure goal for the standard patient is <140/90. Both systolic and diastolic pressures should be below goal in order to achieve optimal blood pressure control.

412. The answer is e. (*NCEP ATP III, pp 19-20.*) Within this group of choices, only exercise has been shown to raise HDL. A low-cholesterol diet actually lowers HDL. Among current lipid-lowering medications, nicotinic acid has the most potent HDL-increasing effect at 15% to 35%, followed by fibric acids and then statins. Alcohol also increases the HDL level (HDL2 and HDL3 subfractions), thereby imparting some cardioprotective effect, but at the risk of cardiomyopathy, sudden death, hemorrhagic stroke, and other noncardiovascular problems among heavy drinkers. The cardiovascular system may benefit from aspirin (because of antiplatelet effects) but it has no effect on HDL. After initial enthusiasm for vitamin E, more recent studies have not shown consistent cardiovascular benefit from antioxidant vitamins. None of these raise HDL. DHEA supplements lower HDL values.

413. The answer is a. *(Fauci, pp 2007-2009.)* Hypertriglyceridemia, which is aggravated by poorly controlled diabetes, estrogen, and alcohol, predisposes to pancreatitis. In general, triglyceride levels greater than 1000 mg/dL place the patient at risk and should prompt treatment in order to lower the chance of pancreatitis. The most effective triglyceride lowering agents are nicotinic acid (niacin) and fibrates. The effect of hypertriglyceridemia on coronary and peripheral vascular disease is complicated. Many studies suggest that it is a modest risk factor, but the cardiovascular risk of extreme hypertriglyceridemia is certainly less profound than the risk of pancreatitis. Hypertriglyceridemia does not increase the risk of acute renal failure. Rhabdomyolysis can complicate treatment of hyperlipidemia, particularly when the combination of a fibrate and a statin is employed.

414. The answer is b. *(Fauci, pp 2724-2729.)* This patient has an alcohol use disorder, which is defined as a maladaptive pattern of alcohol use causing clinically significant impairment or distress. Men who consume more than 14 drinks per week or 5 drinks on any one day, and women who consume more than 7 drinks per week or more than 4 drinks on any 1 day are at risk for this disorder. This patient has had significant marital discord, has been unable to cease alcohol use, and has had an arrest for driving while intoxicated. All of these indicate that the patient has clinically significant impairment from alcohol abuse. Alcohol use disorder may or may not be accompanied by alcohol dependence, which is characterized by symptoms and signs of alcohol withdrawal during periods of abstinence. Patients with alcohol use disorder are usually unable to limit the amount of alcohol that they consume, and therefore complete abstinence from alcohol is recommended. Mutual help groups (such as Alcoholics Anonymous) as well as medications (such as acamprosate and naltrexone) can be helpful in maintaining abstinence. Physician advice alone is usually unsuccessful. Alcohol use disorder is frequently accompanied by other psychiatric disorders such as depression. Alcohol use disorder can aggravate hypertension; blood pressure will improve with abstinence. Current understanding of alcohol use disorder suggests that there is a genetic tendency to this illness.

415. The answer is c. *(Fauci, pp 2711-2712)* This patient meets the diagnostic criteria for generalized anxiety disorder (GAD). GAD is characterized by excessive anxiety occurring at least half the time for a minimum of six months and associated with three or more of the following: restlessness, fatigue, difficulty concentrating, irritability, muscle tension, or sleep disturbance. In addition, the symptoms must result in significant impairment and must not be due to another psychiatric disease, substance abuse or medical conditions such as hyperthyroidism. This disorder is common and occurs in up to 5% of patients seen in primary care offices. Many of these patients have additional psychiatric disease such as depression. Cognitive behavioral therapy and treatment with tricyclic antidepressants or selective serotonin reuptake inhibitors are often beneficial in relieving symptoms, which tend to be chronic. Benzodiazepines often improve symptoms, but may result in dependence. Hyperthyroidism would be associated with symptoms (heat intolerance, tremor) and signs (tachycardia, goiter) of this disorder. Hyperparathyroidism causes depression more often than anxiety and should cause hypercalcemia on the chemistry panel. Sleep apnea would cause abnormal daytime somnolence as its cardinal symptom. This patient's difficulty concentrating is a manifestation of her anxiety disorder; dementia would be very uncommon in a 32 year old.

416. The answer is c. *(Fauci, pp 813-818, 937-942, 956-972, 1311-1313.)* Patient with symptomatic *Giardia lamblia* infection typically present with several weeks bloating, loose stools and weight loss. Most patients respond to metronidazole therapy. This parasite is contracted by ingesting contaminated food or water, with the classic zoonotic reservoirs being the freshwater streams of the northern United States and also the water supplies in Russia and developing countries. Bacterial pathogens such as *Campylobacter jejuni*, enterotoxigenic *E coli*, *Salmonella*, and *Shigella* usually cause acute diarrhea, often bloody. They usually respond to fluoroquinolones or azithromycin. Many bacterial pathogens in developing countries are resistant to trimethoprim-sulfamethoxazole. Oral glucose-electrolyte solution rehydration is the mainstay of *Vibrio cholerae* therapy. Hydration rather than antibiotics is also the key for enterohemorrhagic *E coli*.

417. The answer is b. *(http://www.immunize.org)* The Advisory Committee on Immunization Practices (ACIP) is an independent panel of experts and makes evidence-based immunization recommendations for children and adults. Tetanus-diphtheria-acellular pertussis (Tdap) should replace a single dose of tetanus-diphtheria (Td) for all adults less than 65 years of age who have not previously received this vaccine and who have not received Td in the past 10 years. Health care workers who have not received a tetanus-diphtheria (Td) vaccine in the last two years should be vaccinated with the tetanus-diphtheria-acellular pertussis vaccine (Tdap), especially those health care workers who have direct patient contact with infants. Yearly influenza immunization is recommended for all health care workers. A single dose of trivalent influenza vaccine is recommended each year beginning in October. Booster doses for influenza are not recommended. The ACIP recommends pneumococcal vaccination for all adults over 64 years of age, and for younger adults with certain medical illnesses such as chronic obstructive lung disease, diabetes mellitus, HIV infection, or asplenia. Herpes zoster vaccine is recommended for adults 60 years of age or older. Meningococcal vaccine is recommended for adults with anatomic or functional asplenia, complement deficiencies, and first-year college students who live in dormitories. Up-to-date ACIP recommendations can be found on the website of the Immunization Action Coalition (http://www.immunize.org/).

418. The answer is e. *(Fauci, pp 775-781.)* A Td (adult tetanus-diphtheria booster) should be given every 10 years. The new tetanus-diphtheria-acellular pertussis (Tdap) vaccination is not FDA approved for persons 65 years of age or older. A flu shot should be given in this age group, but at the appropriate time in the fall. There is no recommendation to give the *Haemophilus* immunization in adults. This patient is not in one of the high-risk categories for hepatitis B (including health care workers, hemodialysis patients, routine recipients of clotting factors, travelers to endemic areas, persons at elevated risk for sexually transmitted diseases, injection drug users, those in institutions for the mentally retarded, and household contacts of hepatitis B carriers) and therefore has no specific indication to receive this series. The pneumococcal vaccine may be given again to higher-risk individuals at least 5 years after the original, and to older adults who received the initial pneumococcal vaccine before age 65.

419. The answer is d. *(Fauci, pp 489-492.)* In the United States, cancer is the second leading cause of death. Therefore the detection of asymptomatic cancers through screening examinations is an important part of the periodic health examination. There is now a large body of evidence to guide the physician in the appropriate selection of screening tests for cancer in asymptomatic patients. Bayes theorem tells us that, for rare conditions, false positive screening tests are likely even if the screening test has a very high sensitivity and specificity. Therefore, screening tests are most beneficial in populations where the screened condition is common. There is good evidence that screening for colon cancer in persons age 50 or older reduces mortality. The U.S. Preventative Services Task Force (USPSTF) recommends either fecal occult blood testing, flexible sigmoidoscopy, or colonoscopy. Screening for breast cancer with mammography has been demonstrated to improve mortality in women aged 50 years or older. Screening of women between ages 40 and 49 is still somewhat controversial. However, most physicians and official organizations recommend screening mammography every one to two years in women beginning at age 40. Earlier screening is not recommended for women with fibrocystic breast disease, and indeed false positive mammograms are more likely in women with fibrocystic breast disease. Neither the chest x-ray nor any other test has proven to be an effective screen for lung cancer (although spiral chest CT shows some promise). PSA levels, though somewhat controversial, play a role in prostate cancer screening in men under the age of 70. Screening for less common cancers (bladder, ovary, and pancreas) has not proven to reduce mortality or to be cost effective. Even though CA-125 and vaginal ultrasonography can detect ovarian cancer at an early stage, there are many false positives which necessitate more invasive testing with significant morbidity and mortality. The physical examination remains important (e.g., in detection of testicular and skin cancers), although definitive evidence regarding screening is sparse.

420. The answer is b. (*http://wwwn.cdc.gov/travel/default.aspx.*) Travel to developing countries is becoming more common and exposes the traveler to uncommon infectious diseases. The physician can obtain up-to-date professional advice for travelers at the CDC Travel Medicine website (http://wwwn.cdc.gov/travel/default.aspx). For travel to most countries outside of North America and Europe, hepatitis A vaccine and typhoid vaccine are recommended. Polio vaccine is recommended for travel to areas where polio is endemic. This includes a few countries in Africa, Asia, and Southeast Asia. Rabies vaccination is recommended for travelers who will be spending time in rural areas and outdoors where they might encounter rabid animals, especially if it will be several days journey to a major metropolitan area where rabies biologicals would be available. Malaria prophylaxis is recommended for most of Africa, Southeast Asia, the

Middle East, and Central and South America. If traveling to an area reporting chloroquine-resistant malaria, mefloquine or doxycycline are usually the drugs of choice. Meningococcal vaccine is recommended before travel to sub-Saharan Africa and for pilgrims to Mecca. There is no vaccine against dengue.

421. The answer is d. *(Fauci, pp 107-115.)* This patient has acute low back pain. This is a very common complaint seen by primary care physicians and is the most common cause of occupational disability in young persons. In the absence of certain "red flags," patients with acute low back pain can be treated without imaging studies. Clinical "red flags" that would suggest the need for early imaging include recent trauma, age greater than 50 years, fever, weight loss, corticosteroid or illicit drug use, bladder or bowel symptoms, progressive radicular symptoms, and a history of cancer. Evidence-based studies demonstrate that nonsteroidal anti-inflammatories, chiropractic manipulation, massage, cognitive behavioral therapy, and muscle relaxants shorten the duration of symptoms. Bed rest delays recovery. Lumbosacral spine series can identify fractures, but CT scanning and MRI scanning are much more sensitive for detecting herniated discs, if evaluation becomes indicated. Epidural corticosteroids may be used for radicular pain that does not respond to initial modalities but is less effective for pain localized to the low back and paraspinous muscles.

422. The answer is c. *(Fauci, pp 50-52.)* The Cardiac Risk Index (CRI) is an accurate way to assess cardiac risk in the setting of noncardiac surgery. Its six predictive factors for postop cardiac complications are high-risk type of surgery (intraperitoneal, intrathoracic, or suprainguinal vascular), ischemic heart disease, history of congestive heart failure, history of symptomatic cerebrovascular disease, insulin therapy for diabetes, and pre-op serum creatinine >2.0 mg/dL. Only the last of these applies to this case. In general, classic cardiac risk factors (such as cigarette smoking and hypercholesterolemia) are less important than established disease. Although full-blown alcoholic hepatitis and cirrhosis increase surgical risk considerably, asymptomatic transaminase elevation does not. Age is a risk factor in some analyses, but in the Cardiac Risk Index the cardiac risks of aging were explained by the diseases that accompany aging.

423. The answer is d. *(Fauci, pp 1920.)* The CAGE screening tool for alcoholism consists of asking about alcohol-related trouble: cutting down, being annoyed by criticisms, guilt, and use of an eye opener (ie, alcohol consumption upon arising).

424. The answer is a. (*Fauci, pp 2715-2718.*) Depression is commonly encountered in the outpatient setting. Fatigue commonly accompanies depression and is often the complaint that brings the patient to the physician. Criteria for diagnosis include at least 5 of 9 specific symptoms (occurring during the same 2-week period). The nine symptoms are: depressed mood, fatigue, weight gain or loss, loss of interest, sleep disturbance, difficulty concentrating, psychomotor agitation or retardation, feelings of worthlessness, and recurrent thoughts of death (or suicidal ideation). Thus psychotherapy and antidepressant medication would be the basic treatment. Insomnia and loss of interest in outside activities should suggest depression even if other features are worrisome for a dementing illness. Iron deficiency causes fatigue but not neurocognitive symptoms unless the anemia is very severe, in which case pallor should be evident on the physical examination. There is no evidence of a steroid-responsive condition in this patient's presentation. Hypothyroidism is a common cause of fatigue but usually causes weight gain and slow relaxation phase of the reflexes.

425. The answer is c. (*Fauci, pp 743-745.*) Many medications can potentiate warfarin (Coumadin), including the fluoroquinolone, ciprofloxacin, and various other broad-spectrum antibiotics. ACE inhibitors, benzodiazepines, and famotidine have no effect on the metabolism of warfarin. Nonsteroidal anti-inflammatory drugs may occasionally enhance warfarin's effect, so discontinuing naproxen, if anything, should lower the INR. If the H_2 blocker cimetidine or the proton pump inhibitor omeprazole had been used for gastric acid reduction in this case, either of these can potentiate warfarin and increase the INR. Of interest is that one other increasingly seen potentiator of warfarin is the over-the-counter herbal product ginkgo biloba.

426. The answer is a. (*Fauci, pp 236, 2733.*) The question of cocaine use must be raised in virtually all young adults with cardiovascular symptoms, despite a professed negative history. Therefore, a urine drug screen should be obtained early on. If this is negative, the patient might well need further cardiac evaluation, such as echocardiogram, ambulatory cardiac monitoring, and/or stress test. In the absence of dyspnea, recent immobilization, or physical examination evidence of venous thrombosis, workup for asthma or DVT would not be warranted. Beta-blockers can be used for symptomatic treatment of PVCs but not until the more serious issue of substance abuse has been addressed. Cardiovascular complications from cocaine abuse include hypertension (which may be severe), arrhythmias, myocardial infarction, and stroke.

427. The answer is d. *(Fauci, p 3.)* The principle of autonomy is an overriding issue in this patient, who is competent to make her own decisions about surgery. Proceeding with elective surgery without the patient's consent would place the surgeon at risk of civil prosecution for malpractice as well as criminal prosecution for assault and battery. Consulting a psychiatrist would be inappropriate unless there is some reason to believe the patient is not competent. No such concern is present in this description of the patient. Since the patient is competent, no friend or relative can give permission for the procedure. A court would not override the medical decision of a competent adult unless other lives (eg, that of a minor or an unborn child) were at risk.

428. The answer is a. *(Fauci, pp 468-473.)* This patient has morbid obesity (BMI over 40) and has comorbidities of hypertension, diabetes, and osteoarthritis of the knees. Two large meta-analyses have established that bariatric surgery is more effective than nonsurgical therapy for achieving sustained weight loss and controlling comorbid conditions for patients with morbid obesity. Surgical mortality is low (less than 1%) and associated with long-term sustained weight loss of 45 to 65 pounds. Several professional organizations, including the American College of Physicians, now recommend bariatric surgery as the treatment of choice for patients with morbid obesity, especially if they have comorbid conditions and have failed dietary therapy. Controlled trials have established that caloric restriction and physical activity can achieve modest weight reduction, usually on the order of 2% to 8%. A review of commercial weight-loss programs demonstrated that Weight Watchers was the most effective with a sustained weight reduction of 3% at 2 years. A number of medications (sibutramine, orlistat, and phentermine) are FDA approved for weight reduction but have demonstrated only modest effectiveness. Sibutramine is associated with dry mouth and can elevate blood pressure and therefore is not a good choice for this patient. This patient has morbid obesity with comorbid conditions and has failed dietary therapy and exercise program. Therefore his physician should discuss the possibility of bariatric surgery for treatment of his obesity.

429. The answer is c. (*Fauci, pp 2736-2739.*) Despite overwhelming evidence of the adverse health effects of cigarette smoking that has accumulated over the last 50 years, more than 20% of Americans still smoke cigarettes. Cigarette smoking is the most common health behavior associated with preventable death in the United States. Physicians can play a major role in encouraging patients to stop smoking. Evidence shows that even very brief counseling (as little as 3 minutes) in the physician's office can improve smoking cessation rates. Even in long-term smokers, smoking cessation has major health benefits. After cessation of smoking, the risk of myocardial infarction declines by over 50% in 1 year and the risk of lung cancer declines by 3% to 5% per year even in long-term cigarette smokers. Many professional organizations (including the American Medical Association) recommend that, at every clinic visit, physicians should ask their patients whether they are smoking, advise them to quit, and assess their willingness to do so. If the patient is willing to consider smoking cessation, the physician should assist them in their attempt to quit and arrange follow-up to assess compliance. Behavioral counseling and drug therapy improve the likelihood of smoking cessation. Nicotine replacement therapy, bupropion, and varenicline are FDA-approved for smoking cessation. Nicotine replacement therapy is contraindicated in patients with recent myocardial infarction, angina, and severe arrhythmias. Bupropion is contraindicated in patients who have preexisting seizures. Varenicline has recently been associated with depression and behavioral abnormalities. Smokeless tobacco carries the risk of oral cancer and is not recommended as treatment for cessation of cigarette smoking.

430. The answer is b. (*Fauci, pp 3, 69-70.*) The patient's autonomy as directed by the living will must be respected. This autonomy is not transferred to a surrogate decision maker, even one who is very credible. A family conference in this case would not change the overriding issue—that a valid living will is in effect. Living wills and other advance directives are completed when patients are competent, and give instructions for their treatment if they become incompetent or unable to express their wishes. A medical power of attorney (POA) assigns decision-making capacity to another person (surrogate) when the patient lacks decisional capacity and when no documentation of the patient's previous wishes is available.

431. The answer is b. (*Fauci, p 2604.*) The administration of epinephrine is the best treatment in the acute setting. Epinephrine provides both α-and β-adrenergic effects. Antihistamines and corticosteroids are frequently given as well; although they have little immediate effect, they help prevent the "second wave" of mediator release that may occur several hours after the initial antigen exposure. The patient should be offered venom immunotherapy after recovery from the systemic reaction. Removal without compression of an insect stinger is worthwhile, but not the primary concern.

432. The answer is b. (*Fauci, pp 2445-2447.*) Asymptomatic hyperuricemia does increase the risk of acute gouty arthritis, but most hyperuricemic individuals never have an episode. The cost of lifelong prophylaxis is high, as is the risk of an adverse reaction to a drug like allopurinol. Prophylactic therapy is reserved for patients with repeated gout attacks. Likewise the risk of urolithiasis is sufficiently low that prophylaxis is not necessary until the development of a stone. Structural kidney damage does not occur before a first gouty attack. Hyperuricemia is associated with but not a cause of arteriosclerotic disease, and there is no proven cardiovascular benefit to reducing the uric acid level. However, an elevated uric level may be a clue to look for diabetes, hypertension, and/or hyperlipidemia. In patients with lymphoproliferative disease, prophylaxis for the prevention of renal impairment is recommended, especially in the face of chemotherapy. This patient, however, has no signs or symptoms of underlying malignancy; a search for underlying cancer is not advised in the asymptomatic patient with hyperuricemia. Measuring urinary uric acid excretion is unnecessary in asymptomatic patients.

433. The answer is e. (*Fauci, p 3.*) The concept being advanced here is medication error. A new emphasis is being placed on reducing all medical errors, including those related to misreading of handwriting, which might include avoidance of certain abbreviations or use of an electronic medical record. In this case the pharmacist and/or nurse mistook the medication orders for one tablet po qd (orally once a day) for one tablet po qid (orally four times a day), such that the patient had received three doses of each antihypertensive by 6 PM. Other abbreviations to avoid include qhs (write "at bedtime" instead), QOD (write "every other day"), U ("write "unit"), and MS (write "morphine sulfate"). There is no particular clue to the other listed answers. For example, an allergic reaction would seem unlikely with medications previously well tolerated; there are no symptoms or signs of acute pulmonary embolism, and a prophylactic anticoagulant is in use.

Hypovolemia would be unlikely to develop after admission in a patient receiving IV fluids. Vasovagal reaction would be associated with bradycardia.

434. The answer is d. (*NCEP ATP III, pp 15-17.*) The metabolic syndrome represents a cluster of metabolic risk factors for coronary heart disease, closely linked to insulin resistance. It can be identified when any three of the following five items are present: abdominal obesity (waist circumference in women >88 cm (>35 in) or in men >102 cm [40 in]), hypertriglyceridemia (>150 mg/dL) low HDL (<50 mg/dL in women or <40 in men), blood pressure greater than or equal to 130/85, and fasting glucose >110 mg/dL. In this case, four risk factors are present, all except abdominal obesity. In addition, hyperinsulinemia decreases the renal excretion of uric acid, resulting in hyperuricemia, although this finding is not part of the metabolic syndrome definition. Persons with metabolic syndrome are at risk for developing diabetes.

435 to 437. The answers are 435-a, 436-d, 437-b. (*Fauci, pp 600, 15601448-1451.*) Alpha-blockers such as terazosin or doxazosin improve urinary outflow and might benefit a male with benign prostatic hypertrophy with urinary retention when used as an addition to another antihypertensive; use of this class as a single agent has been discouraged due to concerns about an increased risk of congestive heart failure. ACE inhibitors give renal protective effect in diabetics with proteinuria, are helpful in CHF, and are likely protective post-MI. Evidence is accumulating that angiotensin II receptor blockers provide these same benefits. Beta-blockers are indicated post-MI, often in CHF, and in various tachyarrhythmia settings; they may help prevent migraines and treat essential tremor.

438 to 440. The answers are 438-d, 439-b, 440-a. (*JNC 7 Express, pp 18-19.*) Diuretics predispose to hyperuricemia and therefore acute gout, the condition described in the first of these three questions; they can exacerbate hyperglycemia and must be used carefully in diabetics. Noncardioselective beta-blockers are contraindicated in asthma/COPD and may adversely affect peripheral vascular disease, which the patient in the second of these three scenarios is describing with his symptom of claudication; other cautions include decompensated CHF, bradyarrhythmias, and type 1 diabetes (because inhibition of the usual sympathetic responses to hypoglycemia makes it difficult for diabetics to detect hypoglycemia). ACE inhibitors and angiotensin II receptor blockers are contraindicated in pregnancy, the underlying situation in the third of these three questions, due to the potential for fetal anomalies and death.

441 to 444.   The answers are 441-a, 442-c, 443-b, 444-b. *(http://www. ahrq.gov/clinic/USpstfix.htm#Recommendations.)* Screening tests are employed to detect the presence of latent or asymptomatic diseases or conditions. In order to be cost effective a screening test should (1) detect a disease which has significant morbidity and/or mortality, (2) detect a disease for which therapy in the asymptomatic stage improves outcome, (3) be acceptable to the public, and (4) detect a disease that is relatively common. There is now a large literature on the effectiveness of screening tests for a number of diseases. The US Preventative Services Task Force (USPSTF) is an independent panel of experts, which regularly reviews the literature and issues evidence-based recommendations. Their most recent recommendations can be found on the Agency for Healthcare Research and Quality website (http://www.ahrq.gov/clinic/USpstfix.htm#Recommendations).

Current recommendations include screening all pregnant and sexually active women age 24 and younger for chlamydia infection, the most common bacterial sexually transmitted disease in the United States. In women, genital chlamydia infection may cause pelvic inflammatory disease, infertility, ectopic pregnancy, and chronic pelvic pain. Chlamydial infection during pregnancy is associated with adverse pregnancy outcomes, including miscarriage, premature rupture of membranes, preterm labor, low birth weight, and infant mortality.

The USPSTF also recommends that all men aged 65 to 75 who have ever smoked (current and former smokers) receive abdominal ultrasonography to detect asymptomatic abdominal aortic aneurysms, because early detection and treatment of abdominal aortic aneurysm has been shown to decrease mortality. Chest x-ray as a screening test for lung cancer is not recommended.

The USPSTF and the Centers for Disease Control and Prevention (CDC) recommend targeted screening for the detection of latent tuberculosis infection in persons who are at risk for being infected or developing active tuberculosis. This includes persons who live in congregant settings (such as prisons, homeless shelters, and nursing homes), persons who are severely immunocompromised (such as those with HIV infection), persons recently exposed to an acute case of tuberculosis, and healthcare workers. Healthcare workers and persons entering congregant settings are tested initially and, if negative, then yearly thereafter to detect the acquisition of infection.

Allergy and Immunology

Questions

445. A 20-year-old female develops urticaria that lasts for 6 weeks and then resolves spontaneously. She gives no history of weight loss, fever, rash, or tremulousness. Physical examination shows no abnormalities. Which of the following is the most likely cause of the urticaria?

a. Connective tissue disease
b. Hyperthyroidism
c. Chronic infection
d. Food allergy
e. Not likely to be determined

446. A 20-year-old male is found to have weight loss and generalized lymphadenopathy. He has hypogammaglobulinemia with a normal distribution of immunoglobulin isotypes. Histologic examination of lymphoid tissue shows germinal center hyperplasia. A diagnosis of common variable immunodeficiency is made. Which of the following statements is correct?

a. The patient likely had symptoms in childhood.
b. At least one parent is also afflicted with the disease.
c. The patient may develop recurrent bronchitis and chronic idiopathic diarrhea.
d. The patient should receive the standard vaccine protocol.
e. The patient should receive trimethoprim-sulfamethoxazole as prophylaxis against *Pneumocystis* infections.

447. A 25-year-old female complains of watery rhinorrhea and pruritus of the eyes and nose that occurs around the same season each year. Symptoms are not exacerbated by weather changes, emotion, or irritants. She is on no medications and is not pregnant. Which of the following statements is correct?

a. Her symptoms are likely produced by an IgE antibody against a specific allergen.
b. She has vasomotor rhinitis.
c. The patient's nasal turbinates are likely to be very red.
d. Avoidance measures alone are almost always effective.
e. Decongestant nasal sprays can suppress her symptoms.

448. A 20-year-old nursing student complains of asthma while on her surgical rotation. She has developed dermatitis of her hands. Symptoms are worse when she is in the operating room. Which of the following statements is correct?

a. This allergic reaction is always benign.
b. The patient should be evaluated for latex allergy by skin testing.
c. This syndrome is less common now than 10 years ago.
d. Oral corticosteroid is indicated.
e. She will have to change her career since there is no substitute for latex gloves.

449. A 30-year-old male develops skin rash, pruritus, and mild wheezing about 20 minutes after an intravenous pyelogram performed for the evaluation of renal stone symptoms. Which of the following is the best approach to diagnosis of this patient?

a. Perform 24-hour urinary histamine measurement.
b. Measure immunoglobulin E to radiocontrast media.
c. Diagnose radiocontrast media sensitivity by history.
d. Recommend intradermal skin testing.
e. The patient cannot be exposed to iodinated contrast agents in the future.

450. A 16-year-old woman develops wheezing and shortness of breath minutes after receiving ceftriaxone for gonorrhea. Her blood pressure is 110/65, her pulse rate is 92, and her respiratory rate is 32. She is anxious, but she is well-perfused peripherally. Which of the following is the treatment of choice for this patient?

a. Subcutaneous epinephrine for bronchospasm
b. Intravenous fluids
c. Prophylactic atropine
d. Diazepam to prevent seizures
e. Antihistamines

451. A 32-year-old woman complains of severe seasonal allergies. Every year from April through July she is miserable with sneezing, nasal congestion, and watery itchy eyes. Antihistamines, nasal corticosteroids, nasal saline washes, eye drops, and attempts to avoid potential antigens have proven unsuccessful. She requests referral to an allergist for "allergy shots." What advice should you give her about immunotherapy (hyposensitization) for her allergic symptoms?

a. Immunotherapy is useful is asthma but not in allergic rhinitis.
b. Immunotherapy can be used in allergic rhinitis because there is no risk.
c. The beneficial effect of immunotherapy goes away as soon as the shots are discontinued.
d. Immunotherapy against respiratory organisms can decrease the incidence of bacterial sinusitis.
e. Immunotherapy requires the identification of specific antigen by dermal or serum testing.

452. A 55-year-old farmer develops recurrent cough, dyspnea, fever, and myalgia several hours after entering his barn. He has had similar reactions several times previously, especially when he feeds hay to his cattle. Which of the following statements is true?

a. The presence of fever and myalgia indicates that this is an infectious process.
b. Immediate-type IgE hypersensitivity is involved in the pathogenesis of his illness.
c. The etiological agents are often thermophilic actinomycete antigens.
d. Demonstrating precipitable antibodies to the offending antigen confirms the diagnosis of hypersensitivity pneumonitis.
e. Chronic lung disease does not occur in this setting.

453. A 35-year-old woman is concerned that she may be allergic to certain foods. She believes that she gets a rash several hours after eating small amounts of peanuts. In evaluating this concern, which of the following is correct?

a. At least 30% of the adult population is allergic to some food substance.
b. Symptoms occur hours after ingestion of the food substance.
c. The foods most likely to cause allergic reactions include egg, milk, seafood, nuts, and soybeans.
d. The organ systems most frequently involved in allergic reactions to foods in adults are the respiratory and cardiovascular systems.
e. Immunotherapy is a proven therapy for food allergies.

454. A 32-year-old woman experiences a severe anaphylactic reaction following a sting from a hornet. Which of the following statements is correct?

a. She would not have a similar reaction to a sting from a yellow jacket.
b. She would have a prior history of an adverse reaction to an insect sting.
c. Adults are less likely to die as a result of an insect sting than children with the same history.
d. She should be skin-tested with venom antigens and, if positive, immunotherapy should be started.
e. She cannot use an epinephrine self-injector because of her age.

455. A 62-year-old man is diagnosed with neurosyphilis. Seven years ago he had an anaphylactic reaction to a penicillin shot which was administered for streptococcal pharyngitis. He required treatment with epinephrine and reports that he "almost died." What is the best approach to the management of his neurosyphilis?

a. Oral doxycycline
b. Intravenous ceftriaxone
c. Oral erythromycin
d. No treatment available
e. Penicillin desensitization followed by parenteral penicillin G

Questions 456 to 458

For each clinical description, select the one most likely immunologic deficiency. Each lettered option may be used once, more than once, or not at all.

a. Wiskott-Aldrich syndrome
b. Ataxia telangiectasia
c. DiGeorge syndrome
d. Immunoglobulin A deficiency
e. Severe combined immunodeficiency
f. C1 inhibitor deficiency
g. Adenosine deaminase deficiency

456. A 16-year-old male has recurrent episodes of nonpruritic, nonerythematous angioedema. There is a family history of angioedema. The patient has also complained of recurring abdominal pain.

457. A 42-year-old man requires transfusion for blood loss resulting from an automobile accident. During the infusion, he develops urticaria, stridor, and hypotension requiring IV epinephrine. Further history reveals frequent episodes of sinusitis and bronchitis.

458. A 24-year-old female develops bronchiectasis after recurrent episodes of severe bronchitis and pneumonia. She has prominent blood vessels on the ocular sclera and across the bridge of the nose. Her sister had a similar illness and died of lymphoma at age 29.

Questions 459 and 460

For each patient, select the most likely immunologic deficiency. Each lettered option may be used once, more than once, or not at all.

a. Complement deficiency C5-C9
b. Selective IgA deficiency
c. Postsplenectomy
d. Neutropenia
e. Interleukin-12 receptor deficit
f. Microbicidal leukocyte defect
g. Phagocyte immune deficit
h. Congenital T-cell deficit

459. A 30-year-old male has developed fever, chills, and neck stiffness. Cerebrospinal fluid shows gram-negative diplococci. He has had a past episode of sepsis with meningococcemia.

460. A 22-year-old male has been healthy except for abdominal surgery after an auto accident. He is admitted with clinical signs of pneumonia and meningitis. Cultures of blood, sputum, and cerebrospinal fluid grow gram-positive diplococci.

Allergy and Immunology

Answers

445. The answer is e. (*Fauci pp 2065-2067.*) Urticaria (hives) presents as well-circumscribed wheals with raised serpiginous borders. Individual lesions usually persist less than 24 hours, only to be replaced by other hives at other locations. The process may be triggered by a specific antigen such as food, drugs, or pollen. It may also be bradykinin mediated, such as in hereditary angioedema, or complement mediated, as in necrotizing vasculitis. However, in the great majority of patients with urticaria, a cause is never found. Very rarely, urticaria accompanies illnesses such as chronic infection, myeloproliferative disease, collagen vascular disease, or hyperthyroidism. Usually, however, the patient with one of these illnesses displays clinical evidence of the underlying process.

446. The answer is c. (*Fauci, pp 2058-2060.*) Patients with common variable immunodeficiency syndrome usually develop recurrent or chronic infections of the respiratory or gastrointestinal tract. The fundamental feature is hypogammaglobulinemia, often with associated T-cell abnormalities. Diarrhea can be idiopathic, with malabsorption, or secondary to chronic infection such as giardiasis. There is no Mendelian genetic inheritance, although clusters in families do occur. Symptoms generally do not occur until the second or third decade of life, but also may first present in the older patient. Patients with common variable immunodeficiency syndrome should not receive live vaccines such as MMR, varicella, or oral polio vaccines. Despite their subtle T-cell defects, patients with common variable immunodeficiency are rarely infected with organisms that afflict T-cell deficient patients (such as patients with HIV).

447. The answer is a. (*Fauci pp 2068-2070.*) Allergic rhinitis is caused by allergens that trigger a local hypersensitivity reaction. Specific IgE antibodies attach to circulating mast cells or basophils. Mast cell degranulation leads to a cascade of inflammatory mediators. Vasomotor rhinitis, the second most common cause of rhinitis after allergic disease, is usually perennial and is not associated with itching. In allergic rhinitis, nasal turbinates appear pale and boggy (rather than red and inflamed as in infectious rhinitis). Avoidance measures alone are often ineffective. Antihistamines and intranasal corticosteroids are usually necessary for adequate symptom relief. Chronic use of nasal decongestants should be avoided, since it often causes rhinitis medicamentosa and can perpetuate her nasal congestion.

448. The answer is b. *(Fauci pp 2063, 2069.)* Latex allergy has become an increasingly recognized problem. This is an IgE-mediated sensitivity to latex products, particularly surgical gloves. Patients present with localized urticaria at the site of contact, but can also have generalized urticaria, flushing, wheezing, laryngeal edema, and hypotension. A scratch test with latex extract is the most sensitive approach to diagnosis. The test must be done with caution since anaphylaxis can occur. Education and avoidance of latex products is the best approach to management. Vinyl gloves can be substituted for latex, although she will need to be cautious because latex is present in so many medical devices (including mundane objects such as enema tubes). Corticosteroids might be used in severe asthma or anaphylaxis but, because of long-term side effects, would not be part of routine management.

449. The answer is c. *(Fauci, pp 1405, 2493.)* Signs and symptoms of radiocontrast media sensitivity include tachycardia, wheezing, urticaria, facial edema, bradycardia, and hypotension. When these occur within 20 minutes of the injection of a radiocontrast agent, the diagnosis is made by history. No routine laboratory abnormalities are diagnostic or predictive. Urinary histamine studies are used in the diagnosis of systemic mastocytosis but would be unnecessary in this case. Iodinated agents are direct mast cell degranulators; immunoglobulin E antibodies have not been identified, and no specific skin test is available. If the patient needs IV contrast dye in the future (as, for instance, for a CT scan or left heart catheterization), he can be premedicated with antihistamines and corticosteroids with an acceptable degree of safety.

450. The answer is a. *(Fauci pp 2063-2065.)* Subcutaneous epinephrine is recommended for bronchospasm and anaphylaxis. (For severe bronchospasm or shock, intravenous epinephrine might be used if the patient does not have contraindications.) Intravenous fluids would be recommended only when hypotension is present. Atropine is given only in the setting of bradycardia. Diazepam is used when seizures occur acutely as part of the hypersensitivity reaction but not as a prophylactic measure. Antihistamines, useful in urticaria, are not helpful for the anaphylactic reaction.

451. The answer is e. (*Fauci pp 2068-2070.*) Antigen immunotherapy has been proven to be more effective than placebo in the management of severe allergic rhinitis, but the specific antigen must be identified before allergy shots are begun. Ideally, the test result should correlate with the patient's symptoms (time of year of attacks, exposure history, etc). Immunotherapy requires a long-term commitment; treatment duration of less than a year is ineffective. Once a 3 to 5 year course is completed, however, the beneficial effect can persist for years. Immunotherapy is probably effective in asthma, although the evidence for benefit is less compelling than in allergic rhinitis. The chief drawbacks to allergy shots are the time commitment, expense, and the risk of severe allergic reaction to the injected immunogen. Thirty to fifty deaths are reported each year from anaphylaxis to allergy shots. There is no evidence that specific immunotherapy to bacterial pathogens decreases the incidence of sinusitis or respiratory infections.

452. The answer is c. (*Fauci pp 1607-1610.*) Hypersensitivity pneumonitis is characterized by an immunologic inflammatory reaction in response to inhaled organic dusts, the most common of which are thermophilic actinomycetes, fungi, and avian proteins. In the acute form of the illness, exposure to the offending antigen is intense. Cough, dyspnea, fever, chills, and myalgia, which typically occur 4 to 8 hours after exposure, are the presenting symptoms. Patients are often suspected of having an infection, especially pneumonia, but the history of previous similar symptoms on antigen exposure would be very uncommon in a bacterial or viral process. In the subacute form, antigen exposure is moderate, chills and fever are usually absent, and cough, anorexia, weight loss, and dyspnea dominate the presentation. In the chronic form of hypersensitivity pneumonitis, progressive dyspnea, weight loss, and anorexia are seen; pulmonary fibrosis is a permanent and sometimes fatal complication. The finding of IgG antibody to the offending antigen is universal, although it may be present in asymptomatic patients as well and is therefore not diagnostic. While peripheral T cell, B cell, and monocyte counts are normal, a suppressor cell functional defect can be demonstrated in these patients. Inhalation challenge with the suspected antigen and concomitant testing of pulmonary function can confirm the diagnosis but are seldom used. Therapy involves avoidance; steroids are administered in severe cases. Bronchodilators and antihistamines are not effective.

453. The answer is c. *(Fauci pp 2063, 2065, 2069.)* Food allergy is an IgE-mediated reaction to antigens in food. It is caused by glycoproteins found in shellfish, peanuts, eggs, milk, nuts, and soybeans. Symptoms occur within minutes (not hours) of ingestion in most patients. The incidence of true food allergy in the general population is uncertain but is likely to be about 1% of patients—less than might be generally perceived. Studies have demonstrated that breastfeeding can decrease the incidence of allergies to food in infants genetically predisposed to developing them. Food allergy symptoms most commonly expressed in the gastrointestinal tract and the skin. Respiratory and (in severe reactions) cardiovascular symptoms may occur but are rare. Food allergic reactions are diagnosed by the medical history, skin or radioallergosorbent tests (RASTs), and elimination diets. The best test, however, remains the double-blind, placebo-controlled food challenge. If the diagnosis of a food allergy is confirmed, the only proven therapy is avoidance of the offending food. At present, there is no proven role for immunotherapy in the treatment of food allergy.

454. The answer is d. *(Fauci p 2752.)* The incidence of insect sting allergy is difficult to determine. Approximately 40 deaths per year occur as a result of *Hymenoptera* stings. Additional fatalities undoubtedly occur and are unknowingly attributed to other causes. Both atopic and nonatopic persons experience reactions to insect stings. The responses range from large local reactions with erythema and swelling at the sting site to acute anaphylaxis. The majority of fatal reactions occur in adults, with most persons having had no previous reaction to a stinging insect. Reactions can occur with the first sting and usually begin within 15 minutes. Enzymes, biogenic amines, and peptides present in the insects' venom are the sensitizing allergens. Venoms are commercially available for testing and treatment. Within the *Vespidae* family, which consists of hornets, yellow jackets, and wasps, cross-sensitivity to the various insect venoms occurs. The honeybee, which belongs to the *Apis* family, does not show cross-reactivity with the vespids. Venom immunotherapy is indicated for patients with a history of sting anaphylaxis and positive skin tests. Epinephrine self-injectors can be lifesaving; they are contraindicated in the presence of ischemic heart disease.

455. The answer is e. (*Fauci, pp 1044-1045, 2065-2065.*) As a general rule, a history of respiratory distress or anaphylactic shock associated with an antibiotic use precludes the use of that or similar agents. However, in circumstances where penicillin is the clearly superior therapy and the consequences of treatment failure are dire (as in this case), desensitization is recommended. First, skin testing with several penicillin-related antigens is performed to confirm the diagnosis. Then, gradually increasing doses of penicillin are administered, starting with low oral doses and finally progressing to parenteral doses. IV access and epinephrine must be available, as even in the most meticulous hands, anaphylaxis can occur. Remember that there is 20% cross-reactivity between penicillins and cephalosporins. A history of severe reaction to one class generally contraindicates use of other beta-lactams. Oral antibiotics are of no use in the treatment of neurosyphilis; only high-dose IV penicillin is effective. Syphilis in the pregnant, penicillin-allergic patient also requires desensitization rather than alternative antibiotics.

456 to 458. The answers are 456-f, 457-d, 458-b. (*Fauci, pp 2053-2061.*) C1 inhibitor deficiency prevents the proper regulation of activated C1. As a consequence, levels of C2 and C4—substrates of C1—are also low. Recurrent angioedema is the result of uncontrolled action of other serum proteins normally controlled by C1 inhibitor. The disease may be acquired but is usually inherited in an autosomal dominant pattern as a result of a deficiency of C1 inhibitor. There is no pruritus or urticarial lesions. Recurrent gastrointestinal attacks of colic commonly occur.

Immunoglobulin A deficiency is the commonest immunodeficiency syndrome, occurring in 1 in 600 patients. It is especially common in Caucasians. The most well-defined aspect of the syndrome is the development of severe allergic reactions to the IgA contained in transfused blood. Patients probably have an increased incidence of sinopulmonary infections and chronic diarrheal illness, although the increased susceptibility may be attributed to concomitant IgG subclass (especially IgG2 and IgG4) deficiency. There is no effective treatment for the IgA deficiency although those with IgG subclass deficiency and recurrent bacterial infections may benefit from immunoglobulin infusions.

Ataxia-telangiectasia is an uncommon genetic syndrome of immunodeficiency, cerebellar ataxia, and facial and ocular telangiectasias. The patients have abnormal DNA repair and suffer from an increased incidence of cancer, especially lymphomas. The abnormal gene is called the ATM gene;

approximately 1% of the population is deficient in one allele. Interestingly, heterozygotes, although otherwise normal, are susceptible to increased radiation damage because of the abnormal DNA repair mechanism.

459 and 460. The answers are 459-a, 460-c. (*Fauci pp 534, 763, 911.*) Patients who have a deficiency of one of the terminal components of complement have a remarkable susceptibility to disseminated *Neisseria* infection, particularly meningococcal disease. This association with meningococcal disease is related to the host inability to assemble the membrane attack complex—a single molecule of complement components that creates a discontinuity in the bacteria's membrane lipid bilayer. The complement deficiency results in inability to express complement-dependent bactericidal activity.

The pneumococcus is the most important cause of postsplenectomy sepsis, making up about 67% of all cases. (*Haemophilus influenzae* is the second most common organism.) The spleen serves a variety of immunologic functions, but, as the main production site for opsonizing antibody, it is especially important for the clearance of encapsulated bacteria. A polysaccharide capsule surrounds all invasive pneumococci, and a deficiency in opsonizing antibody post-splenectomy can result in overwhelming sepsis with pneumonia, bacteremia, meningitis, and death.

Geriatrics

Questions

461. A 75-year-old woman is accompanied by her daughter to your clinic. The daughter reports that her mother fell in her yard last week while watering flowers. Her mother suffered scratches and bruises but no serious injury. The daughter is concerned that her mother might fall again with serious injury. The patient has hypertension and osteoarthritis of the knees. She takes HCTZ, lisinopril, naproxen, and occasional diphenhydramine for sleep. The daughter reports some mild forgetfulness over the past 2 years. The patient gets up frequently at night to urinate.

Blood pressure is 142/78 lying and 136/74 standing. Pulse is 64 lying and standing. Except for some patellofemoral crepitance of the knees, her physical examination is normal. A Folstein mini-mental status testing is normal except that she only remembers two of three objects after 3 minutes (29/30). She takes 14 seconds to rise from sitting in a hard backed chair, walk 10 ft, turn, return to the chair, and sit down (timed up-and-go test, normal less than 10 seconds). A CBC, chemistry profile, and thyroid tests are normal.

What is the next best step?

a. CT scan of the brain.
b. Holter monitor.
c. Discontinue hydrochlorothiazide and prescribe donepezil.
d. Discontinue diphenhydramine, assess her home for fall risks, and prescribe physical therapy.
e. EEG.

462. A 78-year-old woman with mild renal insufficiency complains of pain in the right knee on walking. The pain interferes with her day-to-day activities and is relieved by rest. There is no redness or swelling. There is minimal joint effusion. An x-ray of the knee shows osteophytes and asymmetric loss of joint space. ESR and white blood cell count are normal. Which of the following is the best initial management of this patient?

a. Naproxen
b. Indomethacin
c. Intra-articular corticosteroids
d. Acetaminophen
e. Total arthroplasty

463. An 82-year-old man is admitted to a long-term care facility after a right hemiplegic stroke. He is unable to walk and has limited ability to move himself in bed. He is frequently incontinent of urine. He has a past history of type 2 diabetes mellitus. On examination you note a 3-cm area of persistent erythema on the right buttock. Which of the following treatments would you recommend at this time?

a. Sharp surgical débridement to remove the area of erythema
b. Application of a hydrocolloid dressing (such as Duoderm) to be left in place for 5 days
c. Placement of a Foley catheter
d. Use of a foam mattress, repositioning at least every 2 hours, and scheduled voidings
e. Admission to the hospital for IV antibiotics

464. A 65-year-old man has had symptoms of progressive cognitive dysfunction over a 1-year period. Memory and calculation ability are worsening. The patient has also had episodes of paranoia and delusions. Antipsychotic medication resulted in extrapyramidal signs and was stopped. The patient has recently complained of several months of visual hallucinations. There is no history of alcohol abuse. Which of the following is the most likely diagnosis?

a. Lewy body dementia
b. Alzheimer disease
c. Early parkinsonism
d. Delirium
e. Vascular dementia

465. An 80-year-old nursing home patient has become increasingly confused and unstable on her feet. On one occasion she has wandered outside the nursing home. In considering the issue of restraints for this individual, which of the following is correct?

a. A geri-chair would provide the best approach to safety and restraint.
b. Physical restraints are the best method to prevent falls.
c. Restraints cause many complications and increase the risk of falls.
d. Sedative medication should be used instead of restraints.
e. Wrist restraints are more effective than ankle restraints.

466. A 75-year-old woman seeks advice about exercise programs. She has mild hypertension but is otherwise in good health with no other risk factors for cardiovascular disease. Which of the following statements is supported by current data?

a. Walking can reduce mortality from cardiovascular disease and help prevent falls.
b. Tai chi has become popular in the elderly but results in falls.
c. Bicycling is the most common form of exercise among adults age 65 and older.
d. Only high-intensity exercise has been shown to have long-standing benefits.
e. Exercise has not been shown to prevent disease in persons aged 65 and older.

467. A frail 80-year-old nursing home resident has had several episodes of syncope, all of which have occurred while she was returning to her room after breakfast. She complains of light-headedness and states she feels cold and weak. She takes nitroglycerin in the morning for a history of chest pain, but denies recent chest pain or shortness of breath. Which of the following is the best initial test?

a. Cardiac catheterization
b. Postprandial blood pressure monitoring
c. Holter monitoring
d. CT scan
e. EEG

468. A 78-year-old woman with mild Alzheimer disease falls at home and suffers a left hip fracture. She is admitted to the hospital and undergoes a left total hip replacement. Postoperatively she is given D5W and treated with meperidine for pain, diphenhydramine for sleep, and given prophylactic ranitidine. On the second postoperative day, she pulls out her Foley catheter and her IV. On examination blood pressure is 150/90, pulse rate is 80, and temperature 36.7°C (98°F). Oxygen saturation on room air is 92%. She is markedly confused and appears agitated. She has no focal neurologic findings. Laboratory testing reveals WBC = 7500, hemoglobin = 10.2, Na = 132, potassium = 3.2, BUN = 6, creatinine = 0.9. CXR, ECG, and liver tests are normal. What is the next best step in her management?

a. Order CT scan of the brain.
b. Order ventilation perfusion lung scan.
c. Obtain blood cultures and begin broad-spectrum antibiotics.
d. Restrain the patient and order lorazepam for agitation.
e. Remove Foley catheter, change fluids to NS with KCL, and discontinue meperidine, diphenhydramine, and ranitidine.

469. A 78-year-old male complains of slowly progressive hearing loss. He finds it particularly difficult to hear his grandchildren and to appreciate conversation in a crowded restaurant. On examination, ear canal and tympanic membranes are normal. Audiology testing finds bilateral upper-frequency hearing loss with difficulty in speech discrimination. Which of the following is the most likely diagnosis?

a. Presbycusis
b. Cerumen impaction
c. Ménière disease
d. Chronic otitis media
e. Acoustic neuroma

470. A 90-year-old male complains of weakness, some shortness of breath on exertion, and poor sleep. In evaluating this patient, which of the following physiologic parameters does not change with age?

a. Creatinine clearance
b. Forced expiratory volume
c. Hematocrit
d. Heart rate response to stress
e. Hours of REM sleep

471. A 65-year-old male who has not had routine medical care presents for a physical examination and is found to have a blood pressure of 165/80. He has no other risk factors for heart disease. He is not obese and walks 1 mile a day. Physical examination shows no retinopathy, normal cardiac examination including point of maximal impulse, and normal pulses. There is no abdominal bruit, and neurological examination is normal. ECG, electrolytes, blood sugar, and urinalysis are also normal. Repeat visit 2 weeks later shows blood pressure to be unchanged. Which of the following is the best next step in management?

a. Intravenous pyelogram.
b. Begin therapy with a low-dose diuretic.
c. Follow patient; avoid toxicity of antihypertensive agents.
d. Begin therapy with a beta-blocker.
e. Begin therapy with a short-acting calcium-channel blocker.

472. A 65-year-old male inquires about the pneumonia vaccine. He had a friend who died of pneumonia. The patient is in good health without underlying disease. Which of the following is the most appropriate management of this patient?

a. Recommend the pneumococcal vaccine and check on the status of other immunizations, particularly tetanus vaccination.
b. Inform the patient that he has no risk factors for pneumonia.
c. Report that the present pneumonia vaccine does not work.
d. Emphasize that the influenza vaccine is more important.
e. Give pneumonia vaccine and influenza vaccine 4 weeks apart.

473. An 80-year-old white male is being evaluated as part of an annual physical examination. Examination reveals a large plaque on the left shoulder that is well demarcated, hyperkeratotic, and oily to palpation. It appears to be "stuck on." Its surface includes keratin plugs. Which of the following is the most appropriate next step?

a. Biopsy to rule out melanoma
b. Advice about sun exposure and actinic keratosis
c. Reassurance of the benign nature of this seborrheic keratosis
d. Removal of basal cell carcinoma
e. Treatment with topical steroids for psoriasis

474. A 67-year-old male is brought by his wife for evaluation of memory loss. Over the last 2 years he has had difficulty recalling the names of friends. On two occasions he has become lost in his own neighborhood. Recently, he has become suspicious that his wife may be trying to put him in a nursing home.

He has hypertension. He has never used alcohol. He does not have urinary incontinence. His only medication is hydrochlorothiazide 25 mg daily. His mother was diagnosed with Alzheimer disease at age 60.

Blood pressure is 130/76. There are no focal neurologic findings and gait is normal. He is not oriented to date and cannot recall any of three objects at 3 minutes. He cannot speak the name of common objects such as a pen or watch. His clock drawing test is abnormal. A complete blood count, blood chemistries, liver function tests, serologic test for syphilis, thyroid stimulating hormone, and vitamin B_{12} levels are all normal. A CT scan of the brain reveals age-related atrophic changes but is otherwise normal.

Of the following choices, which is the next best step?

a. Begin treatment with donepezil 5 mg daily.
b. Order APOE gene testing.
c. Refer the patient for neuro cognitive testing.
d. Begin treatment with ginkgo biloba.
e. Begin treatment with an antipsychotic.

Questions 475 to 477

Match the patient with the most likely type of urinary incontinence. Each lettered option may be used once, more than once, or not at all.

a. Stress incontinence
b. Urge incontinence
c. Overflow incontinence
d. Functional incontinence
e. Mixed incontinence
f. Normal physiologic functioning of old age

475. A 70-year-old woman complains of leakage of urine in small amounts. This occurs when laughing or coughing. It has also occurred while bending or exercising. The patient has five children who are concerned about her urinary problems.

476. An 80-year-old male has been admitted to a nursing home after a stroke. He has a hemiparesis and expressive aphasia. After 2 weeks he is still unable to make it to the bathroom. Urodynamic testing shows no abnormalities.

477. An 85-year-old male has a history of long-standing diabetes mellitus and prostatic hypertrophy. He complains of dribbling urine. There is a sense of incomplete voiding and of a decrease in urinary stream. Postvoiding residual is 300 mL.

Geriatrics

Answers

461. The answer is d. (*Fauci, pp 57-58.*) Falls in the elderly are common. Nearly one-third of community dwelling adults over 65 years of age fall at least once yearly. Minor imbalances are common in everyday life. Falling in the elderly is usually associated with decreased ability of the elderly to compensate for these imbalances. Age-related declines in vestibular function, autonomic function, hearing and eyesight, and muscular strength all contribute to the inability of the elderly to correct for minor imbalances. Medical illnesses and medications may also contribute to this difficulty. The evaluation of falling in the elderly includes a careful history to exclude syncope, a careful medication history, and a review of medical conditions, which may aggravate falling. Persons who have fallen more than once in the last 6 months are at high risk of falling again. The timed up-and-go (TUG) test also predicts who is likely to fall again in the next year. In an elderly person who presents with falling, evidence-based literature supports three measures to prevent future falls: elimination of medications with sedating and anticholinergic properties, elimination of environmental and structural hazards in the home, and physical therapy. Diphenhydramine has both sedating and anticholinergic effects.

In the absence of syncope and focal neurologic findings, CNS imaging, EEG and Holter monitoring are unnecessary. Since the patient does not have orthostatic hypotension, discontinuing HCTZ is not indicated. Donepezil is indicated for dementia but not just forgetfulness.

462. The answer is d. (*Kane, pp 267-268.*) This patient has osteoarthritis. In addition to physical therapy, the best symptomatic treatment would be acetaminophen because it is frequently effective in providing pain relief and has an excellent safety profile in the elderly. Nonsteroidals should be avoided, at least initially, because they tend to cause gastrointestinal upset and impairment of renal function. Indomethacin is relatively contraindicated in the elderly because of its long half-life and central nervous system side effects. Intraarticular steroids are indicated for large effusions in joints unresponsive to first-line therapy. Arthroplasty is highly effective in treating osteoarthritis of a single joint and is not contraindicated in the elderly. Such surgery is usually considered if attempts at physical therapy, education, and pain control with pharmacotherapy do not provide adequate symptom relief.

463. The answer is d. *(Fauci, pp 59-60.)* Pressure ulcers are a serious problem in the elderly. They result when skin is damaged by compression between a bony prominence and hard surface for prolonged periods. Pressure ulcers are classified using a standard staging system. A Stage I ulcer consists of persistent erythema. A Stage II ulcer is characterized by partial thickness skin loss involving the epidermis or dermis or both. These ulcers are superficial. A stage III ulcer is characterized by full thickness skin loss involving subcutaneous tissue but not extending through underlying fascia. A stage IV ulcer is a stage III ulcer that extends through fascia and results in damage to underlying structures such as muscle or bone. The treatment of all pressure ulcers includes frequent monitoring of the ulcer, modifying the support surface (such as prescribing a foam mattress), frequent repositioning, and keeping the skin dry and clean from urine and stool. Scheduled urinary voidings are preferable to Foley catheters, which increase risk for urinary tract infection. In order to remove devitalized tissue, debridement is recommended for stage II, III, and IV ulcers. Hydrocolloid gels are recommended for stage II and III ulcers. Neither of these interventions would be indicated for this patient's stage I ulcer. All pressure ulcers eventually become colonized with bacteria. Local wound care is the first management of these infections. Topical antibiotics are reasonable if the ulcer is unimproved after 2 weeks of local wound care. Intravenous antibiotics are reserved for patients with cellulitis, sepsis, or underlying osteomyelitis.

464. The answer is a. *(Kasper, pp 52, 2402-2403.)* Lewy body dementia has been recently recognized as a specific type of dementia different from Alzheimer disease or Parkinson disease. On autopsy Lewy bodies are present throughout the brain, including the cortex. Mild parkinsonism may or may not be present. Paranoia and delusions are more common than in Alzheimer disease, and treatment with antipsychotic drugs characteristically worsens the underlying condition. Visual hallucinations are characteristic of Lewy body dementia and uncommon in Alzheimer disease. Parkinson disease causes dementia late in its course, when the characteristic tremor, bradykinesia, and balance disturbance are easily recognized. Delirium is an acute confusional state that would not present with progressive cognitive deterioration or repeated hallucinations over time. Vascular dementia is characterized by stepwise progression (due to numerous lacunar strokes) and upper motor neuron signs.

465. The answer is c. *(Kane, p 438.)* Restraints are being used less and less in nursing homes as their complications and alternatives become more appreciated. The four Ds—deconditioning, depression, disorientation, and decubiti—are all complications of restraints. A geri-chair is just another form of physical restraint and promotes the same difficulties. Effective alternatives to restraints usually require an individual care plan. In this case, alarm bells for the institution's exits and evaluation of the patient's gait would be important. All physical restraints, either wrist or ankle restraints, should be avoided if possible. Sedation leads to complications such as pneumonia and may, in fact, also promote falls.

466. The answer is a. *(Kasper, p 53.)* Walking is the most common exercise in the elderly and has been shown to reduce mortality from coronary artery disease and decrease the incidence of falls. In one study, a rigorous walking program of 2 miles a day reduced coronary events by 50%. Tai chi exercises, which consist of a sequence of movements used in martial arts, have actually been shown to reduce the incidence of falls in older patients. Exercise need not be high-intensity to have benefits; moderate-intensity activity for 30 minutes produces most of the health benefits of daily exercise.

467. The answer is b. *(Kasper, p 50.)* Postprandial hypotension has been increasingly recognized in the frail elderly. Postprandial reduction in systolic blood pressure in the elderly is common. In one study, a quarter of all patients had a reduction in systolic blood pressure of greater than 20 mm Hg. Much of the decrease is attributed to splanchnic blood pooling. Those on nitrates and other drugs that cause postural hypotension are at greatest risk. Older patients with this condition should avoid large meals. Diagnosis is confirmed by monitoring blood pressure after eating. Cardiac ischemia or arrhythmia are less likely to cause the symptoms described. Arrhythmia is more likely to be of sudden onset and is typically NOT preceded by warning symptoms such as coldness and lightheadedness. A Holter monitor could be obtained, however, if initial workup is negative.. CT scan is rarely helpful in the evaluation of syncope in a patient without focal neurologic findings. In the absence of clinical features to suggest seizure, EEG is not recommended in the diagnostic workup of syncope.

468. The answer is e. *(Fauci, pp 158-162.)* This patient has postoperative delirium, characterized by confusion and agitation that develops abruptly.

Frequently the level of consciousness fluctuates. Postoperative delirium is common in the elderly. Males are affected more commonly than females. Delirium occurs more frequently in elderly patients with preexisting dementia, history of alcohol abuse, and memory impairment. Persons with postoperative delirium should receive a careful history that includes medication review, a physical examination, and laboratory testing. Laboratory testing should be directed toward excluding electrolyte disturbance, infection, and hypoxemia. The most common treatable causes of delirium are related to medications and electrolyte disturbances.. Medicines with anticholinergic and sedating property should be avoided. Commonly prescribed drugs with anticholinergic properties include diphenhydramine, tricyclic antidepressants, oxybutynin, and H_2 blocking agents. Management of postoperative delirium includes looking for underlying precipitating factors, correcting electrolyte disturbances, discontinuing aggravating medications, removing indwelling devices, avoiding physical or pharmacologic restraints, early mobilization, and the use the orienting stimuli such as clocks and calendars. Postoperative delirium is a serious condition and has been associated with an increased mortality, prolonged hospital stay, and chance of nursing home placement after hospitalization.

Structural central nervous system disease is an uncommon cause of postoperative delirium; so CT scanning would not be the first test ordered. Pulmonary embolism can cause delirium by causing hypoxia; since this patient's oxygen saturation is normal, lung scan would not be indicated. Infection can cause postoperative delirium, but this patient's normal temperature and white blood cell count militate against an infectious cause. Restraints and benzodiazepines often make delirium worse. If pharmacotherapy is required, haloperidol or an atypical antipsychotic is usually the first choice.

469. The answer is a. *(Kane, pp 345-351.)* Presbycusis is the most common cause of sensorineural hearing loss in the elderly. Probably the result of cochlear damage over time, it is characterized by bilateral high-frequency hearing loss above 2000 Hz. Diminished speech discrimination is more apparent compared to other causes of hearing loss. Both Ménière disease and chronic otitis media are causes of hearing loss in the elderly; they usually present as unilateral hearing loss. Acoustic neuroma is uncommon and also causes unilateral neurosensory hearing loss. Otoscopy should always be used to rule out hearing loss associated with cerumen impaction in the elderly patient.

470. The answer is c. *(Kasper, pp 43-49.)* Hematocrit does not vary with age, and elderly patients with anemia require workup to define the disease process. Lung elasticity decreases with age, resulting a normal age-related decline in FEV_1. Creatinine clearance decreases with age although serum creatinine does not. This is because muscle mass declines, and the decrease in creatinine produced matches the diminished GFR. Therefore, a "normal" serum creatinine in the elderly can mask significant renal dysfunction. Heart rate response to stress and number of hours of REM sleep both decrease with the aging process..

471. The answer is b. *(Kane, pp 284-289.)* There is now general agreement that systolic hypertension in the elderly should be treated and that low-dose thiazide diuretic is the initial regimen of choice in the elderly. Treatment reduces the risk of stroke and cardiovascular events, and side effects appear to be minimal. Beta-blockers or ACE-inhibitors are generally recommended as second-step therapy. Short-acting calcium-channel blockers should be avoided. Workup for secondary causes is not indicated, as they are less common in the elderly; such a workup may be appropriate if hypertension is refractory to medication. An intravenous pyelogram (IVP), however, is no longer used as a screening test for renovascular hypertension. Weight loss and exercise might be initiated prior to antihypertensive medication in a patient with mild systolic hypertension who is obese or sedentary.

472. The answer is a. *(Kasper, pp 813-814.)* The pneumococcal vaccine is currently recommended for all patients over the age of 65 because age per se is a risk factor for mortality due to pneumococcal infection. The vaccine is safe, and the vaccination program for the elderly is cost effective. The importance of the annual influenza vaccine should also be explained to the patient. All patients over the age of 65 are high priority to receive the influenza and pneumococcal vaccine whether they have underlying disease or not. Most deaths from influenza occur in the over-65 age group. Currently, the live attenuated intranasal vaccine is not approved in the elderly patient population. If the visit is during influenza season, both vaccines should be given at the same time. Tetanus vaccination booster is also recommended in the elderly patient who has not had a booster vaccine in 10 years.

473. The answer is c. *(Kasper, pp 285, 502.)* The lesion described is characteristic of seborrheic keratosis, which is extremely common in older patients. The waxy, stuck-on-appearing lesion with keratin plugs is so identifiable that it requires no further workup. It is a benign growth of normal epithelial cells. Melanomas are usually asymmetric with irregular borders and color variegation. Basal cell carcinoma usually presents as a pearly translucent nodule with telangiectasia. Actinic keratoses, a precursor to squamous cell carcinoma, appear as reddish papules or plaques. Psoriasis causes scaling lesions, particularly over the elbows and knees.

474. The answer is a. *(Kane, pp 97, 98, 101.)* This patient meets the diagnostic criteria for Alzheimer disease: the gradual development of multiple cognitive defects, (which must include memory impairment) resulting in significant social impairment and not explained by another physical or psychiatric disease. Neurocognitive testing may confirm the diagnosis but is not necessary. The primary treatment is an acholinesterase inhibitor. Many clinicians initiate therapy with donepezil. The APOE gene on chromosome 19 influences the risk for late onset Alzheimer disease but it is not a clinically useful test for influencing diagnosis or treatment. In prospective trials, ginkgo biloba has been demonstrated to be ineffective in the treatment of Alzheimer dementia. Antipsychotics do not affect the course of Alzheimer disease and are reserved for severe behavioral disturbances, which have not responded to nonpharmacological therapy.

475 to 477. The answers are 475-a, 476-d, 477-c. *(Kane, pp 188-195, 500-507.)* The 70-year-old woman with episodes of leaking small amounts of urine while laughing or coughing has stress incontinence. Stress incontinence occurs when the internal urethral sphincter fails to remain closed in response to increasing intraabdominal pressure caused by laughing, coughing, or lifting. The problem is usually seen in postmenopausal women who have weakening of their pubococcygeus muscle after multiple childbirths.

The 80-year-old male with a stroke history is most likely to have functional incontinence. This often occurs after a major illness or after transfer to a nursing home. The patient cannot notify caregivers about urge to urinate. The patient just cannot make it to the bathroom because of debility, confusion, poor vision, or poor hearing. Sometimes sedative medications contribute to the problem.

Diabetes and prostatic hypertrophy may be contributing to this 85-year-old man's overflow incontinence. Overflow incontinence occurs when there is a mechanical or functional obstruction at the bladder outlet. This leads to overfill of the bladder and leakage with detrusor contraction. A similar picture can occur in a diabetic with an atonic bladder.

Women's Health

Questions

478. A 23-year-old G0 smoker wonders if she is a candidate for the quadrivalent HPV vaccine. She has been sexually active for 5 years with three partners. Her recent first pap smear was normal, but her examination revealed two nontender vaginal lesions which resemble flesh-colored cauliflower. You first educate her that quitting smoking will help her immune system fight the strain of HPV that she already has acquired. What advice should you give her?

a. She is already infected with one strain, but the vaccine will still be effective against acquiring the other three strains.
b. The vaccine will protect her from every HPV strain.
c. If she receives the vaccine, she will never have to have another pap smear.
d. She is already infected with one strain, and there is no benefit in vaccination against the others.
e. The vaccine will help cure her vaginal warts.

479. An 18-year-old G1P1 presents to your office with the results of an abnormal pap smear dated 1 month ago. She tells you that she had one pap smear prior to this one and it was normal. She reports having had four sexual partners since beginning sexual activity at age 15. Upon reviewing the pap smear result you find it is reported as low-grade squamous intraepithelial lesion (LSIL). What is the most appropriate next step in the management of this patient with the abnormal pap smear?

a. Recommend loop electrosurgical excision.
b. Repeat pap at 12 months.
c. Repeat pap smear if and when she changes sexual partners.
d. Repeat pap smear every 3 years.
e. Repeat the pap at this visit and perform HPV DNA testing.

480. A 60-year-old white female presents for an office visit. Her mother recently broke her hip, and the patient is concerned about her own risk for osteoporosis. She weighs 165 lb and is 5 ft 6 inches tall. She has a 50-pack-year history of tobacco use. Medications include a multivitamin and levothyroxine 50 μg/d. Her exercise regimen includes mowing the lawn and taking care of the garden. She took hormone replacement therapy for 6 years after menopause, which occurred at age 49. Which recommendation for osteoporosis screening is most appropriate for this patient?

a. Nuclear medicine bone scan.
b. Dual x-ray absorptiometry (DXA scan).
c. Quantitative CT bone densitometry.
d. Peripheral bone densitometry.
e. No testing is recommended at this time.

481. A 21-year-old female presents for her annual examination. She enjoys drinking to excess on the weekends with her friends and smokes cigarettes to "keep her weight down." She avoids dairy products because they cause bloating and diarrhea. Her medications include birth control pills and OTC antihistamine. She runs 3 miles per day at least 5 days per week. She is 5 ft 2 in and 105 lb. In addition to counseling her on using a barrier method for avoidance of sexually transmitted diseases, what other advice should you give?

a. Binge drinking has no adverse health repercussions
b. She shouldn't start vitamin D or calcium until after menopause.
c. She should change her current exercise routine to water aerobics.
d. She has several significant factors contributing to a low peak bone mass.
c. Smoking is an acceptable form of weight control.

482. An orthopedic surgeon asks you to help him manage an 82-year-old female who just received a hip replacement as a result of a hip fracture. The patient was watering her flowers when she tripped on the water hose and heard her hip crack as she fell to the ground. She has a history of hypothyroidism, mild CVA, and hypertension. Her mother had lost about 5 inches of height in her older years. She believes that she has lost "a few inches" in comparison to her husband. On review of systems, she admits to chronic diarrhea. Her only home medication is metoprolol. On physical examination, her blood pressure is 158/90; pulse 88 and regular; the hip is tender to palpation. Labs show normal calcium, renal function, and alkaline phosphatase. You send a TSH, celiac panel, and 25-OH vitamin D level. Which of the following medications would be most effective in preventing another fracture?

a. Raloxifene
b. Calcitonin-salmon nasal spray
c. Estradiol
d. Hydrochlorothiazide
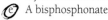 A bisphosphonate

483. A 50-year-old woman presents with fatigue for 2 months. She has recently started having shortness of breath, dizziness, and nausea while walking up the stairs at work. She feels normal after resting at the top of the stairs for a moment. She denies chest pain, orthopnea, paroxysmal nocturnal dyspnea, or recent respiratory infection. Past medical history is significant for hypertension for 10 years and hyperlipidemia for 5 years. She denies tobacco use and exercises regularly. Family history is positive for heart attacks and strokes in her mother's family, but she cannot give details. On physical examination, her waist circumference is 38 in, lungs are clear, and cardiovascular examination is unremarkable and without murmurs. ECG reveals poor R wave progression in V_1 through V_2 and nonspecific ST-T wave changes in the anterolateral leads. Chest x-ray is normal. Pulse oximetry is 99%. Laboratory evaluation shows a normal complete blood count, cholesterol 250, HDL 29 mg/dL, LDL 160 mg/dL, and a random glucose of 250 mg/dL. Which medication(s) should you recommend?

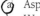 Aspirin and statin
b. Warfarin
c. Selective serotonin reuptake inhibitor
d. Proton pump inhibitor and over-the-counter antacid
e. Albuterol

484. A 25-year-old female presents to your office with complaints of pain during intercourse for 2 months. She states the pain occurs with initial penetration and continues throughout the entire episode. She relates that she and her husband have been married for a year and previously had a pleasurable, pain free relationship. She tells you that she has been to several area doctors, and had a "full workup" without a diagnosis, including a pelvic examination, pap smear with cultures, and sonogram. When you examine her, she has a normal pelvic examination with no pain. You are unsure of the differential diagnosis, so you continue taking more history. She admits to vaginal dryness and low libido during this same timeframe. You ask if anything in her life changed 2 months ago. She suddenly begins to cry and states she found evidence of her husband's infidelity 2 months ago. What is the most appropriate recommendation for your patient?

a. Marriage counseling
b. Estrogen vaginal cream for vaginal dryness
c. Vaginal dilators for treatment of vaginismus
d. Antidepressant therapy
e. Physical therapy for pelvic floor spasms

485. A 38-year-old female present to your office with complaints of fatigue and generalized weakness for 6 weeks. She experiences stiffness in her hands and wrists for an hour after waking, and has taken nonsteroidal anti-inflammatory medication with some relief. Two weeks ago, she noticed that her knuckles were red and tender. Her past medical history is unremarkable, and she takes no medications. On examination, her temperature is 100°F. Erythema with edema is present at most MCP joints. She has minimally decreased muscle strength. Her labs include

WBC: 12,000
Hemoglobin: 10.6 g/dL
Rheumatoid factor: negative
Antibodies to citrulline-containing proteins (anti-CCP): positive
ESR: 62
Hand x-ray: juxtaarticular osteopenia of the MCP joints

Scheduled nonsteroidal anti-inflammatories are started with appropriate monitoring. After one month her pain is unchanged. What is the most appropriate next step in her treatment?

a. Physical therapy.
b. Referral to a rheumatologist.
c. Begin IV TNF monoclonal antibodies.
d. Begin allopurinol.
e. Begin doxycycline 100mg twice daily for 30 days.

486. A 33-year-old female presents to your office with complaints of inability to become pregnant. She and her husband have been having regular intercourse for 10 years without contraception. Her husband has normal sperm count and motility. Her menses are irregular, occurring every 28 to 60 days. She has noticed some facial and upper back acne, as well as increased amount of pubic hair. On examination, her waist circumference is 36 in and she has cystic acne on her neck, forehead, and upper back. She also has acanthosis nigricans in her groin and posterior neck.

Labs: fasting blood glucose: 106
Urine glucose: absent
DHEAS: 360 µg/dL (follicular 32.2-308 µg/dL) (luteal 29.5-269 µg/dL)
Total testosterone: 1.1 ng/mL (0.1-0.6 ng/mL)
Pelvic sonogram: normal

What is the best plan for the initial management of this patient?

a. Weight loss through diet and exercise
b. Metformin
c. Isotretinoin
d. OTC appetite suppressants
e. Gastric bypass surgery

487. A 28-year-old female complains of fatigue and a sense of fullness at the base of her neck. She has no significant past medical history, gave birth to a healthy infant 4 months ago, and is only taking oral contraceptives. On examination, vital signs are pulse 88, blood pressure 110/66, temperature 98.6°F, and respirations 12. Her thyroid gland is homogeneously enlarged and she has a very mild tremor of the outstretched hands. The rest of the examination is within normal limits. Laboratory evaluation reveals the following:

WBC: 7800/μL
Hgb: 12.3 g/dL
Hct: 36%
Plt: 220,000/μL
Na: 138 mEq/L
K: 4.0 mEq/L
Cl: 106 mEq/L
CO_2: 26 mEq/L
BUN: 12 mg/dL
Creatinine: 0.7 mg/dL
TSH: 0.01 mIU/L (normal 0.4-4)
T_4: 19 nmol/L (normal 5-12)
Antithyroid antibody test (TPO antibodies): elevated

What is the most likely diagnosis?

a. Thyrotoxicosis factitia
b. Subacute thyroiditis
c. Toxic multinodular goiter
d. Postpartum thyroiditis
e. Struma ovarii

488. A 51-year-old female presents to your office with questions about whether postmenopausal hormone therapy (HT) is "dangerous." She heard this on the news and read about it in a women's magazine. She denies hot flushes, irregular menses, emotional lability, or vaginal dryness. She has hypertension, but is otherwise healthy. Her family history is negative for breast cancer and cardiovascular disease. According to data from the Women's Health Initiative study, what advice should you give her?

a. Start HT for cardiovascular protection.
b. HT is not indicated for this patient.
c. Start vaginal estrogen cream.
d. Start HT for breast cancer risk reduction.
e. Hormone therapy is too risky to give to any woman.

489. A 25-year-old white female presents to your office for an annual examination. She is a G2P2 and had a bilateral tubal ligation after her last child was born (3 years ago). Her menstrual periods are regular; her LMP was 2 weeks before her visit. On review of systems she describes two to three headaches per month for the past year, usually unilateral and occasionally associated with nausea. The headaches last for several hours. She denies visual changes or other neurological changes when the headaches occur. She had migraine headaches in high school, but they stopped when she was about 20. She has not noted that foods, alcohol, stress, or fatigue trigger the headaches. Her headaches usually happen within the same several-day period and are not spread out over the month. Her last bout with the headaches occurred about 2½ weeks ago. What is the most likely diagnosis?

a. Tension headache
b. Cluster headache
c. Sinus headache
d. Classic migraine
e. Menstrual migraine

490. A 21-year-old female complains of fatigue and difficulty swallowing. She describes the difficulty swallowing as a choking sensation that occurs randomly and not with eating. She denies fever, chills, nausea or vomiting. She notes some difficulty sleeping at night. She is 28 weeks pregnant with her first child. You note that she is wearing long sleeves in warm weather to cover up bruising on her forearms; she also has a bruise on her left lateral thoracic area. How would you most appropriately introduce your concern about domestic violence?

a. "Those bruises look uncomfortable. Do you want to talk about how you got them?"
b. "Who hit you?"
c. "How long has your partner been abusing you?"
d. "I will have to report these injuries to the appropriate authorities if you can't explain them."
e. "Ran into the door again, huh?"

491. A 28-year-old nonsmoking woman presents to discuss birth control methods. She requests a contraceptive option that is not associated with weight gain. She and her husband agree that they desire no children for the next few years. Her periods are regular, but heavy and painful. She frequently stays home from work on the first day due to severe lower abdominal cramping and back pain. She changes her pad every 4 hours. This pattern of bleeding has been present since she was 15 years old. For a week before her period begins, she is uncharacteristically tearful, irritable, and depressed. Her behavior change before her period is beginning to affect her work relationships. Her physical examination reveals blood pressure 110/75, BMI 22, and moderate acne on her face and neck. What recommendation will best address her mood, skin, and contraceptive needs?

a. Tubal ligation
b. Drosperinone and estrogen combination pill
c. Progesterone-infused intrauterine device
d. Progesterone shots every 3 months
e. Condoms

492. Four months after an unremarkable vaginal delivery, a previously healthy 34-year-old G1P1 develops fatigue, dyspnea on minimal exertion, and paroxysmal nocturnal dyspnea. She is no longer breastfeeding. Physical examination reveals a fatigued appearing woman, with normal heart sounds and minimal bibasilar crackles in her lungs. She has no evidence of lower extremity edema, calf tenderness, or ascites. Echocardiogram shows global systolic dysfunction without hypertrophy and an ejection fraction of 40%. Which of the following statements regarding her condition is correct?

a. Peripartum cardiomyopathy may occur unexpectedly years after pregnancy and delivery.
b. The postpartum state will require a different therapeutic approach than typical treatment for dilated cardiomyopathy.
c. For patients with persistent LV dysfunction, future pregnancy carries no increased risk of cardiac decompensation.
d. Fifty percent of patients will recover with normal ejection fraction.
e. Intravenous immune globulin (IVIG) is the cornerstone of treatment.

493. A 68-year-old female presents to your office for follow-up. She has a history of paroxysmal atrial fibrillation and takes warfarin and digoxin for this problem. She has noted 5-lb weight loss, daily fatigue, and loss of interest in her usual activities over the past 6 weeks. She states she doesn't feel like getting up in the morning. She has started taking some alternative therapies from the health food store in an attempt to boost her energy level and mood. On examination, the patient is less animated than usual, and her pulse is irregular at 120/minutes. She has clear lungs and no edema of the lower extremities. What supplement is most likely contributing to the patient's rapid heart rate?

a. Ginkgo biloba
b. Multivitamin with minerals
c. St John's wort
d. Vitamin D
e. Ginseng

494. A 40-year-old female presents to your office regarding a breast lump she found on self-examination 2 weeks ago. The patient does not regularly examine her breasts. Her last clinical breast examination was 2 years ago; mammogram 9 months ago was normal with recommendation for follow-up mammogram in 1 year. She has no family members with breast cancer. Her father had colon cancer diagnosed 10 years ago. She takes no medications regularly. On examination, she has a well-localized nontender nodule in the left breast at 2 o'clock. It is approximately 1.5 cm in diameter with irregular borders. Diagnostic breast imaging includes a negative mammogram and a sonogram that reveals a solid area in the left breast at the site of the palpable abnormality. Which of the following is the most appropriate next step?

a. Reassure your patient and follow-up in 6 months.
b. Refer the patient for needle biopsy.
c. Tell the patient to discontinue caffeine and wear a supportive bra.
d. Schedule a CT scan of the thorax.
e. Start the patient on NSAIDs and vitamin E.

495. A 57-year-old white female with a past medical history of breast cancer stage 2, ER+, PR+, presents to the emergency room complaining of the sudden onset of chest pain and shortness of breath. The pain is sharp and stabbing in the left posterior lung area. The pain does not increase on exertion but increases with deep breathing. The patient denies any history of cardiovascular or pulmonary disease. Her only medication is tamoxifen for 2 years and OTC vitamins. Pulse is 110, RR 26, BP 150/94; lungs are clear bilaterally; cardiovascular examination shows regular rate and rhythm with fixed splitting of S2. ECG shows S wave in lead I, Q wave in lead III, and inverted T in lead III.

Pulse oximetry is 90% on room air. Chest x-ray is unremarkable. Which factor is most likely to be contributing to this patient's respiratory distress?

a. Myocardial infarction
b. Asthma
c. Tamoxifen use
d. Anxiety
e. Pneumonia

496. A 46-year-old woman presents for her annual examination. Her main complaint is frequent sweating episodes with a sensation of intense heat starting at her upper chest and spreading up to her head. These have been intermittent for the past 6 to 9 months but are gradually worsening. She has three to four flushing/sweating episodes during the day and two to three at night. She occasionally feels her heart race for about a second, but when she checks her pulse it is normal. She reports feeling more tired and has difficulty with sleep due to sweating. She denies major life stressors. She also denies weight loss, weight gain, or change in bowel habits. Her last menstrual cycle was 3 months ago. Physical examination is normal.

Which treatments is the most effective choice to alleviate this woman's symptoms?

a. Levothyroxine
b. Estrogen
c. Estrogen plus progesterone
d. Fluoxetine
e. Gabapentin

497. A 47-year-old diabetic female presents to the emergency room with a 45-minute history of chest pain with radiation to the arms and jaw. The pain is relieved with nitroglycerin and morphine. She has ECG changes of ischemia; her second serum troponin level (obtained 6 hours after onset of pain) is elevated. Compared to a similar male patient, which of the following is more likely to occur in this female patient?

a. Death during this hospitalization
b. Percutaneous transluminal coronary angioplasty
c. Hypertension during initial presentation
d. High triglycerides contributing to cardiac risk
e. Less depression after MI than her male counterparts

498. A 60-year-old woman presents with complaints of pain during intercourse. She describes the pain as sharp and constant during sexual activity, and there is a lack of lubrication. This discomfort is very bothersome to her because she wishes to continue an active sex life. She underwent surgical menopause at age 44 due to uterine fibroids and heavy bleeding. She used oral estrogen until age 50; she has used no hormonal therapy since then. On physical examination you note significant urethral and vaginal atrophy. Which of the following is the best treatment option for this patient?

a. Commercial lubricant (K-Y lubricating jelly)
b. Oral estrogen
c. Vaginal estrogen preparation
d. Sildenafil
e. Topical antifungal therapy

499. A 43-year-old woman presents to your office as a new patient for musculoskeletal pain and weight gain. Over the past 6 months, she has noted generalized aches and pains of muscles and joints, fatigue, and poor sleep quality. She admits to wanting to stay in bed rather than socialize with her friends and family. She denies fever, night sweats, morning stiffness, joint redness, blood loss, easy bruising, or daytime somnolence. Her physical examination is significant for a normal BMI, normal thyroid, normal cardiovascular examination, normal joints, and no tenderness to palpation. CBC, TSH, ESR, ANA, RF, electrolytes, liver enzymes, and kidney function tests are normal. She wants pain control. Which treatment is most likely to relieve her symptoms?

a. Long-acting opiates
b. Oral acetaminophen/hydrocodone combination
c. Prednisone
d. Methotrexate
e. An antidepressant

500. A 58-year-old female presents to your office for a sinus infection. She takes no medications except a "baby aspirin." When you inquire why she is taking the 81-mg aspirin, she says "to prevent heart attacks." Her history is negative for hypertension, hyperlipidemia, smoking, diabetes, obesity, or family history of cardiovascular disease. What would you advise this patient about the use of aspirin for heart attack prevention?

a. She should take a full-dose aspirin for primary prevention of heart attacks.
b. She does not need to take aspirin for cardiovascular protection.
c. She should take an 81 mg-dose of aspirin every other day.
d. She should take an aspirin only if she experiences chest pain.
e. A nonsteroidal anti-inflammatory has the same cardiovascular benefits as aspirin.

Women's Health

Answers

478. The answer is a. *(Fauci, pp 608, 1119-1120.)* Human papillomavirus (especially subtypes 16, 18, 33, and 45) has an established relationship to genital warts and cervical cancer. The current multivalent vaccines are highly effective in establishing immunity to the subtypes included in the vaccine, even if one or more of the subtypes is already acquired. It is yet to be proven how much cross-reactive protection exists to subtypes not included in the vaccine. The vaccine is not effective in treatment of any disease (ie, vaginal warts) caused from prior infection. Because over 40 sexually transmitted HPV subtypes exist and the vaccine includes the types responsible for about 70% of cervical cancer, there is still a risk of cervical dysplasia caused from other subtypes not covered in the vaccine. Therefore, continued pap screening is needed. This patient's likelihood of clearing her current HPV infection increases with tobacco cessation.

479. The answer is b. *(Williams, Chapter 29.)* In adolescents (aged 20 years and younger) with low-grade squamous intraepithelial lesions (LSIL), follow-up with annual cytologic testing is recommended. At the 12-month follow-up, only adolescents with high-grade SIL or greater on the repeat cytology should be referred for colposcopy. Reflex HPV DNA testing is not recommended for adolescents. Abnormal cytologies (ASC-US, LSIL) are evaluated differently in adolescents age 20 years and younger due to a higher rate of HPV positivity, the rarity of cervical cancer, and the high rates of spontaneous regression of cervical neoplasia in this group. Reflex HPV testing should not be done. Instead, annual repeat cytology should be obtained and colposcopy performed only with a high-grade cytology result or if any cytologic abnormality persists at 2 years. If DNA testing is performed, the results should not influence management. For women after age 30, a pap smear every 2-3 years is acceptable for low-risk patients with three consecutive negative annual pap smears in a row, or every 3 years with an HPV DNA test plus a pap. There is no recommendation for early repeat pap smear if a patient has a new sexual partner. Most newly acquired HPV infections clear spontaneously.

480. The answer is b. *(Fauci, p 2401)* Accepted indications for bone mineral density testing include estrogen-deficient women at clinical risk of osteoporosis and all women over age 65. This patient's risk factors include estrogen deficiency, low calcium intake, family history, and previous tobacco use; therefore peripheral bone densitometry, such as a heel quantitative ultrasound, would not be sufficient. The heel ultrasound, which does predict fracture risk in women over 65, is less accurate than DXA and is useful for population-wide screening programs, not individual treatment recommendations. A nuclear medicine bone scan has no role in the diagnosis of osteoporosis. Quantitative CT allows for adequate prediction of vertebral fractures, but is not considered standard of care at this time, and exposes the patient to greater radiation than DXA.

481. The answer is d. *(Fauci, pp 2397-2400.)* Peak bone mass is achieved around age 30, and is largely determined by genetics, nutrition, endocrine health, and physical activity. Cigarettes are a known toxin to bone metabolism. This patient's weight bearing exercise should be continued, not replaced by nonweight bearing activities such as swimming or water aerobics. This patient should be advised to ingest, preferably through calcium-rich foods, the USDA recommended 1000 mg of calcium per day. Excessive alcohol intake increases her risk of sexual assault, fatal automobile accident, and alcohol poisoning. Other, less risky methods of weight maintenance should be recommended.

482. The answer is e. *(Fauci, pp 2404-2406.)* This patient has a diagnosis of osteoporosis based on the occurrence of the hip fracture, regardless of her T-score. Bisphosphonate therapy is proven to reduce the high risk of subsequent hip and vertebral fractures. Raloxifene is less appropriate for this patient with her history of a CVA, as it has been associated with increased incidence of thromboembolic events and stroke. The effect of nasal calcitonin on fracture risk is unknown. Estrogen therapy is approved by the FDA for the prevention of osteoporosis, but not for treatment. Hydrochlorothiazide decreases urine calcium loss and helps maintain bone density. Epidemiologic data suggest decreased first fracture risk with long-term use, but it is not proven to decrease risk of subsequent fractures.

483. The answer is a. *(Fauci, p 41, 1508, 2427.)* This patient has exercise-induced symptoms worrisome for angina. Women with vascular disease commonly present with vague symptoms, such as shortness of breath, nausea, vomiting, indigestion, and upper back pain, as compared with the classic symptoms of chest pain, tightness, or pain radiating to the arms or jaw. This patient has untreated hyperlipidemia and undiagnosed type 2 diabetes mellitus with a random glucose greater than 200 mg/dL. For this high-risk patient, the current American Heart Association guidelines recommend a goal LDL of < 70, Triglycerides < 150, HDL > 50. Primary prevention of myocardial infarction with aspirin may not be effective in low-risk women but is still considered standard of care for high-risk women. (See more about aspirin in the answer to question 500.) Warfarin is not indicated for treatment of angina. The history is not suggestive of anxiety or panic disorder. Asthma and gastroesophageal reflux disease may be present, but coronary disease must be ruled out urgently.

484. The answer is a. *(Bieber, pp 61-66.)* An organic cause of this patient's sexual dysfunctions is unlikely. Her pain during intercourse, poor desire, and lack of sufficient lubrication probably stem from the psychological stress from her husband's infidelity. Marital counseling may aid in resolving the issues that resulted in the infidelity, and the aftermath. Female sexual dysfunction consists of four broad categories: dyspareunia, orgasmic disorder, arousal disorder, and impaired sexual drive. Sexual dysfunction results from physical conditions, such as neuropathy or sleep deprivation, or from psychological conditions, such as depression or a history of abuse. A thorough evaluation should include medical conditions as well as psychosocial questions pertaining to the health of her relationship with her partner and personal issues that contribute to her sexual well-being. The other answers are effective treatments for specific types of sexual dysfunctions; however, they will not address the cause of this woman's distress.

485. The answer is b. *(Fauci, pp 2083-92, 2149-58.)* Despite the negative rheumatoid factor, this patient has rheumatoid arthritis. Rheumatoid factors, which are autoantibodies reactive with the Fc portion of IgG, are present in more than 2/3 of adults with the disease, but are not specific for rheumatoid arthritis. Anti-CCP is found in most patients with RA, and has a higher specificity than the measurement of rheumatoid factor. Vague musculoskeletal complaints are common early manifestations of RA. Early diagnosis and treatment are key to slowing the irreversible bony destruction caused by synovial inflammation. While physical therapy maintains joint strength and mobility, it will not mitigate the disease. Disease modifying antirheumatic drugs (DMARDs) are appropriate for early use, but their use requires experienced and well-educated practitioners. Therefore, the most appropriate next step in this patient who has failed nonsteroidal anti-inflammatory drugs is referral to a rheumatologist for DMARD initiation. There is no indication for allopurinol without the diagnosis of gout, or for doxycycline without the diagnosis of Lyme disease.

486. The answer is a. (*Fauci pp 42, 43,306,467-468.*) This woman has polycystic ovarian syndrome (PCOS), the most common cause of infertility in women. Although the precise definition of PCOS is controversial, most agree it may be diagnosed in women with at least some combination of oligomenorrhea, clinical or biochemical evidence of hyperandrogenism (excluding other causes of hyperandrogenemia), and polycystic ovaries by ultrasound. (Polycystic ovaries on ultrasound are not required in the diagnosis of PCOS.) High levels of androgens, either from the ovaries or the adrenal glands, interfere with ovulation, and result in ovarian cyst formation, excess facial and body hair, and acne. Most women with PCOS will have an elevated serum androgen concentration. Hyperinsulinemia and insulin resistance, seen clinically as acanthosis nigricans, are also common findings. Women with PCOS are at increased risk of metabolic syndrome, diabetes, and cardiovascular disease. Exercise and weight loss are first-line recommendations, and may restore normal ovulation without medications. Treatment for women not pursuing pregnancy include oral contraceptives or metformin. Spironolactone has clinical efficacy but is not FDA approved for this use. Rapid weight loss through gastric bypass is not the best option for this patient due to her mild obesity and her desire to become pregnant immediately. Isotretinoin for acne treatment should not be used in women actively trying to conceive due to the extremely high risk of birth defect.

487. The answer is d. (*Williams, Ch 53.*) The patient's clinical presentation is most consistent with postpartum thyroiditis, a form of autoimmune-induced thyrotoxicosis that occurs 3 to 6 months after delivery. The hyperthyroid state usually lasts for 1 to 3 months and is generally followed by a hypothyroid state of limited duration. The patient's thyroid gland would not be enlarged if she were taking exogenous thyroid medications. Subacute thyroiditis usually presents with a tender, enlarged thyroid gland. The patient's thyroid gland is described as homogeneous, not nodular, which would be inconsistent with toxic multinodular goiter. Struma ovarii is unlikely because of the enlargement of the thyroid gland. Struma ovarii is the name given to the approximately 3% of ovarian dermoid tumors or teratomas that contain thyroid tissue. This tissue may autonomously secrete thyroid hormone. Postpartum thyroiditis can be distinguished from Graves disease with thyroid uptake scan; uptake will be suppressed in thyroiditis but normal to increased in Graves disease.

488. The answer is b. *(Fauci, pp 2334-2338.)* Data from the Women's Health Initiative randomized trial of estrogen and progesterone in healthy post-menopausal women found a 26% increase in the risk of breast cancer over a mean follow-up of 5.2 years. This trial confirmed the benefit of HT in pre-vention of osteoporotic fractures, but did not show a benefit in prevention of coronary heart disease. Routine use of postmenopausal HT for prevention of coronary heart disease is no longer recommended. Short-term use of HT (< 5 years) for relief of menopausal symptoms in a healthy perimenopausal woman remains a reasonable and highly effective option.

489. The answer is e. *(Legato, pp 131, 134.)* This patient's headache pattern is typical of menstrual migraines, occurring within several days of menses. She denies that fatigue or stress contributes to the headache; therefore, tension headache is not likely. She has no aura associated with the headache; therefore, classic migraine (migraine with aura) is not correct. Sinus headaches would not occur cyclically. Cluster headaches tend to occur in brief, sharp bursts and are more common in men than women. Migraine is precipitated by menstruation in 24% to 68% of women. Although this patient's history points to menstrual migraine, before initiating treatment a headache diary should be recorded for 2 to 3 months to ensure that the migraines occur exclusively or primarily within 3 days of the onset of menses.

490. The answer is a. *(Marx, pp 2408-2409.)* Since a woman rarely sponta-neously reports domestic abuse to her doctor, recognizing signs and symptoms of domestic abuse may be the only opportunity the physician has to intervene. It is also important to recognize the increased risk of domestic abuse during pregnancy. An abused woman can have vague physical symptoms, including headache, fatigue, insomnia, choking sensations, gastrointestinal complaints, and pelvic pain. Inviting the patient to discuss the situation in a caring and sensitive fashion will create a trusting environment and may encourage the patient to accept help. However, opening the conversation with a joke, or jumping to the conclusion that the patient's spouse caused her apparent injuries is not appropriate or effective. A compassionate and yet professional approach may open the door to help, even if the abused patient is unwilling to accept intervention at her first visit.

491. The answer is b. *(Bieber, pp 31, 831-840.)* While each of the options will provide contraception, only the combination pill fulfills all of her requests. Tubal ligations are permanent sterilization. Progesterone-infused IUDs provide convenient and effective reversible contraception; they usually decrease menstrual flow and do not cause significant weight gain. IUDs, however, are not effective in treating acne or premenstrual dysphoric disorder (PMDD). Progesterone intramuscular injections are associated with weight gain. Condoms do not provide benefits beyond contraception and protection against sexually transmitted infections. The only FDA approved contraceptive pill for PMDD is a drospirenone/ethinyl estradiol combination.

492. The answer is d. *(Fauci 45, 1482)* By definition, peripartum cardiomyopathy is cardiac dilatation and dysfunction of unexplained cause occurring during the last trimester of pregnancy or within 6 months of delivery. Half of patients will completely recover normal cardiac size and function. However, further pregnancies in women with persistent left ventricular dysfunction frequently produce increasing myocardial damage and increased mortality, and patients should be counseled to avoid future pregnancies. Treatment is the same as for other types of dilated cardiomyopathies and includes salt restriction, angiotensin-converting enzyme inhibitors, diuretics, and digitalis and/or beta-blockers for symptomatic treatment. Intravenous immunoglobulin therapy has shown some benefit in small studies, but has not been established as first-line therapy.

493. The answer is c. *(Gaster, pp 152-156.)* The patient is attempting to self-treat her depressive symptoms with St John's wort, which has been reported to interact with certain prescription medications, including digoxin. St John's wort may lower levels of digoxin by 25%. Another interaction that could be important in this case is bleeding, which has been reported in patients taking warfarin and ginkgo biloba. Patients often forget to include their "nutritional supplements" on their list of medications; several alternative and complementary therapies have significant pharmacological effects.

494. The answer is b. *(Fauci, pp 564-565.)* Evaluation of a breast nodule should determine whether the patient has a true mass or prominent physiologic glandular tissue. The next step is to determine whether the dominant mass represents a cyst, a benign solid mass, or cancer. Worrisome characteristics of this patient's mass include irregular borders, size larger than 1 cm, and location in the upper outer quadrant of the breast. Her age (> 35) also places her at slightly higher risk. Therefore, repeat imaging including mammogram and ultrasound is warranted. Even if the mammogram is negative, a noncystic mass on ultrasound should be examined by a breast surgeon or a comprehensive breast radiologist and biopsy performed. Six months is too long to wait for reevaluation. In a younger woman (< 35), repeat examination after the next menstrual cycle might be warranted (ie, < 1-month reevaluation). To assume breast changes are benign without further investigation is not appropriate. CT scanning does not provide useful information in the evaluation of palpable breast mass.

495. The answer is c. *(Fauci, 1652-1654.)* This patient's history and physical are consistent with a diagnosis of pulmonary embolus. The combination of respiratory distress, mild hypoxia, sinus tachycardia, clear chest x-ray, and typical ECG changes warrants emergent treatment and testing to confirm the diagnosis. A myocardial infarction is less likely with this ECG pattern. Asthma rarely presents as pleuritic chest pain. There is no evidence on chest x-ray suggesting an infiltrate. An anxiety attack would not cause hypoxia or these ECG changes. Tamoxifen, a selective estrogen receptor modulator, is associated with an increased risk of thromboembolic events.

496. The answer is c. *(Stenchever, pp 1227-1228.)* The differential diagnosis for palpitations and sweating is broad but major consideration should be given to hyperthyroidism, panic attacks, cardiac arrhythmias, malignancy, and vasomotor instability. This patient denies symptoms of malignancy such as weight loss. She does not have symptoms of clinical depression such as decreased concentration, apathy, weight changes, sleep changes, sadness, irritability, or suicidal thoughts. She reports no change in bowel habits or weight, which would indicate the diagnosis of thyroid disorder. The most likely diagnosis for this patient is vasomotor symptoms associated with the menopause transition. The best treatment option for this patient is a combination estrogen and progesterone low-dose oral contraceptive. Her symptoms are more suggestive of hyperthyroidism than hypothyroidism; so levothyroxine would be of no benefit. Estrogen alone would increase the risk of endometrial hyperplasia and cancer. Fluoxetine and gabapentin have been used to treat hot flushes but are much less effective than hormone replacement.

497. The answer is a. *(Fauci p 41. Naqvi T. et al.)* Women have higher rates of mortality during hospitalization for MI than men. In the setting of an acute MI, women are also more likely to present with cardiac arrest, hypotension, or cardiogenic shock. In addition, women are less likely to receive diagnostic and therapeutic cardiac procedures, such as angioplasty, thrombolytic therapy, coronary artery bypass grafts, beta-blocker therapy, or aspirin. The incidence of depression is higher among women in general, and evidence has surfaced that women suffer from depression after MI more than men. Hypertriglyceridemia exerts an equally deleterious effect toward cardiovascular disease in women and men.

498. The answer is c. *(Fauci, p 300.)* This patient has dyspareunia, or pain during intercourse. She has been postmenopausal for many years without hormone (estrogen) replacement. A commercial lubricant would be helpful for vaginal dryness but will not treat the underlying cause of her urogenital atrophy, which is hypoestrogenemia. She has no other symptoms of menopause (such as vasomotor symptoms or sleep disturbance) that impair quality of life. Therefore oral estrogen is not required. She denies depressive symptoms. The best treatment option for this patient is to treat the underlying disorder of urogenital atrophy with topical estrogen applied to the vagina. A commercial lubricant could be used as needed, but would be in addition to the vaginal hormone cream. Though sildenafil has been shown to be efficacious in the treatment of antidepressant-associated sexual dysfunction, it is not FDA-approved for use in women. Nothing on examination suggests fungal vaginitis.

499. The answer is e. *(Fauci, pp 2717-2718.)* This patient is suffering from the emotional and physical symptoms of depression. Her weight gain is due to her sedentary lifestyle. Initiation of an antidepressant is the most appropriate pharmacologic management, either with a selective serotonin reuptake inhibitor, or with a serotonin-norepinephrine reuptake inhibitor. The SNRI may provide more relief from her physical symptoms than SSRI therapy. Opiate therapy for the pain of depression is inappropriate and exposes the patient unnecessarily to potential addiction. Steroids are not clinically indicated. DMARDs are reserved for specific rheumatologic diseases, not nonspecific musculoskeletal symptoms.

500. The answer is b. *(Fauci, p 1508.)* This patient is at low risk for cardiovascular disease. Her only listed major cardiovascular risk factor is age > 55. Aspirin prophylaxis should be used for women at high risk for CVD. In intermediate-risk women aspirin should be taken if blood pressure is controlled and benefit exceeds gastrointestinal risk. In low-risk individuals, aspirin prophylaxis is not recommended. Nonsteroidal anti-inflammatory drugs (NSAID's) do not have cardioprotective effects, and some NSAIDs (such as rofecoxib) raise the risk of myocardial infarction.

Bibliography

Books

Bieber EJ, Sanfilippo JS, Horowitz IR. *Clinical Gynecology*. Philadelphia, PA: Churchill-Livingstone Elsevier; 2006.

Chen MY, Pope TL, Ott DJ. *Basic Radiology*. New York, NY: McGraw-Hill; 2004.

Fauci AS, Braunwald E, Kasper DL, et al. *Harrison's Principles of Internal Medicine*, 17th ed. New York: McGraw-Hill; 2008.

Gardner DG, Shobock DM. *Greenspan's Basic and Clinical Endocrinology*, 8th ed. New York, NY: McGraw-Hill; 2007.

Ho AC, Brown G, McNamara JA, Recchia F, Regillo CD, Vander JF. *Retina: Color Atlas and Synopsis of Clinical Ophthalmology*. New York, NY: McGraw-Hill; 2003.

Kane RL, Ouslander JG, Abrass IB. *Essentials of Clinical Geriatrics*, 5th ed. New York, NY: McGraw-Hill; 2003.

Legato MJ. *Principles of Gender-Specific Medicine*. London: Elsevier; 2004.

Marx JA, Hockberger RS, Walls RM. *Principles and Practice of Infectious Diseases*, 5th ed. St Louis, MO: Mosby; 2002.

McPhee SJ, Lingappa VR, Ganong WF. *Pathophysiology of Disease: An Introduction to Clinical Medicine*. New York, NY: McGraw-Hill; 2005.

Schorge JO, Schaffer JI, Halvorson LM, Hoffman BL, Bradshaw KD, Cunningham FG. *Williams' Gynecology*. New York, NY: McGraw-Hill; 2008.

Stobo JD, Traill TA, Hekkman DB, Ladenson DW, Petty BG. *The Principles and Practice of Medicine*. New York: McGraw-Hill; 1996.

Wolff K, Johnson RA, Suurmond R. *Fitzpatrick's Color Atlas and Synopsis of Dermatology*. New York, NY: McGraw-Hill; 2005.

Journal articles

American Diabetes Association. Nutrition Recommendations and Interventions for Diabetes. *Diabetes Care*. 2008;31:S61-S78.

Anderson JL, Adams CD, Antman EM, et al. ACC/AHA 2007 guidelines for the management of patients with unstable angina/non-ST-elevation myocardial infarction. *J Am Coll Cardiol*. 2007;50:e1-e157.

Chobanian AV, et al. The seventh report of the joint national committee on prevention, detection, evaluation, and treatment of high blood pressure: The JNC 7 report. *JAMA*. 2003;289:2560-2572.

Gaster B, Holroyd J. St. John's wort for depression. *Arch Int Med.* 2000;160: 152-156.

King MD, Humphrey BJ, Wang YF, et al. Emergence of community acquired methicillin-resistant Staphylococcus aureus USA 300 clone as the predominant cause of skin and soft tissue infections. *Ann Int Med.* 2006; 144:309-317.

Naqvi TZ, Naqvi SA, Bairey Merz CN. Gender differences in the link between depression and cardiovascular disease. *Psychosomatic Medicine.* 2005;67(suppl):S15-S18.

National Cholesterol Education Program. Executive summary of the third report of the National Cholesterol Education Program (NCEP) expert panel on detection, evaluation, and treatment of high blood cholesterol in adults (Adult Treatment Panel III). *JAMA.* 2001;285:2486-2497.

US Preventive Services Task Force. Screening for abdominal aortic aneurysm: Recommendation statement. *Ann Int Med.* 2005;142:198-202.

Wilson W, Taubert KA, Gewitz M, et al. Prevention of infective endocarditis: Guidelines from the American Heart Association. *Circulation.* 2007;116:1736-1754.

Websites

http://www.immunize.org/
http://www.cdc.gov/travel/default/aspx.
http://www.ahrq.gov/clinic/USpstfix.htm#Recommendations.
JNC 7 express, available at http://www.nhlbi.nih.gov/guidelines/hypertension/express.pdf.

Index

Notes